Open Season

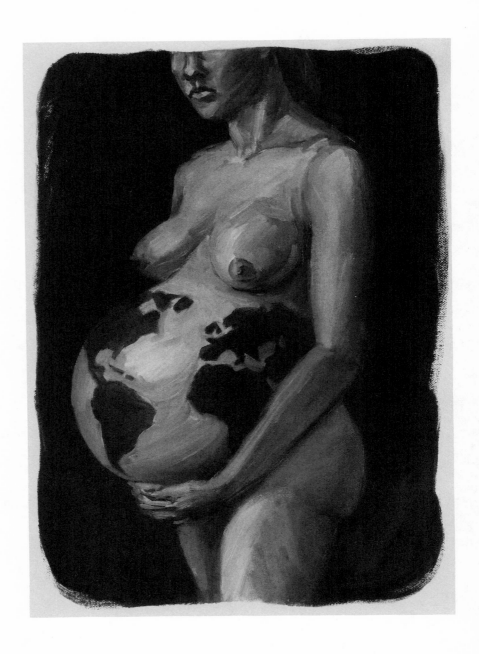

OPEN SEASON

A Survival Guide for
Natural Childbirth and VBAC
in the 90s

Nancy Wainer Cohen

Bergin & Garvey
New York · Westport, Connecticut · London

Library of Congress Cataloging-in-Publication Data

Cohen, Nancy Wainer.
    Open season : a survival guide for natural childbirth and VBAC in the 90s /
Nancy Wainer Cohen.
        p.   cm.
    Includes bibliographical references and index.
    ISBN 0–89789–252–6 (alk. paper).—ISBN 0–89789–272–0 (pbk. :
alk. paper)
    1. Natural childbirth—Miscellanea.   I. Title.
RG661.C65   1991
362.1'984'0973—dc20   91–10569

British Library Cataloguing in Publication Data is available.

Library of Congress Catalog Card Number: 91–10569
ISBN: 0–89789–252–6
         0–89789–272–0 (pbk.)

First published in 1991

Bergin & Garvey, One Madison Avenue, New York, NY   10010
An imprint of Greenwood Publishing Group, Inc.

Printed in the United States of America

The paper used in this book complies with the
Permanent Paper Standard issued by the National
Information Standards Organization (Z39.48–1984).

10   9   8   7   6   5   4   3   2   1

To summer camp
another senior prom
a peach dress, accessorized
and
To my Ben

Time does not bring relief. you all have lied
who told me time would ease me of my pain!
—Edna St. Vincent Millay

There should have been quatrains and cellos instead of silence and
discords. . . . There should have been castles, I do believe.
—Herman Raucher

IN MEMORIAM

Merton Wainer, O.D.

You stapled this book, too, Dad. You made my life rich. You were soooo tall! These pages are my tribute to you: how alive you are inside of me!

> "When wealth is lost, little is lost;
> When health is lost, much is lost;
> When character is lost, all is lost."

Robert Mendelsohn, M.D.

"Each time a man stands up for an ideal, or acts to improve the lot of others, or strikes out against injustice, he sends forth a tiny ripple of hope, and crossing each other from a million different centers of energy and caring, those ripples build a current that can sweep down the mightiest walls of oppression and resistance."

—Robert Kennedy

Mary Sorrento Ripple

You said it yourself: "I am strong, I can see the sky." Peace, my friend.

Fredelle Brusser Maynard

Your hat sat on top of my computer from the first word until the last, but then, you know that, don't you. I remember your own words:

I tell them, truthfully, that I write almost as I breathe—all the time, compelled, because writing is the way I make sense of my experience. . . . 'How do I know what I think till I see what I say?' . . .

Dayna Marie Hagen

I never met you, sweetie, but you taught me something very important: "A goal is a dream with feet." Thank you.

Contents

Special Acknowledgments

Lynn and Esther:

To my special VBAC sisters, Esther Booth Zorn and Lynn Baptiste Richards: For your continual involvement and total commitment to cesarean prevention and VBAC, I thank you. To use your own words; Lynn, you *are* Very Beautiful And Courageous; Esther, you *do* make a difference. Both of you are a source of inspiration and strength to me and to thousands of others as well.

Acknowledgments

You've held me, you've supported me, you've caught my tears. You've listened to me when I've made sense, and when I haven't. You've encouraged me, you've believed in me. Always, you have loved me. Never once have you turned away through all these crazy years. We've walked, we've talked, we've laughed, we've despaired. You have been the cradle I have needed so that I could birth this child. I have much to learn; you all teach me love.

> You are helping me to make
> Of the lumber of my life
> Not a tavern
> But a temple;
> Out of the works
> Of my every day
> Not a reproach
> But a song.

—Roy Croft

Ethel Wainer—I love you, Mom. You teach me strength and organization. (Hi Maury!)

Joyce Kisner—my F.S. What do people do, who don't have a sister? You teach me unconditional love and how to be silly.

Alzero Fleabag—You teach me faith, endurance, and passion. In twenty-five words or less?: Evergreen.

Scott Kisner—Ya'll is my brother. You teach me respect.

Cathy Romeo—By your shining example, you teach me to grow beyond what I believe I am capable. You teach me peace and grace. You're the best.

John Romeo—You are the King of Hearts. You teach me integrity.

Lori Bass Howard—I wished upon a star for you. You teach me Spirit. You are a miracle.

Shirly Zarin—You teach me total acceptance and support. How do you put up with me?

Neil Zarin—You teach me perseverance. You save me from Roche Brothers. What a neighborhood!

Bonnie Poole Robinson—You teach me patience. You show me Spring. What would I do without you?

Patricia Varon—You teach me courage. You are beautiful on the outside and on the inside.

Sylvia Olkin—You teach me wisdom, healing, and depth. You are so precious to me!

Bob Olkin—You teach me politics (—and bocce!)

Laurie Ure—You teach me gentleness and an appreciation of Nature. You teach me to listen.

Nancy Gore—You teach me friendship and the true meaning of abundance.

Heather Laier—You teach me caring and independence. *You walk the path.*

Jini and Michael Fairley—You teach me hope.

Yahara Katseff—You show me my inner child.

Mary Elizabeth Carrero—You teach me "letting go."

June Levy—You teach me constancy.

Norma Shulman and Beth Shearer—You teach me commitment.

Holly Hausmann—You teach me adventure!

Karen Riem—You teach me upliftment!

Sylvia and Bernie Cohen—You teach me tradition.

Rena and Frank Shear—You teach me sensitivity.

Debra and Joel Kaplan—You teach me openness.

Miriam Van Orman—You teach me to strive.

Carol Gras—You teach me the value in honesty and communication.

Laine Sohier and Roland Juli—You teach me about space and boundaries and about sharing.

Susie Smits—You teach me faith.

Susan Coronis—You teach me color.

Caroline Sufrin—You teach me expression.

Maryah Antonellis—You teach me feisty-ness!

Terri and Daniel Youssi—You teach me generosity.

Bob Tuck—You teach me humor.

Fred Kresse—You teach me conviction.

Stephen Stern—You teach me to sing!

Alison Rausch—You teach me thought.

Janna Hodges—You teach me to be outrageous!

Janet Parker—You teach me softness, power, and equality.

Barbara Yardley—You teach me selflessness.

Charles Yardley—You teach me humility.

Marilyn Brier—You teach me trust.

Sue Driehaus—You teach me calm.

Judy Cohen—You teach me warmth.

Julie Beckwith—You teach me compassion.

Marla Hirsch—You teach me reflection.

Aaron Ogilvie—You teach me fearlessness!

Judy, Jeff, and Jessica Ogilvie—You teach me kindness.

Ilene Horvitz, Layne Lepes, Gail Epstein, Barbara Lippiello, Jami Osborne—You give me memories.

Added thanks to Janet Leigh, Kathleen Matthews, Valerie Elhalta, Nan Koehler, Lisa Gery, Nancy Hinchey, Ruth Boyd, Pam Murphy, Tom Brewer, Gail Brewer Krebs, Kim Price-Wen, Leo Sorger, Elizabeth Noble, Mitchell Levine, Fran Ventre, Mary Cooper, Michalene Bratton, Chris Sternberg, Wintergreen, Edmund Lundberg, Dorothy and Ralph Johnson, Archie Brodsky, Jody McLaughlin, John Gibb, Karen Murphy, Maureen Murphy, Lois Estner (I missed you!), and Wendy Maier. Special thanks to Cheryl Rowen, April Asquith and the reference librarians at the Needham Public Library, Sophy Craze, Jim Bergin, Jim Sabin, Margaret Brezicki Maybury, Teresa R. Metz, Betty Pessagno, Nora Kisch, Denise Van Acker, and Kathy Gray Farthing.

And to my family: Very few people know, nor would they understand, the sacrifices that you have had to make—not once, now, but twice. You have lost a wife—or mother—for weeks, months, at a time. (You lived through it—did it make you strong, independent, and capable—or did it just make you crazy?) Your understanding and love are blessings in my life. You teach me boundless energy, wonder and joy. I love you all with my heart, my spirit, and my soul.

Paul, my lifetime friend, you teach me honesty and forgiveness, support, and understanding. It's been quite a trip, huh?: never (never!) dull. Do you remember the roller coaster ride we took at Lincoln Park when we were in eighth grade? Good preparation, wouldn't you say?!!? As were the "Scrambler" and especially "The Nut House", too. You teach me excellence, integrity, and non-judgment. I hope your neuronal pathways are ok: Moo. You're an incredible man.

Eric, my firstborn. You're all grown up! Will I ever get over missing you? You teach me strength of character and dedication. You teach me that it's okay to be me. You teach me to follow my dreams. You stand up for what you believe. You make me soooo proud. You were the "little guy" who's birth rocked a nation. I am so glad to be your mother.

You were my Poosey-Chicken. Now you are one handsome dude. You'll be a famous musician someday. Awwwwwwc' mon.

Elissa, my incredible, beautiful, sweet Elissa. You teach me truth, laughter, and to listen. Your smile warms my heart. You were my VBAC: "Aim for the stars; You may not reach them, but you will fly far higher than you ever did before." Your birth inspired a nation. You were my Bunny Rabbit. I am so lucky to have a daughter like you. Your sensitivity and constant reach toward the Light are astonishing. (I only wish you'd come with instructions!) You are the prime example that wonderful things come in small packages. Now you are quickly fleeting through your teens, almost a woman. I want to make the world better for you, for us all.

And Andrea, always my baby. But no, a baby no more. You are growing too fast! In many ways, you taught me everything I needed to know. You were my Poosey-Goose. You are a beautiful, bright, creative person. You fill my heart. You were the fulfillment of an "impossible dream." You helped me find 'the blueprints'—now I bequeath them to you—and to your brother, sister, and any one who wishes them, as well. You remembered how to be born; you did it gently and easily, but with determination and focus. You own those qualities, and so many other wonderful ones, as well. Your birth showed us all. I am eternally grateful to you, Sweet Potato. I promise that tonight I will sit on your bed *for as long as you want*!

To my other children, Aki Nishida (it is *inconceivable* to me that you are so far away!) and Peter Moodie (I'm still workin' on bread; how's your ear?!): *How I miss you*! I carry you *every minute of every day* in my heart. Each day, I thank your parents, too, for believing in this world enough to let you cross the oceans and be "ours" for those years.

Introduction

Dear Reader,

Hi! I know this looks like a book, but it's actually a letter, to you, from me. I wanted to tell you some of the things that I've learned about birth since *Silent Knife* was published seven years ago. I wanted to put, under one cover, the answers to so many questions you've asked me when you've written to me or called me. I wanted to help counteract the growing indifference toward cesarean section, to increase the enthusiasm for VBAC, and to help eliminate the emotional anesthesia that surrounds natural childbirth these days. I wanted a book that excited you and helped us all to heal.

It is 6:30 A.M. on a Sunday morning. In another few hours, the manuscript will be ready to send to the publisher. I feel a jumble of contrary emotions—excited, scared; exhausted, animated; peaceful, anxious; confident, not confident. This book, more than anything else in my life, has required sacrifices that I am not certain I was ready to make—and yet I must have been willing because it is written. A dear friend encouraged me to "push through the fear and just keep trusting"—which is precisely what most women do when they give birth naturally.

Already, it is warm and sunny outside; just yesterday, it was cold, grey, and snowy: New England weather. Maybe, just maybe the birth situation in this country can change that quickly. Maybe it will be a precipitous birthing, like my third. I realize that in less time than it has been since *Silent Knife* was written, two of my children will be older than I was when I had my first baby.

Things have to change quickly: Pregnancy in this country is one big American bellyache; birth here is one of the saddest, most unnatural disasters on the planet.

One of the burning reasons why I felt compelled to "get this out" was a feeling of responsibility. *Silent Knife* was an angry book, though the anger was both justified and appropriate. But one of the things I have learned is that both personally and globally, anger does not work in the long run. Now I wanted to give the world something that was healing. This is not to say that *Open Season* is any less strong or powerful than its predecessor. There are bursts of anger and more than a few irreverant or "uncalled-for" remarks; I think you will find here the feistiness, humor, and "bite" that you have come to expect after reading *Silent Knife*. But underneath all of this is my desire to help women and my plea for a healed birth community. Nothing less will do.

Someone once told me that the uglier the truth, the truer the friend who tells you. While this saying may not hold in all circumstances, in *Open Season* I have told you my Truth. It is often no prettier than the scars left on women after their births. I have also been told, "When you tell me your truth, I know that you love me," and "you'll know quickly if my words are misleading or wise by listening to the voice of your own heart, whispering in your ear."[1]

We live in a world in which, despite their best intentions, people sometimes hurt each other. My intention in *Open Season* is not to offend or to hurt. When eyes and hearts have been closed for a while, they may "smart" to some degree as they gently open up. More than one person, upon hearing that I was completing OS, has said to me, "Oh good! You'll give us another shot! We need that now!" No, no more "shots". Women have had enough of them in labor rooms, birthing rooms, and operating rooms to last an eternity. The only thing infiltrating our veins from now on must be a measure of uncockeyed optimism and unwavering belief—along with kindness, caring, and love. If I have pleased you, happily may you remember; If I have offended, easily may you forget. "Don't bite my finger, look where I'm pointing."[2]

Open Season is a semi-sequel to *Silent Knife*. That means that a portion of it can be read on its own but that each of the chapters also refers back to information and concepts in the earlier work. I have tried not to repeat myself, although in a few places I have used previous information to reemphasize a point that needs to be said one more time. So most of the "overlap" is quite intentional. If you find a term that isn't defined, or if you feel a little "lost" while reading a particular section, you will find what you need in a corresponding chapter in *Silent Knife*. One important note: I quoted very little from sources such as the *Cesarean Prevention Movement Newspaper* (The Clarion), the C/ SEC (Cesarean/Support Education and Concern) newsletter, *Mothering* magazine, *The Compleat Mother*, *The Doula*, and NAPSAC (National Association of Parents and Professionals for Safe Alternatives in Childbirth) News. I didn't use these works because anyone involved in childbirth should be reading those publications for themselves.

Now that *Open Season* is completed, I have so many feelings, and many of them are similar to those I felt after my natural birth—excitement, relief, fullness, loss, pride, astonishment! I feel strong and invincible—and at the same time I feel so vulnerable! I feel extremely "inside-out," too—but definitely not in the same way I did after my cesarean. There is a freedom and a joy that comes from having pushed through the myriad of fears, insecurities, and sadnesses that I had to get through in order to write this letter to you.

I began writing when the snow was a foot deep around my house and now there are flowers and the birds are singing—

> i thank you god for most this amazing
> day: for the leaping greenly spirits of trees
> and a blue true dream of sky; and for everything
> which is natural which is infinite which is yes[3]

I'm going out for a walk . . . Daffodils!

Love,
Nancy

May 1990

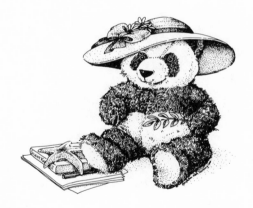

Open Season

1 *Hello Again!*

A story is told of a girl who was walking along a beach, throwing objects into the ocean. "What are you doing?" an old man asked the girl. The girl answered, "These starfish have washed ashore and if they don't get back in the water they'll die." Pointing to the thousands of starfish lying stranded, the man said, "You'll never be able to save all of them, so what does it matter?" The girl looked at the starfish in her hand. "Well, sir," she said, "It matters to this one."[1]

Someone once told me that when you feel passionately about a subject, you never really finish writing about it. You just temporarily abandon the writing, only to begin again when you can no longer contain the words that form inside and literally beg to be freed.

In 1983, when Lois Estner and I finished writing *Silent Knife: Cesarean Prevention and Vaginal Birth After Cesarean*, I felt finished. I filed the hundreds of research articles that had been strewn all over the dining room, shoved the dictionary and the thesaurus back into the bookshelf, and washed the ink marks off the woodwork. Last but not least, I dusted myself off and knit the last sleeve of a sweater I had begun several years earlier. I'd done it. I'd written my book. I felt a tremendous sense of accomplishment and espoused a definite belief that one book per human being per lifetime was enough!

Lois went on to work in the field of early childhood development and then had her third baby (second VBAC, first son, a wonderful purebirth). Our family got a puppy, Mischief (third dog, a girl). On occasion, Lois and I would joke about writing again. "In my next marriage!" she would say. "In my next *life!*" I'd reply. We were proud, we were depleted, we were done.

As for me, I continued to research cesarean prevention and VBAC. I presented workshops and lectures and worked individually with pregnant women. I spent most of my time answering letters from cesarean mothers and counseling women from all over the world by telephone.

Some days, after receiving a number of calls from women who were filled with pain about their childbirth experiences, I'd wonder if I'd not drown in the tears. I'd often try to numb myself to the pain, and for periods of time I could continue to work without "losing it." I knew that I was helpful, and that was most satisfying, but the intense sadness returned time and again. As I listened to their stories, I sometimes thought that my own heart would break as well. I was extremely discouraged by the lack of change in the field of childbirth, despite the efforts of so many outstanding people.

It was at such times that I thought about leaving the field of childbirth—a decision that wouldn't exactly upset most of the obstetricians in my area. I simply felt worn out. I found, however, that when women would ask me for help, I could never quite muster the words, "I'm sorry. I can't help you. I'm not doing this work any more." I read an article on "burn-out" and realized that *Silent Knife* had been my latest "baby." I needed a little time to rest from what had been, in some ways, an eleven-year labor with her: I believe now that she was conceived the moment I had my first child by cesarean. I realized that the support I was able to give to the women who contacted me was very important to me; it helped counteract the sadness and frustration I felt regarding the unconscionable way our culture reacts to birth. In that sense, it was vital to my own well-being and my ability to "recover." I began to reaffirm what I had known all along: that being involved with birth was in my blood, and that my "earthly path" was routed in my being able to make a contribution to childbirth.

After *Silent Knife*, Lois and I received hundreds of thank-you letters from women all over the world. Letters continue to arrive weekly. Among the letters I most cherish was one that said, "I cried buckets through the first few chapters, threw-up through the next few, chuckled on occasion, and then felt like smashing the pages a good portion of the rest of the time. I got so angry, in fact, that I had to put the book down for quite a while. I picked it up six months later and it changed my life."

I look at the papers mounting up on my dining room table and I think I hear Webster and Roget beckoning to me in my sleep. Could it be? It couldn't. *Am I really writing another book?* Goodness gracious, I am.

I began *Open Season* over four years ago. Hundreds of times, I allowed feelings of fear to interfere with my progress. First I'd worry that it wouldn't be good enough. Then I'd get anxious looking at the stacks of articles I would need to wade through. At one point, I even began thinking that this work wasn't really that important anyway. Having been introduced to organizations like Beyond War and Operation Clean Sweep, which had total planetary survival as their goals, it seemed pretty lame to help women have vaginal deliveries instead of cesarean sections or avoid an episiotomy. What difference did it make? It all seemed so insignificant.

One day, however, as I attended a meeting on preventing nuclear war, I realized that everything is connected. How one woman births *does* matter because in a very real sense, we are all one, and the process or the mind-set that creates a natural birth in one woman, when understood and imitated by the next, has the power to change everything. Grace Akinyi Ogot, a political activist from Kenya, as well as a nurse, midwife, teacher, and writer, says, "We have an expression: Educate a woman and you educate a nation."[2] Alice Walker writes, "But one day when I was quiet, it come to me: that feeling of being part of everything, not separate at all. I knew that if I cut a tree, my arm would bleed. And I laughed and I cried and I run all around the house."[3]

Around the same time I saw a video about midwives entitled "Push, A Women's Western" in which Suzanne Arms, author of *Immaculate Deception*, interviews midwives Raven Lang and Kate Boland. Suzanne asks: "As we approach the turn of the century, this planet seems to be facing very crucial issues. Not just unemployment, but world starvation, violence, crimes against women and children—interpersonal violence is at an all time high—and so on. And perhaps the biggest threat of all: the shadow of total destruction under nuclear war. Given these parameters, do you still believe that birth is a major issue?" Kate's reply: "My feeling is that when people birth, when we make our rites of passage beautiful and deep and meaningful, you get a different, a deeper respect for life, a different commitment to each other. My feeling, my hope, my belief is that better births will make a better world . . . deeper relationships, stronger bonds, and a sounder family, and if we start there, we can begin to effect on a larger scale." Raven's reply: "It's a beginning. It's a metaphor for all of Life. When you go to a birth to be with a couple, you see their daily life—how they love, how they eat, how they work together. And it's all there. It is a very, very powerful time. Everybody is born once and everybody dies once—it's really the only thing we all do. It's pain and joy and sensual and aggressive and ecstasy all in one. And who can say whether it hurts or it is exquisite pleasure at that moment?"[4]

It was at that moment that I knew I was in this work for the duration. And so, today, my head is filled with words that need to be pounded out on this keyboard, words that might be valuable to someone who is pregnant or involved with birth. I've been daydreaming and having difficulty sleeping. I feel very emotional. Those close to me know the signs. Forget dinner: she's serving air tonight. New sheets on the bed? Naw, they were changed in March. I don't answer the telephone or the doorbell. Anything that takes me away from my writing is completely superfluous.

Many people remarked that *Silent Knife* was a strong, angry book. Evidently, it wasn't strong enough. The cesarean rate continues to climb, and the rate of VBAC is just over 2 percent. What a disgrace! New gadgets are being developed every month to "assist" women as they birth (i.e., to do it for them). If you thought birth was technology-oriented before, just wait. I am reminded of a scene from *Alice Through the Looking Glass*. The White Queen is crying, and when asked why, she replies, "Because I am going to hurt soon."[5] An almost anticipatory kind of grieving seems to be going on during many pregnancies, a sort of nebulous emotional overcast that arises as if, on some intuitive level, women know that it is going to be difficult to have a natural delivery. The fear crosses socioeconomic lines, and, as Kenneth Keyes, author of *The Hundredth Monkey*, could have predicted, it has even begun to pass from us to other countries. Although the exact number may vary, the hundredth monkey phenomenon means that when only a limited number of people know of a new way, it may remain the conscious property of these people only. But there is a point at which if one more person tunes in to a new awareness, a field is strengthened so that this awareness reaches almost everyone.[6]

Most of you have heard of cellular consciousness, or mass consciousness. Which of you would want to be "the hundredth woman"—the one whose fear of birth furnished the added consciousness energy to create an entire planet of women who no longer felt capable—or interested—in giving birth to their babies? Which of you would rather be "the hundredth woman" who furnished the added consciousness to create a world in which women embraced this aspect of their lives, confident, and eager.

Because we wanted to have an impact on birth in this country, Lois and I hoped that *Silent Knife* would appeal to obstetricians and obstetrical staffs as well as to birthing women. In fact, a number of obstetricians wrote to us telling us they had enjoyed the book and had learned from it. It seems clear to me now, however, that in trying to speak to both women and medical professionals, neither is truly serviced. *Open Season* is therefore written for women, for those who have asked for a sequel of sorts to *Silent Knife*. I particularly recall the words of Janet Leigh, a wonderful midwife, who wrote to me:

> I read your words and I read my truth, the truth so many of us have known, have preached, have practiced, in the face of powerful opposition, of unbelievers and "unsee-ers." We who have felt ourselves "voices crying in the wilderness", we hear your voice as ours, and are so grateful for it. . . . I have realized so often, after some years of not understanding the problem, that even with sympathetic or potentially sympathetic supporters, the great difficulty is that we are simply speaking another language . . . and there is simply no translation dictionary. I do not know how to bridge the gap. We can show them if they care to watch, but we cannot tell them. Perhaps, as you speak words of truth, those words will partially bridge that gap—if they have the hearts to hear.

One woman wrote, "Your first book got my goat (and the whole rest of the zoo besides). You rattled my cage. . . . Like an angry tigress, I became vicious, violent, furious . . . and broke out of the cage. And now, I understand you are writing again. You are definitely going to continue to rattle a lot of cages. A LOT. . . . You can't open the doors. No one can. [But] you dare to rattle cages. . . . Some say that is cruel. Is it? The beasts will be furious at YOU. Some will even lash around with such fury that they will break out of their cages. And then, having earned their own freedom, they will be free to explore the infinite boundaries of their own souls." I look at my copy of *Silent Knife*. Hi, Book. I thought you were going to be my only opus. You're going to have a friend.

In the years since *Silent Knife* was published, I have learned a thousand lessons: I have kicked and screamed through a number of them, been numbed by others (only to find them staring me straight in the face as soon as the "thaw" began), and leaped for joy at the few that were cemented in my brain without too much of a struggle. What it takes to grow! Two close friends have died, one came close, and another lost her daughter in a car accident. I held my father's hand as he died and my cousin's as she birthed. I've grounded my teenagers and slept outside under the stars. Horror of horrors, I turned forty, then forty-one and more—at this rate, who knows how old I could get?! "Life. If we knew what was going to happen, we might not have shown up."[7] Well, I didn't and I did. I'm still here, and I'm mostly glad—and I bring all that I am to you in this endeavor.

I no longer defend my desire to write this book, my need to put into complete sentences the fragments of feelings and thousands of thoughts that have been filling my head and my heart. It may sound trite, but if I can help one more woman birth joyfully, if I can help one more couple move from the operating room into their bedroom for birth, I will have done something good. I'm tired of passing out bandaids! (At the seminars I lead, I ask those who have unresolved hurt about their childbirth experiences to come up and get a bandaid, and to wear it on their heart until the healing begins. In every seminar, almost every single woman, and not just those who have had cesarean sections, but most of the women who have had hospital vaginal deliveries, too, rush to get a bandaid. What a sad commentary—an entire generation of women with birth-related broken hearts.)

I also have a more personal reason for writing this book: I have children who will be of childbearing age in this decade, and I must contribute in whatever way I can toward making childbirth better for them. As Judy Herzfeld said to her daughters after she wrote her childbirth book: "It is my fervent hope that by the time they are old enough to be reading books on the subject, I hope it will seem unfathomable that it ever had to be written."[8]

Welcome to *Open Season!*

2 *The Cutting Edge*

Years from now, parents and doctors are going to look back on the 1900's
and wonder, "How could they possibly have practiced childbirth like that?"
They'll wonder how any civilization could tolerate the perversion of such
a natural process. They'll wonder how any "modern" technological society
could accept such unbelievable levels of iatrogenic [doctor-caused] mental
illness and death. They'll wonder how any group of people with such an
advanced educational system, let alone the wisdom of the ages, could be so
stupid as to accept, practice and perpetuate the childbirth practices which
take place in our hospitals today. . . . And we'll have no answers; only excuses. . . . We have deviated from the natural process to such an extent that
it has become irrecognizable as a natural function. . . .

—Sue Roberts[1]

The Monty Python movie, *The Meaning of Life*, includes a birth scene, in which
a woman ready to give birth is wheeled into a delivery room. She is lying on
her back on a narrow table, her legs up in stirrups. "Doctor, Doctor, what do
I do now?" she asks. "You? YOU???" replies the doctor. "*You* don't do anything.
You aren't qualified."

It has been seven years since *Silent Knife* was written. Naively, I believed that
within a short time our book, and the many others that had also been published
on the subjects of cesarean prevention, VBAC, and assertive birth would help
to turn the tide. I believed that the cesarean rate would decline, that the rate of
medical intervention would decrease, and that everyone—obstetricians and anesthesiologists notwithstanding—would live happily ever after.

In actuality, the cesarean section rate continued to increase. Granted, a fair
amount of 'lip-service' was given to VBAC, but in a larger number of situations

those VBACs somehow "failed." In many areas, VBAC isn't even an option yet, and in most places, it isn't even a minor "threat." Women are being re-sectioned to death, literally and figuratively speaking. Hospitals that proudly boast about lower section rates have only to look at their increased forceps deliveries and increased vacuum extractions to remind themselves that "their" babies are simply being tugged out and sucked out rather than cut out.

Many of the letters that continue to arrive at my door are from women who are still unable to locate a doctor who truly understands and supports purebirth (see *SK*, Chapter 6) or VBAC. Many are unable to find midwives to attend them, due to difficult, "sticky," political factors and impossible "birth climates." Most birthing centers still refuse to admit VBAC "aspirants," and those that do continue to camouflage their IV poles with flowering plants and to hide the instruments behind oak cabinets. Scare tactics—not just about VBAC but about all aspects of birth—still abound. Throughout the country, far too many women are still unquestioningly praising their cesareans: "I can't imagine wanting to have a vaginal birth. I'm glad that all my babies can be born this way." Some women continue to be grateful for fetal monitors, drugs, episiotomies, and the whole gamut of technological devices and interventions that have become routine at birth in this culture. Home birth? Forget it, most say—too dangerous.

So many of us had hoped that by the end of the eighties childbearing practices in the United States would have dramatically improved. What we meant by improvement was resurrecting truly natural birth, and putting a stop to the continued barrage of tests, interferences, fear tactics, and "The doctor knows best, dear" platitudes. Thanks to the efforts of many courageous and determined women and to a number of birth organizations, yes, some improvements were made—but they were so slow, painstaking, and isolated that one often began to wonder if the efforts were worth the results. Perhaps we should all simply forget "the fight" and go back to birthing our babies the way the majority of women in our mothers' generation did. We could all just lie down and temporarily "check out." In fact, many American women coast to coast still do it this way.

As we enter the 1990s, it seems that more and more women in this country are being labeled unqualified. "If I was given a tee-shirt to wear at my labor," remarked Lori, "it could have sported a giant "U": Unclothed, Unfed, Un-questioning, Unenlightened, and later, mercy, most Ungrateful. Of course, I ended up with a section, which I now know was absolutely Unnecessary." As are most of them.

The typical American pregnant woman has only to step foot into an obste-trician's office and she is transformed in an astonishing, deeply disturbing way. These active, creative, household-organizing, career-balancing wonderwomen become reserved, shrinking violets. Poked and prodded, primed and prostrate, they wilt. Faster than magic wands turn toads into princes, these princesses become asses. As they are semi-drained of blood, urine, and/or amniotic fluid, they reassure themselves that this is all for the good. Often, they blushingly admit that they even love their "assailants." As they are stripped, prepped, examined, and all but "de-fleaed," they affirm their womanhood and their choice of caretakers. Their brains remain in the waiting room, their natural instincts in the parking lot. On their way out of the 2 x 4 cubby hole, also known as the examining room, they stop at the receptionist's desk to make another appointment, for which a fair number of them will starve themselves (lest they put on too much weight and be chastised). They are gluttons for punishment, the lot of them, but they just don't know it yet.

A professor and chairman of an obstetrics and gynecology department in the Midwest recently made the following amazing statement: "The vagina is not made for having babies any more than the penis is," he said. "I'm speaking as the head of the ob/gyn department here. I want to come across as the voice of reason in this."[2] Another obstetrician, also the head of a department, remarked, "If I could give all men vasectomies, I would. No wives should have to go through birth more than twice, at the most." And a third: "I'd section all women if I could. It's the 'way to go'." Sadly, these physicians represent the views of a large portion of the obstetricians in our country, as you will see.

This week I received a letter from a woman who had just had a cesarean section. "I was too chicken to go through much labor," she wrote, "but I am writing to tell you that I hope other women like me won't be too chicken." Unfortunately, the vast majority of pregnant women in our culture do feel "chicken." With the prevailing attitudes in this culture that birth is unsafe, that women aren't physiologically or psychologically designed to have babies anyway, and that the total management of labor and delivery is essential, it is no wonder that women find their instincts blocked, their hormones confused, their confidence disintegrating, their dignity stripped. We are part of one big obstetrical disgrace. One mammoth maternity mess.

And it is a mess. This year alone over a million healthy pregnant women will wind up on an operating table. Countless others will just barely make it through without surgery. The majority of those who manage to have their babies with no talk of cesarean section will be the recipients of modern obstetrics' greatest "gifts" to womankind—including but certainly not limited to—catheters, fetal monitors, IVs, drugs, uterine stimulants, forceps, and/or vacuum extractors—all in an effort to try-and-get-that-baby-out. Many women believe that these "gifts" and procedures are necessary to ensure the well-being of their infants, and their obstetricians will expend a great deal of energy instilling the belief that these interferences are indeed essential. But they are no more necessary than they would be at the *conception* of the baby, to get the baby *in*.

So many people have done so much to humanize the childbirth experience, to make birth more natural (which is surely a redundancy: what could be more human than childbirth or more natural than giving birth?), and to spread the truth that women are fully capable of birthing the infants they have carried. Despite all this effort we continue to injure far more mothers and babies than necessary and to have to tend to those who arrive in halfway decent condition, *because* of our methods of delivery, not in spite of them. If women are in any way "chicken," it is perhaps because of the many (far-too-many) roosters who strut and meander around the hen house, ready to spring at any moment and ruffle unsuspecting feathers. (This has been better said: "You don't set a fox to watching chickens just because he has a lot of experience in the hen house.")[3] It may also be due in part to the number of females who don rooster headdresses, including the many female ob/gyns who have learned how to "think, cut, drag, and sew with the rest of the boys." It is doubtful that even a real chicken could lay her eggs in a maternity unit in this country. Sadly, each day in the American obstetrical system, many eggs are laid.

The rate of prenatal testing, drugs, IVs, monitoring equipment, induction agents, and vacuum extractions, for example, has increased in the past ten years, despite the vast amounts of information cautioning against them and despite the high percentage of couples in this country who go through "prepared-childbirth" classes. This is a joke. Couples taught in hospitals are rarely *prepared* to have their babies; rather, they are prepared for induced labors and pain-killers, for having their water broken, and for episiotomies, all of which are invasive, unnecessary, and complicate the birth process. These couples are alternately courted, humored, intimidated, and patronized. They're *lied to*. Not surprisingly, cesarean sections among hospital-trained couples also continue to increase, turning the illness into a plague. Babies are drugged out, forced out, pulled, pushed, sucked, or sliced out of their mothers' "prepared" bodies, and both parties are left to "recover" from the experience.

If childbirth classes really "worked," more women would be having babies without interference. More women would recognize the complete naturalness of birth and would remain at home, delivering their infants with feelings of confidence and trust. More and more, midwives would be demanded. The names of those hospitals and doctors who treated women and babies with anything less than absolute respect would be public knowledge, and childbirth classes would be the first place these names would be discussed. "You're seeing What's-His-Face? He's a pig! *In my opinion*, of course," I tell people who come to my classes. I then proceed to give them the names of people who have used Pig-face. They can always ask Dr. P. for the names of people who have used him and been satisfied with their births, for balance.

If childbirth classes worked, birth "paraphernalia" would be used less and less rather than more and more. If the classes worked, if they truly prepared women to deliver their babies, then women would be delivering them. Instead, women are delivered of their infants through the "wonders" of medical technology, by the wielders of those technologies. For all the good that hospital childbirth classes may have set out to do, few have done much, and little has changed. Thousands of naive pregnant couples, listen to unqualified childbirth educators teaching nothing more than a glorified biology lesson, dishing out misleading and unenlightening information, and who thus deliver their couples into the waiting hands of equally unqualified members of the obstetrical establishment. Few American women survive "prepared childbirth" without suffering indignities that leave them scarred for years to come.

It is not only childbirth educators that bear responsibility. Medical schools and nursing schools are also at fault. Ginny Cassidy-Brinn, one of the authors of *Woman-Centered Pregnancy and Birth*, remarks that she has become thoroughly convinced that her nursing instructors were "abysmally ignorant" about normal childbirth.[4] Most students finish their obstetrical rotations no longer believing in the process of birth. In fact, few have ever even seen a purebirth. I was not surprised, but nonetheless appalled, to learn that not one of the nursing students to whom I spoke had seen a natural birth. (Two thought they had, but when I reminded them that enemas, IVs, and episiotomies do not constitute a natural birth, they realized that natural births did not take place in their institutions.) Most were horrified or repulsed by their obstetrical rotation and were extremely fearful of giving birth themselves. Obstetrical students rarely understand or experience the broad variations that may occur in normal birth. They are severely limited by what they are taught is within "safe" boundaries. Their "boundaries" become our barbed-wire fences, leaving each of us little freedom to do our own births in our own ways. Few medically trained students yet know what roles herbs, chiropractic care, acupuncture, homeopathy, or a change in beliefs, for example, can play in helping a woman have her baby.

Pediatricians, neonatologists, anesthesiologists, and physical therapists are responsible. They have long known the damaging effects of many of the tests and drugs—as well as cesarean section—on the infant. As a rule, they know the obstetricians who get "good babies" and those whose results are lethargic and floppy. Their silence has been an embarrassment to their profession and a veritable shame to the babies they attend. Since these people often depend on obstetricians for referrals, it is not surprising that we have heard so little from so few. Of course, you don't bite the hand that feeds you.

Hospital administrations are equally responsible. It is time that physicians be required to make their statistics public. A woman should be able to know the number of births a particular care-provider has attended and, of these, the number of cesareans performed. In addition, she should be able to ascertain how many of the women were monitored, had IVS, drugs, forceps, vacuum extractions, episiotomies. You don't eat at the restaurant if you don't like the menu. Hospital administrations often protect their obstetricians in ways that ultimately shortchange the general public.

Politicians, legislators, and insurance companies are responsible. Cesarean section remains an enormous political, legal, and economic football. Many decisions that affect mother/baby/family are made, perhaps unconsciously, for personal, institutional, and bureaucratic gain.

The media are responsible. I am constantly amazed at the number of people quoted as "experts" in the field of obstetrics who have never been pregnant, never felt a contraction, never had a baby; many of them don't even have a vagina! (Would you want a person to teach you how to swim who'd never been in the water?) Women all over the country who are truly the experts are frequently not considered a reliable or knowledgeable source of information. The "expert" OB is called to corroborate or to refute information.

Television is little help. Soap operas haven't changed since Lois and I first reported to you, and they continue to give us erroneous insights into present cultural attitudes about birth. On Friday afternoon, viewers are still left hanging by a thread. Will the emergency cesarean save her baby? The "natural" births that have been shown in the last few years have been good for nothing more than a belly laugh. Mother, holding her breath, turning beet red. Father, dressed in green, looking like part of the anesthesiology staff, secretly wishing someone would put *him* out. Nurse, instructing mother to PUUUUUUUSH with all her might. Everyone draped, instruments readied, doctor in control. These scenes bear no resemblance to what normal birth is and no understanding of what childbirth can or should be. The newborn that emerges is generally big enough to wear twelve-month "jammykins" and has a vocabulary of ten words. Recently, a new daddy on a soap looked at his newborn and said, "Look what you did to your momma, big boy. She'll never forgive you for that. You should be ashamed." Meanwhile, the new mother is moaning, "Oh, I hurt! I hurt everywhere!" and the nurse replies, "Well, it's only been three days, and he wasn't exactly a peanut, you know." Birth is not supposed to be a battle from which women must recover, nor are babies supposed to be "peanuts."

Some childbirth organizations are also responsible for the mess we're in. Wanting to be respected by the medical community at large, they have continually copped out and sold out. They have smiled, given in, compromised, given up. They have little respect for doctors, less for themselves perhaps, but a great deal of fear. Until these organizations begin to exert their power over the medical and obstetrical groups that rule them, they haven't established a proper "pecking order." Until they help turn public ignorance and apathy into concern and are clear as to what they have contributed to the way our society "does" birth, they continue to be among those who do our sweet little "chicks" a grave injustice.

Of course, in the end we are all responsible! Drug companies, the government, fetal monitoring companies, lawyers. "Who is responsible?" asked the Cesarean Prevention Movement of Southeast Florida. "As the cesarean rate continues to climb, we are left with that nagging question. Many of us have played the game; have felt the frustration; have felt the intimidation. Many of us have felt the fear, the pain, the grief. Who is responsible? 'Am I responsible for what is happening?' Well, let's make sure the answer is YES."[5] Philosopher-teacher-writer Virginia Sandlin says, "How can we expect results to happen in the world if we don't regard ourselves as the source of those results?" *We are responsible!*

Childbirth educator and co-author Cathy Romeo comments, "Instead of encouraging women to feel capable and powerful during the birth experience, most people contribute to the woman's feeling helpless and frightened. If a man were giving birth, would we say, 'Don't worry about a thing, dear, everything will be

taken care of.'? No. We'd say, 'GO GET 'EM, TIGER!!! Go have that baby!'[6]
Midwife Janet Leigh reminds us that 90 percent of modern obstetrical practice
is based on fear and folklore. "But the beliefs are stubborn. They run deep."[7]
Cassidy-Brinn says, "Since 1977 we have seen women's options in childbirth
shrink [emphasis mine] dramatically. What was considered normal twenty years
ago became high risk ten years ago, and what was considered normal ten years
ago is high risk today." She reminds us that women have the right to refuse
technology "without punishment."[8] She echoes Sue Roberts, whose quote began
this chapter: "How did an event which was considered normal for thousands of
years become such a crisis?"

3 *Open Season?*

Go now, not to kill beasts or to find minerals—
Not to grow coffee, cotton, or bananas,
But to open, whilst there is yet time,
The windows of your own souls,
And let in the light that floods the forest of the valleys and the hills;
The light that is law of the jungle,
The law of nature
And the law of God.
And try to understand.[1]

A hologram is a form of lensless photography that, using laser beams, interprets seemingly meaningless swirls and images and reconstructs them as a three-dimensional picture. Surprisingly, it can construct the whole picture from any fragment of the swirls.[2]

According to Sheila Kitzinger, we can know almost everything we need to know about a culture by observing the way the majority of women in that culture birth their babies.[3] If that is true, and I believe it is, then we're in trouble deep. The vast majority of women in this culture birth their babies either as if they were stars in a science fiction movie or casualties of war. They are attached to beds by means of tubes, beeping machines, and inserted needles. They are observed, much like laboratory mice, by fearful, unfamiliar, white-coated technicians. Increasingly, "normal" birth in our country has come to mean drugged women, slashed perinea, sluggish babies, forceps deliveries, vacuum extractions, cesarean sections. "The medical profession has such a huge ego that if they can't fix something, they make it normal. That way they don't have to admit their

failure."[4] Childbirth activist Beverly Beech remarks that birth, the normal, physiological result of pregnancy, is often viewed as unsafe until after the event. She
says that doctors are so adept at concealing their errors that injured patients even
end up thanking them for the mischief they have done.[5] Natalie Shainess tells
us that often, giving birth, instead of being "a moment of pure ecstasy and the
beginning of greatly enhanced sense of self-worth"[6] is a shock from which some
women never fully recover. Some cultures respect and honor the childbearing
woman and her baby; others hold the belief that childbirth "is the result of a
carnal sin to be expiated in pain. From pampering to neglect, the treatment of
women in labor seems to parallel their position within their society at that time."[7]
By that criterion, then, the American woman's position stinks.

Many of the women who give birth in our culture have been traumatized,
enraged, and hurt by the experience. I'm certain that the many thousands of
women who have written to me in the past eighteen years are representative of
the hundreds of thousands of other women who have not picked up a pen to
write: they are women in mourning. These women include not only the vast
majority of those who have had cesarean sections, but also a large number who
have given birth vaginally. Their pregnancies, labors, and deliveries are monitored and managed by green-garbed gods and goddesses. They are met by probing
fingers, disapproving glances, and patronizing, paternalistic, condescending attitudes. Their confidence is drained along with their bladders; their strength
diminishes as an assortment of drugs dribble into their veins. Their bodies,
hungry for nourishment, find the menu wanting: "instant dinner on a pole" (a
la carte). Hungry for human touch and soothing voices, they find catheters,
belts, and electrodes wrapped around various body parts and "bleeps" echoing
in their ears. If they cry out for support, they are given a predesignated number
of milligrams of whatever instead. If they choose to birth naturally, they are
"martyrs"; if they succumb to a cesarean section, they've "failed."

I'm certain that aliens, watching from any galaxy in the universe, would be
aghast if they could see into our obstetrical units, even our birthing rooms. They
would draw conclusions about our planet that would make them hesitant to plan
a visit here, or even shake our (IV-implanted) hands.

In the course of this book, we'll continue to look at how women in our culture
birth. I suggest that you take a look at *Silent Knife* first. We'll peek into doctors'
offices, birthing rooms, and operating rooms, and see how things are going.
Prepare yourself.

Last year, my local town newspaper featured an article entitled "Hunting Rare
Animals Morally Wrong Act." The article reminds us that our forests are being
cut down to make way for human development. "With guns and bulldozers we
have killed off hundreds of species of animals that can never be recreated."
Shouldn't the hunting or obliteration of endangered species be a moral issue?
the author asks. "Regardless of how one feels about hunting as a sport, there is
no way to condone those who would help wipe a species of animal off the face
of the earth."[8] Similarly, the pure-birthing American woman has almost become

extinct. It's not just guns or bulldozers that can wipe out an entire species: in this case, it takes knives, amnio hooks, heparin locks, spiral electrodes, and the like—obstetrical bulldozers, if you will.

Most states have a Department of Natural Resources, Division of Wildlife, that issues a pamphlet outlining hunting laws.[9] The rules for hunting animals are clearly defined. At certain times of the year, different types of animals are considered "fair game." The time when the hunting of these animals is permissible by law is called "open season." It is unlawful to hunt these animals except during open season time periods, and there are strict penalties for anyone caught hunting when the season is closed. During closed seasons, the animals are protected: they are free to roam, graze, and exist without fear of harm from humans.

The pamphlet sets forth elaborate rules. For example, there is a limit to the number of animals that individual hunters can "bag"; and hunting is prohibited at certain times of the day and year. No person under the influence of drugs or alcohol is permitted to hunt. It is unlawful to tear open or disturb a beaver house, or to remove any mammal from walls, holes, trees, the ground, or logs. Destroying or disturbing eggs or nests is prohibited by law. All accidents, injuries, or deaths must be reported. Careless or negligent use of instruments is prohibited. The use of artificial lights is prohibited, as well. Those who wish to hunt or fish must obtain a license. In most areas, licenses must be renewed annually. Any careless or negligent behavior is punishable by fine and/or six months' imprisonment, and the loss of one's license for five years. As soon as the season closes, any violation results in strict disciplinary measures. In fact, any violation at all, at any time, results in strict disciplinary measures.

The rules that protect the quail, pheasant, raccoon, opossum, trout, ruffled grouse, and even the chipmunk afford them far more extensive protection than childbearing women are granted. The weasels, foxes, skunks, and turkeys in the obstetrical wards in our country hunt continuously, trapping, mutilating, and destroying the unsuspecting, trusting, not-easily-camouflaged pregnant female. Anyone at any stage of gestation or labor is fair game. Open season on birthing women in the United States runs from January 1 to December 31. Sundays are not only included but are also considered prime time for a kill.

There is no limit to the number of women a doctor can section without being challenged, fined, or jailed. A significant number of U.S. doctors purchase phony medical credentials.[10] Renewal of licenses is automatic upon payment of a fee.[11] Competent or successful work is nowhere a condition for continuing in practice.[12] The AMA itself estimates that 10 percent of all physicians are incompetent, "severely impaired."[13] It is no secret that physicians are high on the list of those who work under the influence of drugs and alcohol, or both. They remove their prey from their chosen "trees and logs." Worst of all, they disturb and/or destroy the "nests of birds and their eggs"—physiologically, psychologically, spiritually, emotionally. And they aren't even required to wear orange hats.

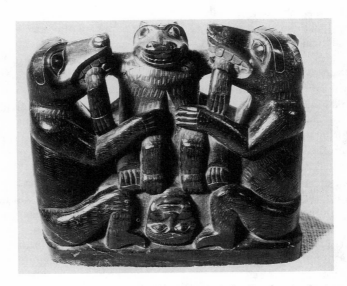

Courtesy of National Museum of the American Indian/Smithsonian Institute.

Women in our culture are "bagged" the minute they walk into a maternity unit. They are welcomed and all but trussed for delivery. (I was astonished to learn that there are still hospitals that give enemas to women in labor.) The pregnant woman often feels confused: while she is being targeted, braceleted, and confined, she may be unsure as to whether she is in the presence of her hunter or her savior.

In the state of Minnesota, there are specific instructions for transporting an "undressed bird." "No more than one hunting party consisting of no more than three hunters shall occupy any such designated hunting station at one time." Most of our maternity units have a number of "hunting stations" these days; teaching units can pack in six or more inexperienced 'marksmen,' and they all have artificial lighting. Most of the women in the units are "undressed birds"; even at two o'clock in the afternoon, most of them are wearing hospital jonnies or nightgowns.

James Prescott, among others, tells us that those societies that give their infants the greatest amount of physical affection and touching experience the lowest incidence of physical violence. Findings overwhelmingly support the thesis that deprivation is closely related to warfare and interpersonal violence. "The world has only limited time to change its custom of deprivation. . . . We do not know how many generations it will take to transform our psychology of violence into one of peace."[14] Most of you are familiar with Ashley Montague's wonderful book, *Touching*, which corroborates our *vital* need—as individuals and as a people—for contact.

The hunters take babies right out of their mothers' arms. Those of you who have been in my classes and seminars have seen the pictures from *Ranger Rick* magazines, depicting a mother gorilla holding her newborn baby. By the look in her eye, we know there is NO WAY anyone could take her infant from her without losing at least an eye. In the next photograph is a picture of her mate, their "security blanket"; just in case momma isn't quite quick enough at that moment to fight off an intruder, dad is ready to protect and defend. After our own deliveries, we are most often so exhausted, weak, and unalert that we allow our natural instincts to fly out the window.

It could take only one generation to turn our world into a haven of peace. It has been said that if each of us went out into the world tomorrow and shared our love with two people, "such that they got it, and they in turn went out the next day and shared it with two more . . . following that progression, in less than 33 days we could reach the entire planet."[15] *Thirty-three days*. It begins at the beginning. At birth. A peaceful birth, where there are no hunters and no game. At this point in time, however,

> The Tiger stalks night and day.
> He strikes with a clawing slash,
> a menacing growl,
> or a snatch with his powerful jaws.
> . . . Like an impaled roast, am I . . .
> The Tiger again tears into my flesh.
> [I feel] the stinging pain of his reinserted teeth . . . [16]

It is time to take another look at cesarean section in the United States and at our birthing practices in general.

4 Caught, Red-Handed!: The Status of Cesarean Section in the United States, Revisited

I was cesarean born. You can't really tell, although when I leave a house, I usually go out by the window.

—Steven Wright, comedian[1]

There is an old Hindu saying about the melon and the knife: "Whether the melon falls on the knife or the knife falls on the melon," the saying goes, "it's the melon that suffers." And so it would appear to me.

—Merle Shaine, writer[2]

I've heard it said a number of times that we may become a nation in which all babies are born—removed—by cesarean section. Don't be ridiculous, you say! That won't happen. How could it? Answer: one cesarean at a time.

Allan Parachini states that in many hospitals in southern California, the section rate is over 30 percent.[3] The article recommends that women ask their obstetricians what their personal section rate is. But what obstetrician is going to admit he or she cuts open every third woman? I'm not picking on California; the section rate is that high or higher in almost every other state. Three counties in Florida, for example, have a rate of almost 50 percent.[4]

In 1987, the Public Citizen Health Research Group, which is part of Ralph Nader's "Raiders," concluded that about 50 percent of the 906,000 cesareans performed that year were unnecessary, resulting in 142 unnecessary maternal deaths.[5] Although the report received a lot of attention when it was released, the furor seems to have died down. After all, it was only 142 (and they were women . . .). For years, childbirth advocates have been telling you that far more than 50 percent of the sections that are done are unnecessary! Most of you know my own opinion; I'm certain that at least 97 percent are preventable and therefore unnecessary.

Nader's report projected that by the year 2000, the rate would be 40 percent. (Some doctors and hospitals are way ahead of that already!) The report made several recommendations for reducing the cesarean rate: (1) Require hospitals to disclose their cesarean rate and rates of successful VBACs. (But the figures are neither honest nor accurate, and by some hospital standards, "successful" VBACs include babies who are tugged out, pulled out, and sucked out, too.) (2) Require obstetricians to attempt a "trial of labor as often as is medically indicated." (But birth is *not* a medical circumstance, so medical indications are invalid. In fact, almost every one of the "contraindications" to VBACs that I have read is not a contradiction in my experience.) (3) Require additional tests. (To supplement the already overused and inaccurate tests that are being done? One inaccurate test times two equals two inaccurate tests.) (4) Obtain a second opinion for all nonemergency c/sections. (A good idea as long as it's not another obstetrician. I'd say a second opinion from Paula in Rhode Island would be good. She had babies 4, 5, and 6 at home after three sections.)

Please understand that I'm glad Nader did something; it's just that it wasn't enough, and it hasn't had the kind of impact we all hoped. It didn't touch the core of the matter: the fears and the lack of understanding about the birth process, some of the issues that must be addressed if doctors are to stop cutting babies out of women's wombs.

And why should they stop cutting? For all the reasons cited in *Silent Knife* and in all others on the subject. Because women and babies are far more hurt than helped by the procedure. Because little baby Kristen in Minnesota wouldn't have lost her two fingers and little baby Sherilyn in Arizona wouldn't have lost her ear if they had been born vaginally. Because maternal deaths are four times greater after cesarean section and the complications for babies are astronomical. We discussed all these reasons in *Silent Knife*. Michele Odent has often said that anyone with two hands and few instruments can do a cesarean section: it frequently requires great intelligence *not* to do it.

By the Authority Vested in Me

From 1972 to 1986 I was a walking compendium of information on the subject of cesarean prevention and VBAC. I knew not only the titles of practically every article that had been written on the subject, but also the authors and journals in which they appeared. I knew the statistics so well that I could rattle off numbers easier than my children's names. When I decided to write *Open Season* a few years ago, I assumed that I would have to be up on all the latest cesarean and birth-related articles. I figured I'd have to resume my bimonthly excursions to the medical library. By my third trip to the library, I realized that my enthusiasm and "drive" were gone. I found myself doing errands and cutting my research time short, or staring out the window. I no longer felt excited and challenged; I only felt impatience and an eagerness to get home.

I also began to feel uneasy and depressed. There were hundreds of new articles coming out. How could I ever keep up with them all? HOW WAS I EVER GOING TO CONVINCE ANYONE if I couldn't locate the articles or didn't have the facts straight?? How could I help pregnant women to stay 'one-up' on their doctors if we didn't know what was in their literature better than they did? I had relied on stored information to spurt out at the appropriate moment and either stun or silence my "attackers"—or to reassure a pregnant woman. And then, in a flash one day something became crystal clear: I didn't have to go to the library to be an expert on birth. I had all the necessary information programmed into my female form: I had been pregnant, and I had given birth. I already was an expert of sorts. Whatever answers I needed wouldn't be found in obstetrical journals or in any scientific research per se.

Now when some people called, expecting me to rattle off some new stuff, I'd tell them I didn't have the foggiest idea. Since I didn't "do" libraries much anymore, I said, they should perhaps check one out themselves if they wanted the information. If they wanted a specific article to convince a doctor, I'd tell them that they probably had the wrong doctor. I kept feeling our whole approach to birth was wrong. Within months of that awakening, I read two books that affirmed my new belief and greatly influenced my thinking: *Woman's Reality* by Anne Schaef and an incredible book that I recommend to everyone, *Going Out of Our Minds: The Metaphysics of Liberation* by Sonia Johnson. The final straw came when I read the title of one of the articles I had xeroxed: "A multicenter prospective randomized controlled trial of induction of labor with an automatic closed-loop feedback controlled oxytocin infusion system." I'd had it. Life was too short. Since that time, I have spent no time whatsoever in a medical library—and have still been learning as much about birth as ever I had.

"Keep Them in Stitches"

Esther Zorn, founder and director of the National Cesarean Prevention Movement, has prepared a "profile of the Cesarean Epidemic."[6] Years ago, cesareans were performed only in rare circumstances: they were a last resort—a "failure," in fact, on the part of the doctor. As new techniques and anesthesias became available, the rate began to climb, albeit slowly at first. As women were anesthetized for vaginal delivery (and almost the entire generation before ours was), the need for forceps and sections rose—paralyzed bodies do not "expel" their "contents" on their own. Zorn reports that the cesarean rate rose from 5 percent in 1970 to 14.7 percent in 1978—and then to 24.1 percent in 1986, 24.4 percent in 1987, and 24.6 percent in 1988. *This rise was not accompanied by a related improvement in the infant mortality and morbidity rates.* A recent article observes that any improvement in perinatal mortality does not necessarily rely on an ever-

Cesarean Birth
(for Gabriel)

I wanted to greet you slowly, in whispers,
with cool light and warm water.
Instead I let them squeeze and push you.
My fault they said.
You were big enough to burst, but not quite ready.
You stayed. I held you, breathing the All,
our rhythm still throbbing, strong.

They stuck us with tentacles,
an insect, a telephone pole.
and poisoned us together,
for our "own good,"
poisoned us forever.

Lost in foggy fear I disappeared.
They pumped the spasms through me,
telling me to spit you out– a bad taste.
I writhed hour by hour
as they pumped more and more,
counting heartbeats on a screen.
heartbeats even and strong,
rating our pain on a scale,
blaming me.
Blaming me, tied to their bed,
believing their Black Magic
instead of the Mother.

I first saw you in a dream,
cut from my belly like my heart
at the Great Sacrifice.
Covered with my blood
you flashed before me,
cringing at the white and icy assault.
Screaming for my warmth
you were wrapped in cotton.
Longing for our 'single' breath
you were whisked away from me.

Green gowns melted into hallway walls.
I wept as I was wheeled to greet you.
You refused their rubber tits and sugar water,
waited for my breast and sucked, strong.
Familiar voices smiled
into our starry silence.
I could not move, I could not cry out

I begged them not to take you again
But my words were weak on jailers ears.
They turned out my lights and closed my door.
Sleep was a handsome paramour.

Your late night cry woke me
to darkness, an empty womb.
Sleep still tugged at my brain
as I recalled the butcher's smile,
the henchman's mask.
Sleep. Sleep reached out a soft hand,
offered to slip me into heaven for awhile.

But you cried
and I called across the hall,
"Bring my baby. My baby!"
You were not a stranger when I held you
and I held you till dawn.

                        Kate Dahlsted

---

increasing cesarean section rate.[7] (*I would say that it depends in full measure on a decreasing rate!*) The article states: "Not infrequently, the rates of cesarean section and perinatal mortality have been considered and presented as reciprocally dependent variables, without taking into consideration many of the other factors or forces that have been at work during this same decade." YOU DO NOT GET BETTER BABIES WITH C-SECTIONS!! We have all been duped; and it is high time for un-duping!

I have several articles on the "underreporting" of cesareans; as we told you in *Silent Knife, maternal deaths may be underreported by "as much as twenty—or possibly even thirty—percent."*[8] Jack Smith, an analyst for the Center for Disease Control, states that the new figures may call into question a major assumption of contemporary public health: that the health effects of procedures such as cesareans have essentially eliminated maternal death from the American scene. Women die three to four times more often with cesareans than with vaginal deliveries. If hospitals are willing to claim a certain percentage of sections, chances are it's even higher than that. What's discouraging is that even many doctors admit that it is unlikely that the trend will be reversed without changes in the legal climate (although fear of malpractice may be just an excuse). More on that later.

Esther says that most doctors just don't understand birth or VBAC. They think that the way you reduce the number of cesareans is by increasing the use of forceps or by using vacuum extractors. In fact, a number of hospitals have "successfully lowered" the section rate because they have instituted these measures. We are definitely not talking improvement here.

Blood Thirsty?

If the number of cesareans were reduced by 50 percent, there would be an excess of $1 billion saved a year in hospital costs alone.[9] Hospitals are having enough money problems already, so why would they want to reduce the section rate at all? Rather, they need to increase it to keep them solvent! Natural childbirth? No, that's not where it's at. Women should utilize their stress-test rooms, nonstress (what a misnomer) rooms, their special care nurseries.

A number of people—health economists, statisticians, and childbirth experts and advocates alike—report that *anything over a 5 percent c-section rate requires justification.* A 5 percent rate would reduce obstetricians' incomes by over $175 million per year. (Do you know any obstetricians interested in a reduced income?) The predicted rate for sections is 29 percent for 1990 and over 35 percent soon after that. By then, all the obstetricians, anesthesiologists, and nurse anesthetists in this country should be happily sunning themselves and their loved ones on the Riviera a few months out of the year. In this materialistic society of ours, "no-frills" births are passé, and at least from the medical point of view, they're a ticket to nowhere. The reduction in c-sections would reduce hospital profits by $1.1 billion. "The new sound of joy heard in delivery rooms is not 'It's a boy' or 'It's a girl,' but 'It's a bonanza!' "[10]

Insurance companies are beginning to get with it, but not fast enough. If they covered the cost of labor support people, they wouldn't have to chalk up the money for nearly as many sections. One woman said that her company dropped her when they found out she was going to have a VBAC after two sections; they considered her a risk. She challenged it and eventually won, but at great emotional cost to her. Another woman's insurance company stopped paying for labor after the first twenty-four hours. Every added hour in the hospital meant several hundred dollars added on her own personal bill; she said that the added tension may have had an influence on her having a cesarean—which, by the way, the insurance company did pay for. It is time that insurance companies begin giving bonuses for vaginal births. The doc who doesn't plug anything in, turn anything on, or stick anything in, wins; he gets the most money for just watching the woman give birth. Insurance companies must begin to cover the cost of homebirths and midwives as well. More on that in future chapters.

Insurance companies pay more for cesarean sections than conventional births partly because of the higher fees charged for cesareans by the doctor. According to Dr. Robert Schneider, "The presumption is that cesareans require greater skill or training, which is not always true." The obstetrician profits when he convinces you to have a questionable cesarean. For your doctor's personal life, Robert Schneider says, the increased acceptance of cesarean section by the "blissfully unaware public" has been a great boon—shorter hours at increased pay with the added bonus of avoiding the inconvenience of waiting for labor to progress. We all know that more cesareans are done on certain days of the week—and right before long weekends and holidays. We have also been told that money that expands medical control "unleashes a nightmare forged with good intentions."[11]

All this increase in sections in spite of the literature that proves beyond any shadow of a doubt that they are unnecessary and dangerous makes you wonder. The National Institutes of Health spent all that money and all that time a few years ago to study the cesarean epidemic and concluded that far too many were being done.[12] In Canada, the Final Statement of the Panel from the National Consensus Conference on Aspects of Cesarean Birth[13] expressed concern over the growing number of sections and suggested how to reduce them. Laurie Brant, VBAC childbirth educator from British Columbia, says that, although the recommendations from the task force were all adopted as "standard of practice," it has made little, if any, difference. The NIH study seems an equal waste of money. Judy Cochrane, director of the Cesarean Options Committee from ICEA, says that the rates of cesareans in some locations in Canada seem to be stabilizing. This is welcome news, but it should have happened a long time ago.

An article entitled "The Mounting Evidence Against Cesareans" states: "If doctors took their own advice, the number of cesareans should fall." Since they aren't even taking their own advice, it is an absolute puzzle to me why women do. I have a cartonload of studies done within the past five years on the epidemic from medical journals, ob/gyn publications, newspapers, and childbirth organizations all over the country: "Doctors Urged to Discourage Cesareans"; "Study Says Cesarean Rate Can Be Halved; "Pros, Cons of C-Sections Debated"; "Many Cesareans Needless"; "A Successful Program to Lower Cesarean Section Rates"; "MDs Question Rising Cesarean-Section Rate." From the *Los Angeles Times* to the *Boston Globe* and back again, from the *New England Journal of Medicine* to the *Lancet* across the sea we find that too many sections are being done. In 1988, *The Wall Street Journal* article "Physicians' Group Seeks to Lower High Rate of Cesarean Deliveries" reported that the American College of Obstetricians and Gynecologists had "announced a fresh effort to bring down the cesarean section rate."[14] What "effort"? Has anything changed? They just keep doing more and more studies and then more and more sections! They tell us there are too many women getting cut and then they cut them anyway! The same mentality that harpoons our seals, nets our dolphins, sprays our grapes, and radiates our vegetables slices our women. So many get on the bandwagon and decry the appalling number of sections, but what do they do to stop them?

It is not, nor does it appear that it will ever be, the "physicians' group" that seeks to lower the rate of unnecessary women's gynecological and obstetrical surgery. It has been, and will always be, the women's groups. "And though it seems impossible," says Sonia Johnson, "most women's organizations are even more in thrall to patriarchy. They stand for reform and yet want respect from those they do not respect. Abandoning the patriarchal mind, we consign it to oblivion. So that, after all, and despite everything, we and all other things may escape with our lives."[15] But I'm getting ahead of myself. We will have more on this in Chapter 7.

Doctors Who Will, Women Who Won't?

By no means can doctors solve the problems alone. They are the problem—but not the entire problem, to be sure. Women themselves are also the problem. If they refused to show up, there'd be no one to cut. Typical are the following letter-writers. In one woman's magazine, a woman wrote that she was glad that her child was born by section: "I discussed the pros and cons with my doctor [I would have liked to sit in on that conversation] but after weighing the pros and cons, I decided to have a repeat cesarean. [No labor for the baby, even!] . . . It is important to keep things in perspective and remember that the actual delivery of a child is really insignificant [you are unconscious, lady] in comparison to the rest of the things he will experience in his lifetime. A woman's ability to be a good mother is not gauged by the method by which ["method"—I sigh, deeply] her child was delivered."[16]

In another article called "Expectant Mom Gives C-Notes," the author says, "I have a friend who knows someone who had a cesarean, she said she could feel the whole thing. Sure. I have a friend who knows someone whose soul leaves her body every night and travels to Atlantic City. Really, the only thing that hurts while a doctor is performing a cesarean delivery [not a delivery, a cesarean operation—it's a major abdominal *operation*!] is the fact that you have a lot of time to reflect on all the dumb remarks leading up to the birth."[17]

Another woman writes that "Like everyone else in this society, my husband and I were led down the garden path and believed that 'natural childbirth' was the only way. Well, three years ago, we brought a 9 lb. baby boy into the world. I say 'we' because my husband was there every minute, I was fully awake and saw him the moment he was born. We could not have been more elated had he been born 'naturally.' [How do you know?] This year, when my doctor said I had a forty % chance of having a vaginal delivery, I chose cesarean. Rather than go with any risk to my baby, I'll take the odds. Isn't a healthy baby the most important thing?"[18]

YES. A healthy baby is important! But it does matter. Many women have bought the whole bag of potatoes! "As long as we get us a fine, strapping young lad, what difference does it make?" For starters, according to a number of studies, child abuse is three to nine times greater among cesarean mothers than among the general population.[19] Those who are battered learn to batter. Recovery time is much longer, which means that the infant is deprived of vital ongoing care those first days and weeks from a mother capable of holding her and taking care of her. Cesarean babies are always at a disadvantage. Those who say it doesn't matter are only fooling themselves. Cesareans matter because they are not only "the problem," but a symptom of a much greater problem, as we will see.

One woman from Canada says, "Every woman having a c-section feels—or wants to feel—that having endured the procedure, it was warranted. There is enough to deal with without having to go over the events that led to the surgery time and time again to (possibly) determine its necessity." True, and yet it is that very journey—the very willingness to open oneself to the possibility that the cesarean could have been prevented—that may foster growth and healing.

I have found that underneath the fear and relief of a large number of women who protest that a cesarean is a perfectly fine way to have a baby lies a devastated womanplace (see Chapter 13). Writer-therapist Shirley Luthman says that denial requires great amounts of energy: the effort occasionally overloads the system, producing physical or emotional symptoms or breakdown.[20] Sarah, a VBAC after two cesareans, says that scheduling a cesarean is like making an appointment to get your leg broken—unnecessary self-inflicted suffering. Pam Brown says that doctors think of scheduled sections as the "Cadillac of c-sections." They must see homebirth as the Edsel of normal deliveries.

Some women have been told that now that they do the "bikini" cut, it isn't major surgery.[21] Talk about heads in the sand. Barbara Katz Rothman, author of a number of books on birth and women's rights, asks, "When a woman 'chooses' to have a cesarean is she gaining or losing control? In part, the answer depends on the accuracy of the information given [to her which influences her decision]. The woman is having major surgery with all of its attendant risks to her health and life—making her sick, weak and dependent as she enters motherhood."[22]

In certain areas of Massachusetts, certain operations are done more often than in other areas, even though the populations are geographically close and homogeneous. Hingham residents, for example, had their gall-bladders removed four times more often than Holyoke residents. There were 15 percent more tonsillectomies west of Boston than south. Cesarean sections ranged from 22 to 48 percent, depending on location. "The crazy-quilt pattern cannot be explained, say the authorities, by differences in age or incidence of disease from one community to another. Rather, the wide range of surgical rates stems largely from differences in physician 'practicing styles.' "[23] Affluent women and women with insurance, it seems, have far more cesareans (up to 75 percent more) than those who are in lower brackets and are not covered—in spite of greater access to "better" health care and to better food.[24] "Women shouldn't have to bring themselves into poverty to lower the section rate," one article states. "Doctors often list non-existent complications to justify doing the procedure, which is more lucrative for themselves and the institutions for which they work."[25]

The media have helped the cause in a few ways but hurt it in others. The papers, for example, give the impression that it was the doctors who uncovered the cesarean epidemic and that they were really concerned for women's well-being. Similarly, newspapers seem to tell us that the idea of VBAC came from the doctors. This is quite a joke, but it's not surprising considering our patriarchal culture. Dr. Sidney Wolfe, head of the Public Citizen Health Research Group, says that cesareans are the number one unnecessary surgery in this country and that "Mothers are not being adequately informed of the risks involved."[26] Instead, we are told that cesareans are "the best route" for the baby and that women should "opt for cesareans."

Gena Corea asks "Will the media continue to write articles uncritically glorifying technology and the miracles of modern medicine?"[27] Are doctors, lawyers, and journalists all in this together? (For more on this question, see Chapter 7). One article states that the newest technologies are "easing the worries of pregnant women."[28] We'll see about that. A film on VBAC produced by a large video broadcasting company had a medical and legal consultant, but no one from the Cesarean Prevention Movement. Those women are the experts on birth—not the doctors and the lawyers. The movies also do their damage. In a number of films in the past few years, pregnant women have ultrasound and amniocentesis. We get to watch the procedures. Such an exposure to birth technology establishes pregnancy as pathology and emphasizes the doctor as saviour. A number of movies here of late have shown couples giving birth "American style." The way birth is shown also has a negative effect on our youth. I overheard a group of local teens discussing birth after they had seen a movie. "I want to be put out!" said one. "Yes!" said another. Obviously, the film had failed to portray birth in a way that would open these young women's hearts to the power and joy of the process.

What we need is one big star who has had a VBAC to speak for us—someone whom the world loves and admires, someone who hated being cut open and finally reached an understanding of birth as a natural function of a woman's body. Someone has to come through for us—what with Sesame Street selling out. (You'll catch that in another chapter.) But, as you know, a large portion of the "stars" out there get washed up on the beach (albeit Malibu) too, along with the rest of us.

Cut and Paste

"Do you have to tie me down?" I asked.

"Yes," said a woman's voice behind the curtain. "You might contaminate yourself." She buckled the restraints tightly around my wrists, and I fanned my fingers in protest.

"I can't see anything," I cried.

"That's right," she said.

The anesthesiologist towered above me and above the curtain. . . . He moved with nonchalance around my table. . . . I hated his freedom, the pivot of his shoulder, his view of the room and my body, his effortless reach over my barrier. . . . his mastery of movement, his stroll.

"Now I am going to touch you with a pin," he said as his hand and arm disappeared behind the curtain. "Tell me if it's sharp."

I felt a prick below my breasts. "It's sharp," I said.

"Now is it?"

"Yes," I said.

"Now?" The pin wandered, coming down near my ribs, near my hips, on my sides, and below my naval. It was random voo-doo.

"Yes," I said.

"Now?" Impatience was creeping into his voice.

"Yes."

"Still sharp? Tell me when it gets less sharp."

"It still is" I said, anxious about the meaning of the word, "sharp," trying to distinguish a pinprick from half a pinprick.

"I can still feel it," I said.

"Now? It should begin to feel less sharp."

"Well, maybe a little."

"Now?"

"Yes, it's getting less sharp," I said, waiting for the next one.

—from "Random Voo Doo," by Chase Collins[29]

In *Silent Knife*, we provided you with a detailed textbook description of a cesarean section operation and the serious complications associated with it. As a little "refresher," some descriptions by a few of the women themselves will show us that it is not relatively minor surgery. The chapter that follows will give us additional "testimonies." But before that, I want to tell you about a young mother in Uganda.

"Akuu Naibi" was a Ugandan woman who was sectioned in 1879. She lay on an inclined bed, the head of which was placed against the side of the hut. She was liberally supplied with banana wine, and

> the operator stood . . . on her left side, holding the knife aloft with his right hand, and muttering an incantation. . . . Then . . . he proceeded to make a rapid cut . . . a few bleeding points were . . . touched with a red-hot iron by an assistant. . . . his assistant held the abdominal walls apart with both hands. . . . The child was next rapidly removed . . . and then the operator. . . . removed the placenta through the abdominal wound. . . . The red-hot iron was used . . . sparingly. . . . No sutures were put into the uterine wall. . . . A porous grass mat was placed over the wound and secured there. . . . Bands that had tied the woman down were cut, and she was gently turned . . . over so that the fluid in the abdominal cavity could drain away on to the floor. . . . She was returned to her former position . . . the edges of the wound were brought into close apposition . . . and seven thin, well-polished, iron spikes were used. . . . and fastened by string made of bark cloth.[30]

A paste was prepared and spread over the wound. The observer noted that the patient had uttered no cry, and an hour after the operation, "she seemed to be comfortable. The baby was placed to breast two hours after the operation. . . . Eleven days later, the wound was entirely healed."

At the end of the article describing the cesarean in Uganda, we are told that we can only wonder what the Ugandan surgical genius would have been able to achieve "had he had access to the resources of the best medical institutions in the world at that time."[31] Well, here are the testimonies of women who did have access to excellent medical institutions, 111 years after Akuu had her cesarean.

Scar Tactics

We'll start "easy."

Valerie (Florida)

I have no memory of the beginning of my son's life and when other mothers recount seeing their baby emerge into the world, of holding their infant moments after birth. . . . I can't help but feel a stinging stab of loss for a joyful human experience I was denied and now may never have. Barely a day has gone by that I have not cried for the few precious first hours of our baby's life that were stolen from my husband and myself. . . .

First and foremost, I should have been awake. I received an epidural hours in advance in preparation for a cesarean. . . . The catheter fell out and was re-inserted. The anesthetic was discontinued and wore off. . . . Ten minutes later, I was given general anesthesia without any consent whatever from me or my husband. I have yet to find out why. Either the obstetrician was not aware of it or had forgotten our agreement that there would be an epidural only. When questioned, he guessed that "we probably couldn't wait for the epidural to take effect." Couldn't wait ten more minutes after I had labored for ten hours with a fluctuating fetal heart rate? . . .

My husband should have been present to tell me about everything I missed. He was scrubbed and waiting outside the OR. I asked to be able to talk to him and I was told it was not permitted. We weren't even allowed to kiss goodbye. . . .

Hours later, I awoke and asked for my baby. They said, "Not now.". . . The nurse looked at me and asked, "Why are you crying? You're supposed to be happy! You just had a baby! Lamaze is fine as far as it goes but at least you have a healthy baby. . . . " I was given a shot to help me sleep—I had just woken up! I still have frequent "pain" in my thigh where this shot was given, each time I am reminded that I was denied the right to refuse medication. . . . This was the first of many insensitive, unnecessary procedures that were inflicted upon me have left two scars—the physical AND the emotional. . . .

George Eliot said, "What do we live for if not to make the world less difficult for each other?" . . . I wish you had known me before. I was happy, confident, loving and healthy: albeit naive and slightly apprehensive about the unknown. Now I am depressed, angry, violated, scarred, and afraid. They probably think they saved my baby's life. I know they ruined mine."

Vivian (California)

Everything went wrong. Absolutely everything. . . . The spinal I desperately wanted so that at least I'd be awake, didn't "take." Then—after some anesthesia had been administered by I.V.—enough so that I couldn't talk or open my eyes, but not enough to keep me from hearing—I felt like I was choking, gagging on something. And evidently I was, on the trach tube they felt was necessary so as to complete the anesthesia with nitrous oxide. I heard them say, "Well hurry up because I am going to take the baby now anyway." . . .

Everything in me fought to open my eyes, to scream, to do anything to let them know I wasn't "under" yet. But I couldn't. I could feel my own gagging. I could hear my heart beat on the monitor, racing. I knew I had to relax to let the trach tube in. I did, it did, and I felt the rush of nitrous—but not before I felt the incision being made into my body!!

Caroline (Toronto)

Wheeled. Narrow table. Chrome. Green. Flourescent. Metal. Arms strapped down like Jesus on the cross. Masked strangers march in, hands up, yellow gloves in the air. My body, the sacrificial animal. . . . Green. Mask. Cap. I don't recognize the stranger—oh, he doesn't have the yellow gloves. Otherwise he looks just like them. Green. Mask. Cap. He holds my strapped-down hand and smiles helplessly. I shake. I can't see beyond the green and screen. I am having a baby. God help me.

A gurgle. He stands up excitedly to look beyond the screen. I'm glad they don't tell him to sit down. At least he can see the birth—surgery—whatever. A lot of uncomfortable tugging and a mask holds up a blue baby. How ugly. More tugging. I fight back tears of . . . ?

I am wheeled to recovery. . . . The body is full of tubes. . . . The body, tubes and all, is taken to its room. I don't know where I am.

The epidural is wearing off. The pain is excruciating. They keep coming to check the body. Morphine. The pain is still excruciating. Dark. Quiet. Pain. Alone.

The hospital stirs to life. Pain. Hunger. Nausea, They bring a bundle. I don't know what to do with it. Too much pain. They take it away. . . . Searing excruciating pain. . . . They bring the bundle again. I must learn to get used to it. . . .

. . . The bundle won't nurse. . . . The body may go home. . . . He comes to pick it up, and the flowers, the gifts, the 5-day old bundle, squalling and screaming, pack into the car. . . . It hurts to stand straight. The sun shines its paradox. Home. Exhausted. Pain. . . . I am confused.

I look into the bundle and see the big wide eyes. I suddenly see how beautiful they are, My eyes fill with tears. . . . I have fallen in love, helplessly in love, with a bundle. My child.

Random Voodoo

Doris (Michigan)

I was never told that there was any chance that I would be operated on without anesthesia. Well, I was subjected to a level of suffering I have only heard of in stories of what the Nazis did to people in concentration camps like Dachau and Bergen-Belsen. I am a nurse, and in all my days, I had never seen the likes of what happened to me. . . .

. . . A medical student came in to start the IV and it quickly became obvious he didn't know what he was doing. He blew two veins trying to go in bevel down at a 90 degree angle, and after blowing the veins he continued digging around in there trying to find the vein he had already blown. As he left he told me that it was really my fault because I . . . had bad veins. . . .

Once the monitor was on, the nurses never again initiated any conversation with me. Instead, they ignored my attempts to talk with them. I began to feel as if I was in a ghost movie in which I was dead, but didn't know it. The nurses felt free to make tactless comments right in front of me as though I couldn't hear.

. . . . They began operating without anesthesia. It never even occurred to me that the doctor would start surgery without saying anything to me. Because of the screen, I couldn't even see when she came to my side to start the operation. I was just sort of dozing on the table when I experienced the sensation of a razor blade slashing the tender skin just above my pubic bone. The initial slash was followed immediately by a deep, pulsating aching pain, like the pain after you get a paper cut. Only this was a seven inch long gash to my abdomen, a thousand times more agonizing than a paper cut. As I tried to call out, I remember thinking, "Oh my God, this can't be happening to me!" I finally managed to scream out, "I can feel you cutting me!" The doctor looked at the anesthesiologist, as though for guidance. He said that I was fine and she should continue the surgery. No one paid any attention to my distress. All I know was that the cutting stopped for a few seconds and she said, "Doris, I'm already down to the faschia. I couldn't have gotten this far unless you were anesthetized."

The next thing that happened after I was told that I had enough anesthesia was that I felt the most horrible slashing sensation. The pain was different and much, much worse than the skin incision. I can't describe it except to say that it felt like razor blades were cutting me deeper and deeper. My whole world turned blood red, and the pain was so terrible I felt as if I couldn't breathe. It felt like a huge monster was clawing at my guts. I screamed for my husband to do something and waved the only part of me that wasn't securely tied down, my left hand. . . . The nurse yelled at Kevin to "get her hand," and he grabbed my hand. I needed his support so badly because of the terrible pain, but he didn't do anything to help me, and it seemed to me he was helping hold me down so they could continue to torture me! He didn't help me, he was helping them. This episode has nearly destroyed our marriage.

As the cutting continued, I lost all hope. This new agony quickly became so great I couldn't even scream. All I could do was gasp and try to hold on. I was trying to hold still because I was intensely aware that a woman was wielding a scalpel less than two inches from my baby and if I moved or jerked by abdomen she might accidentally put it through my baby's head. Somehow, I managed to hold still for my baby's sake. Kevin tells me that I was writhing in pain, grimacing and whipping my head back and forth on the operating table, and grunting and moaning. One nurse in the OR recognized my agony as abnormal and begged the anesthesiologist to do something to help, but he said he had given me everything he could. Why couldn't he have given me general anesthesia? Everyone ignored my agony; nobody made any attempt to comfort me or aid me in any way. Even today, the memory of that horror is so painful, I get sick to my stomach even thinking about it. I have nightmares so terrible, I am afraid to go to sleep, and when I do get to sleep, I often wake up screaming because in my dreams, I relive the pain of that knife being plunged into my belly over and over and over. . . . I felt another slash and I screamed, "My bladder! You're cutting my bladder!" and the doctor said, "No, Doris, I am nowhere near your bladder. I am cutting peritoneum." Then she just went on cutting me.

At some other point, the nurse who had tried to help before asked for help on my behalf again. She was ignored. After the peritoneum was cut, I got delirious with pain. I lost all sense of time and my entire world was reduced to the terrible pain in my gut. I sort of psychologically detached from my body to cope with the pain I guess. The next thing I knew, I heard the doctor yell over the drapes, angrily, "Doris! You have to stop breathing like that! I can't work down here."

. . . Everyone in that room had to know I was being operated on without anesthesia. . . . I felt like I was all alone in green hell. . . . After a while, they hung the baby over the drapes. I didn't care. I totally rejected him. I felt hatred toward him. I heard him cry and I heard a nurse exclaim, "Would you get a load of the size of those big feet?" . . . I had no mothering feeling about him. I didn't care if he was deformed, alive, dead, or what. . . . I felt as if I was an inanimate wrapper for a baby, with no intrinsic worth or value. I wanted to die to get away from . . . my Gestapo torturers.

I have no further clear memories of the operating room. I began hallucinating that I was being attacked by a bear. I became confused and delirious. I vaguely remember "knowing" that I had to hold still and play dead. Years earlier I had read an article by some forest ranger who said that in a bear attack, one must play dead in order for the bear to stop attacking. . . . I felt overwhelmingly weak and I knew that meant I was going into shock and was going to die from the bear attack.

One of the nurses later told me that the surgical staff was extremely rough, pounding and pushing on my uterus. . . . They found it impossible to close the wound because I had tensed my abdominals so much as a response to the pain. The doctor literally couldn't get the edges of my abdominal tissue together enough to put in any sutures. At that point, she angrily said, "I can't do anything down here!" and the anesthesiologist replied, "Well, do you want me to put her under?" The next thing I knew I was waking up in the recovery room. . . .

Doris' letter goes on. It is thirty pages long altogether—typed, single-spaced. Not surprisingly, there were major complications. I just can't bear to type any more of it. My throat is constricted and my stomach hurts. Doris went to court and won her case, but no amount of money could compensate for what had happened. "I wanted someone to say, 'I'm sorry.' " She ended her letter to me by saying, "It was the most cruel, brutal, barbaric experience I have ever heard of. I was abandoned in labor and then treated like a cadaver being chopped up in an autopsy when I was in reality a living, feeling woman having her first baby. I was lied to, abused, and denied appropriate medical care and nursing care. It was bad enough that they viciously and sadistically tortured me, but to hurt an innocent baby is . . . an atrocity." Doris was sexually nonfunctioning for over two years following her cesarean section.

In an article entitled "Cesarean Nightmare," Anne Cooper writes that she, too, could feel the cutting. "It felt like cutting through a roast with a blunt knife." She went through a "black depression" that lasted a long time. "I got the impression that I shouldn't worry about a little pain; the baby was fine and that was all that mattered. They said sometimes these things happen—it's a fine balance between too much and too little anesthesia." Anne still sleeps curled up in a ball so no one can get her stomach. She said she'd rather die than have another section. She's singly amazed at the complacency with which the public has accepted the false notion that cesarean section is an almost innocuous procedure.

Anne is not alone in her sentiments. There were some days when I, too, felt I'd rather die than be sectioned again—and my cesarean, by most standards, was "good." You may have noticed the name Mary Ripple at the beginning of this book, on the page "In Memoriam." Mary once told me that she'd rather die than have another cesarean. Ironically, she died one year after her second child was born by cesarean section. She was 32 years old and never really recovered from the procedure, physically or emotionally. I miss you, Mary.

When I first decided to write *Open Season*, I had planned to quote more of the story, "Random Voodoo." In it, the operation begins before the anesthesia has taken effect: "They started without me! 'I can feel it! I can feel it! I can feel it!' I screamed

> on a cold wind that, rising and rising, carried me up like a thought, snapped me up like an idea, taking no longer than the millisecond of "getting it" in the brain. . . . Yanked and catapulted into airless heights like a Frisbee in a tornado. . . . I shredded like paper in a gale; I shattered like light through a prism; I cracked and came apart. . . . I am being torn open by toothless dogs and I am the deer and I am alive and the hunter has strung me up with my feet tied together and my arms tied together and I am hanging on a wire. . . . My head dangles . . . I see the gorge and the sky and I am open, my entrails quiver in the heat and I am still alive and hideous and gutted and upside down, hanging from the scaffold of my own limbs.

I realized, however, that I didn't have to use as much as I had originally intended: as you see, I had "original manuscripts" of my own to quote.

So, do you think we've come a long way . . . ?

Maybe if they'dda used banana wine. . . .

More Testimonies

Here are just a few more excerpts from letters from cesarean women:

> Laura: I broke down on the operating table just before they started to cut. I cried out, "I don't want this to happen!" The anesthesiologist said, "Oh, just be quiet!"

> Denise: Being young and naive, I listened to the doctor when he said he was sure my pelvis would be too small to deliver. So, two weeks before my due date, with no labor at all, my son was taken by c-section. My beautiful 7 lb. 5 oz. son was delivered, perfectly formed and chubby. Our joy was short-lived, however, because twelve hours after he was born, he died of hyaline membrane disease—the surgery had been done before he was ready to be born. So not only did I have major surgery to recover from, I had to face the death of my first born child. I am angry—

angry for a lot of things. Had we waited until nature took its course, his lungs would have been mature enough to sustain his life. Angry that no one ever gave ME a choice—other than cherry or lime Jell-O.

Peg: Three sections. Don't get me wrong, I am thankful for my children. I just feel so damn cheated and used by the medical profession. I am scarred for life. The physical scars, as ugly as they are, are just something I have to live with. But the emotional scars, the aftermath of all this will haunt me for a long time to come, if not always.

Gloria: I woke up in the recovery room alone in the room with the janitor mopping the floor.

Lynn: There were two surgeons sewing me up. Each took 1/2 of the scar and they each did it differently! So one side is relatively flat and the other side sticks out and is lumpy and GROSS.

Betsy: My body hurt. More than that, I was spiritually stunned.

Roberta: My husband is having a vasectomy tomorrow. Neither of us ever want to go through another cesarean section again.

Elaine: I am a survivor of three cesarean sections. I was humiliated, demeaned, violated, and submissive for the first. The next two were repeats—can you believe it?

Toby: A week after my section, I hemorrhaged. Something had been left "untied." When I got pregnant the next time, I went to get my medical records and was told they couldn't be found.

Fredda: I was dizzy for three months, and I still have a funny feeling when I stand too quickly. I blacked out once but the doctor said that would go away.

Rosie: To whomever can answer my question: I had an emergency cesarean over a year ago and I have noticed that sometimes since then I get tongue tied or I say things backwards or when I try to say unemployment check I say income tax check. I slur my words and stutter sometimes, too. Also, I have problems processing my thoughts in correct order when I speak to someone. I was very drowsy and tired for this whole year as I had never had major surgery before. Do these things have anything to do with the anesthesia used on me, could it have caused some brain damage? Also, I get severe headaches in the back of my head, neck, shoulder— is this caused from stress or the cesarean? It really bothers me, because I never was like this. A lot of times I try to communicate something to my husband or friend and I complete the thought in my head but when I speak it, it comes out backwards or I go blank and can't remember what I'm saying. If you have any information or case studies that could help me, here is my address. . . .

After the Cuttin' . . .

For many women, pain doesn't end after the "recovery" period. Jeanne wrote:

My baby was born over a year ago. . . . We marvel at the love he's brought us. But our happiness has been clouded by my chronic pain ever since the cesarean. . . .

During the first month I had excruciating pain, especially with activity, but I expected it and accepted it. My OB put me on antibiotics at six weeks. . . . When this did not help, I was told to be patient. . . . Beautiful summer, beautiful baby, and I was in such constant pain I could hardly move. We consulted several other doctors, and none had ever heard of such long-term post operative pain.

Jeanne was referred to plastic surgeons and occupational therapists. She went to a pain clinic and a rehabilitation therapist (the only one who really listened Jeanne says, and appreciated the ramifications of this pain in her daily life and in her relationships), tried many techniques and therapies, and followed the suggestions given to her. She ate well, took vitamins, tried to take walks, did isometrics. At night, her husband would gently smooth Vitamin E on the scar. She also tried a session with a therapeutic masseuse who had had two cesareans and who told Jeanne to "breathe into her belly and love the place that had let the baby live."

Jeanne's story is related in the *C/SEC Newsletter* (1988), Volume 14, No. 4, and you might want to take a look at it. She has had two additional surgeries to try to help the pain, and is in a waiting period. She is still in debilitating pain much of the time. While Jeanne's situation is dramatic, and somewhat unique, you will find in this book, as you did in *Silent Knife*, that cesarean section does indeed cause a number of women to become unstrung.

They Cut Our Bodies, but it Still Hurts in Our Hearts

> . . . with her atrophy of spirit [she] degenerates
> into an impersonation of life
>   not demanding to live the dignity
>   that may be born
>   of her own intrinsic wisdom . . .

— Carolyn Kleefeld[32]

Stanislav Grof, states that how one is born seems closely related to one's general attitude toward life, determining, among other things, the ratio of optimism to pessimism, how one relates to other people. It is astounding, he says, that Western psychologists and psychiatrists have almost entirely ignored the nature of birth; that when birth is studied at all, the studies are concerned more about possible prenatal brain damage than the emotional significance of birth. Until recently, he says, only a few studies had explored the psychological significance of cesarean section. "This is alarming in view of the fact that . . . the rate of cesarean birth . . . has skyrocketed. It is imperative that we learn about the psychological and social implications of such a drastic change in childbirth patterns." Grof believes that there are differences between babies who are non-labor cesarean-born and labor cesarean-born, as well as uncomplicated vaginal delivery, difficult vaginal birth, and emergency cesarean section.[33] Childbirth author Judith Goldstein says that cesarean section causes the child to be born in a manner that is completely abnormal for the design of the body. "When it is used to sidestep a vaginal birth or accelerate delivery in a birth that could have been concluded vaginally, it definitely lowers the quality of the birth experience for both the mother and the baby," she says.[34]

Jane English, author of *Different Doorway*, has a lot to say about cesarean babies. If doctors could only appreciate the importance of birth, she says, perhaps they could act differently when performing sections, thereby making the birth experience more positive for the baby. She says that cesarean sections are intense—and that it takes a lot of work to suppress strong feelings. While she agrees that the doctor should focus on the procedure itself, and not on his feelings, "...I wonder if medical people might be trained in the psychological and spiritual aspects of birth in order to come to terms with their gut responses to cutting, the pulling out of the baby, and the emotion."[35] She says that when a baby is coming down the birth canal, the whole body is stimulated at once, giving a sense of wholeness, coherence, and integrity. Vaginal babies have an experience of the body. For a nonlabor cesarean, the suctioning and the wiping of the baby is the first body experience—and it is done impersonally by the doctors and nurses. She believes they might do it differently if they knew they were "laboring" with the child, were actually giving birth to the child. "I think of all the people who handle cesarean babies—giving them what they need on the physical level. But it seems the emotional and spiritual levels are not being nurtured." She reminds us that the hospital staff has been trained medically and scientifically: "Forgive them for shutting down their hearts and acting professional. It is a way of handling their own hurt."[36] If obstetricians were "heart-centered" and trained in meditation, for example, they would handle things much differently.

English claims that when she walks into a room she gets a strong sense of which people are cesarean born. She talks about cesarean birth-learned patterns and a cesarean world view. C-section babies, she says, begin to breathe out of fear, not readiness; rather than "choosing" to breathe, they are forced into it. They have a different way of entering and seeing the world. They are also conscious of their "lack of mom—where is she?": years later, many cesarean-born still find themselves grieving for the hours of separation surgical births generally precipitate. While cesareans do not have to be painful and fragmenting, most of them are "because the people who deliver the woman are . . . unconscious of the transforming power, spiritual nature, and long term effects of the experience—indeed, the mothers themselves are often unconscious." She believes that a doctor-shaman with "not just medical training—but also spiritual wisdom and heart"—should allow all of these to "inform and guide his/her hands."[37] She does not believe that cesareans are necessarily bad or wrong—but a different way of being.

English speaks of a cesarean as creating a chasm: "A woman who is delivered by cesarean section has to be connected with her infant again. And she has to be connected to womankind again." Laboring with a baby lets you know that it is yours, that it came from you. With a normal birth, there is separation but a feeling of connectedness exists. Vaginal birth is a pushing out, whereas cesarean section is being broken into. Babies have a "half-born" feeling, she says, which corresponds to the mother's "not having given birth" feeling.[38]

A number of discussions I've heard link unnatural birth and the child care crisis. The deep connections that begin instinctively at conscious births may be torn when the process is interrupted or denied. Fredelle Maynard, author of *The Child Care Crisis*, believes there is a correlation between negative births and the ability (her word) to leave a baby for many hours each week. Cesareans are, for the most part, negative birth experiences. They are a *dis*-connection. And while attachment certainly doesn't rest solely on "birth hours," there are many who believe that those moments affect the rest of our lives.

One woman wrote, "I was sitting in the dentist's chair and I had been numbed. The dentist had his hands in my mouth, then the assistant was suctioning my saliva. There was a light above me and my heart began to race. I wanted to scream, "Stop!" The only thing being extracted was a tooth—not a baby—and the scars wouldn't show. But I felt as if I was in the operating room all over again, and I found myself blinking back tears."

Lynn Richards says that women often feel angry and confused after a section. They are "supposed" to feel joyful about their baby and grateful that the doctor saved them both from certain death. She says these women feel inadequate and powerless to take care of themselves after the surgery, while they are expected to go home and take care of the baby as well. "This situation is somewhat akin to being required to begin a high pressure job or go mountain climbing after a coronary bypass."[39] Having a cesarean shakes what I call the "womanplace"— the place that knows about birth on a cellular level and aches to know it on this plane. This shakeup is not simple postpartum blues, a momentary imbalance of hormones, Lynn says. "It is a grieving process through which a woman must pass to be able to reorder her beliefs about herself and about life."[40]

In *Birth Without Surgery*, Carl Jones writes that cesarean surgery is followed by "surgical birth trauma—a constellation of physical and emotional problems that can affect the entire family."[41] *The VBAC Experience* says that women who have just experienced a cesarean find that their sense of self-worth and their sexuality have been reduced to zero. They may even feel vaginal pain. This is, of course, perplexing to their husbands and to their doctors, who see no reason why she should feel any pain since the baby didn't come out of her vagina. "NOT TRUE!" says author Lynn Richards. "When the woman has experienced much emotional pain especially regarding her birth and sexuality, if she feels a deep loss at not having been able to push out her baby through her own vagina, her vagina may become a holding place for her emotional pain, which translates into physical pain."[42]

Kimberly Wulfert agrees with Stanislav Grof. Considering the importance and complexity of birth, she says, there has been little interest in the effect of a person's psychological orientation on the process. "Technology is so rampant that it now substitutes for investigation into other approaches which could reduce the number of problems that our society runs into at birth."[43] An article entitled

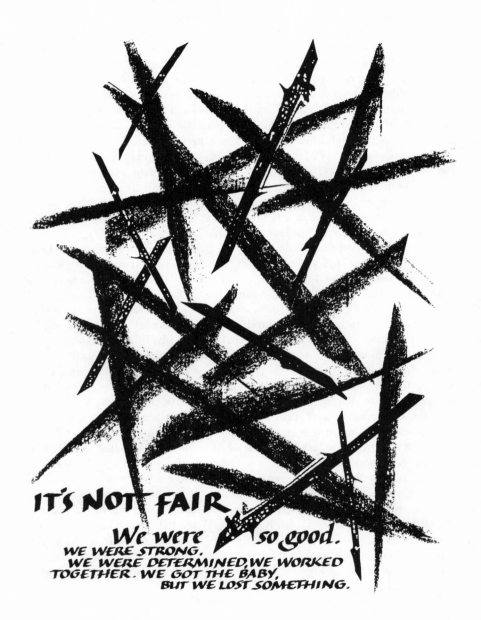

IT'S NOT FAIR.
We were so good.
WE WERE STRONG.
WE WERE DETERMINED, WE WORKED
TOGETHER. WE GOT THE BABY,
BUT WE LOST SOMETHING.

"Women's Perceptions of Vaginal and Cesarean Deliveries" remarks that "if a negative perception of the birth experience influences the woman's view of her infant and her own adequacy as a woman and mother, it would be even more imperative that. . . [positive psychological] intervention be implemented and directed toward modifying the circumstances that influence those perceptions."[44]

Marilyn Moran has said many times that "the commandeering and managing of that other sexual experience, birth, by medical engineers . . . can only be destructive to the psychic and spiritual life of the [woman and man] in the conjugal love dialogue."[45] The vast majority of women who contact me after their sections complain of sexual dysfunction. Since cesareans rob them of one vital aspect of their sexuality, all aspects suffer.

> Orgasm is
>   a state of mind
>   seldom possible
>   after cesarean castration.
> Funny, how they don't warn you about that
> when they ask you to sign the consent paper
> . . . Maybe they don't know.
>
> . . . I don't think they realize
>   those doctors who cut our babies out of us,
> that the soul cannot be anesthetized
> nor can the heart be cauterized
> when dreams of birth have died.
>
> —Caroline Sufrin-Disler

Sleep, Perchance to . . . Listen?

Since banana wine does not seem to be commonly available in the West, many women end up with other forms of anesthesia for their cesareans. As we stated in *Silent Knife*, anesthesia is dangerous and you should avoid it whenever possible. A few years ago the television program "20–20" featured the dangers of anesthesia, as a result of which in the next few weeks people were canceling elective surgery by the busload. I am reminded of a cartoon I once saw. The surgeon is coming out one door marked "Surgery" and entering the door right next to it marked "Unnecessary Surgery." Almost all of the cesareans in this country are preventable—unnecessary.

Russ Rymer says that people under anesthesia do not remember every word that is being said, "but it registers in their brains, and they don't want any remarks like, 'Whoops, I dropped this,' or 'This patient sure is ugly.' "[46] During surgery Dr. Bernie Siegel found that his patients bled less and recovered more quickly when he talked to them. He once told one of his patients, "You've got to help me out right now—stop bleeding immediately, John!" and John, knocked out completely, followed the doctor's instructions.[47] Rymer says that sometimes cardiac arrests during surgery can't be explained "except by their coincidence with off-hand comments made around the operating table."[48] One groggy, over-medicated cesarean mother, whose baby was in a critical state, reported: "The baby started to respond a bit and I said, 'Can I hold him?' Someone snapped at me, 'Are you kidding? It will be quite some time before you'll be able to do that.' My baby died that minute."

Young Blood

Biologically, teenaged women are "prime" for birthing; instead, a good percentage of them get "primed" and double-coated for a section. In an article on "teenage oppression," Eleanor Trawick[49] writes that teenagers, by their very position in society, are easily deprived of their rights of choice in matters of childbearing.

I have received several letters both from teenagers and from older women who were sectioned when they were in their teens. Pam writes, "I was a teenage parent. I had no information on birth. I ended up in the hospital with monitors, IVs, drugs, the whole bit. With only twenty minutes of pushing on my back its no wonder I 'couldn't do it.' I'd like to add that I was told that I had 'cpd'—a label I'm proud to say I overcame. I had to go through a re-learning of attitudes and when my second was born, four years later, I had a homebirth. I think it is very important for high school kids to learn about normal birthing and cesarean prevention. We need to start then, and not wait until the last six weeks for childbirth classes." Even high school may be too late. So many of the views we have are formed far earlier than that. My ten-year-old comes home from school to tell me which of the pregnant teachers are going to have a boy or a girl, or which day their inductions are scheduled for.

Ellen wasn't quite seventeen when she was sectioned. She said,

> The girl in the next room was screaming all night long and I said I didn't want to do that. I was scared, young, a baby myself inside. . . . The operation was a shock! All my illusions were shattered. I was given the spinal anesthetic. It completely terrified me. It was the most frightening experience of my life to be paralyzed, to try to move my toes and have no control. The doctors were chatting about a ball game. Thankfully, my husband was allowed to come in. Just this year, he told me that the doctor made lewd comments about how much better shape my body would be in sexually than after a normal delivery. . . . I was completely unprepared for after the surgery. I was terrified that my insides would spill out. For months afterwards I vowed I would never to do it again.

Another teen mother says,

> They treat you different if you are not married. They think you don't know how to think. If you are older and got pregnant, you made a decision, whereas if you are young and pregnant, you must be irresponsible. It's bad enough you are having sex—but look at you, you got "caught." When I wanted to have my baby natural,

they told me I had to do exactly what the doctor said or they'd take the baby away. I didn't want them to do the cesarean operation, but I had no choice.

Many people believe that a poor birth is the price teenagers have to pay for their wanton ways, as if they deserve punishment. They don't understand that gentle, loving support, adequate information, and the chance to birth consciously can help to empower them, to "grow them" to a new place of decision-making and responsibility.

Maryah had her cesarean at the age of eighteen. Her second child was born two years later, a repeat. Three years later, she had twins, vaginally. She now works with pregnant teenagers, helping them to achieve natural birth. Most people, she says, feel that the teenager can't take care of herself; if she could have, then she wouldn't have gotten herself into such a predicament. With this attitude everyone thinks they have to take over at the birth. Maryah says that when labor begins, all of a sudden the reality "hits"—automatic parenthood—and panic sets in. A cesarean allows these young girls to be taken care of for a while longer. Maryah says, "When I attend a birth, this is the hardest part: You want them—they have to—grow up. Part of you wants to baby them, and part of them needs to be babied—mothered. The other part has to grow up—quick. As the mother is birthing the baby, the baby is birthing a woman. . . . Sometimes, despite all my efforts, there is no way I can seem to help her avoid a section. I can't do a vaginal birth for her. Most of the time, the births go very well. These teens are strong and determined, and come away from their natural births wiser for the effort." Maryah says that a positive birth experience has the potential to transform young mothers and to give them something extraordinary which they can use for the rest of their lives.

Secondary Infertility: Bleeding Hearts

MANY YEARS, SEVEN MONTHS
AND FIVE HOURS LATER

How was I to know, my love,
    my little one?
How was I to know
    when they excised
    your brother
    from my uterus,
    they cut the chance
    that I would carry you,
    first in my womb
    and then in my arms?
How was I to know, my love
    my child,
    you were destined
    to be the one

I would carry only
        in my heart?

—Patricia Newell[50]

Patricia Newell of the Cesarean Prevention Movement says that cesarean section may contribute to secondary infertility and that this may be one of the least recognized and most emotionally devastating long-term aftereffects of cesarean section. It is difficult to assess the degree of influence a cesarean has on subsequent fertility, and it is "almost impossible to get a doctor to admit that there is a causal relationship between [the two]." Newell reports that a cesarean heightens the chance of "one-child" infertility. Although U.S. researchers have ignored the matter, such studies have been done in other countries. For more information on the subject, you can read the *CPM Clarions*. Beth Shearer, co-director of C/SEC, has noted that a significant number of women who have had cesareans have endometritis—up to 50 percent of women are found to have scarring and do not become pregnant.

One woman wrote

> When I couldn't get pregnant again it seemed as though there were pregnant women and nursing babies everywhere! I knew a few women who were pregnant and didn't want to be—or who were ambivalent—and I would gladly have changed places with them. It made me angry to see a pregnant woman abusing her body, smoking for example, because I knew that I'd do everything right to take care of myself and my baby. I asked God "why can they be pregnant and not me?" and I got very angry. I even said, "Okay, okay, I'll have another c-section. Anything!" It just wasn't fair. Few people could understand what I was feeling. As my child got older and older, I realized that even if I did have another baby, the dreams of my two children being within a reasonable age span disappeared. They'd both be like "only" children.
>
> At first I thought, "Well, maybe next month." Then that month would come and go, and I'd cry and say, "Next time." I tried to stay optimistic. Sometimes though, I would get very depressed. Then I tried not to think about it. If my period was late, I'd get so high, thinking I shouldn't get my hopes up, but I did. Once I went 42 days and I thought, "Yes!" I cried every month for the baby I loved that wasn't there. It was hard to make love with my husband and it really hurt our relationship.
>
> Maybe it is easier now to know that I won't be having any others. Easier than hoping, I mean. But even diaper commercials are tough.

Another woman wrote,

> I have had two cesareans. . . . My next pregnancy was something of a nightmare. For about five weeks, I proceeded to bleed. It was always at night. I resisted suggestions that I incarcerate myself in a hospital, until one night when the hemorrhage wouldn't stop. I was seven months pregnant when I had to be delivered again by cesarean section of a beautiful miniature girl, who is now a precious six year old. Exactly two years later, the same thing happened, except that the ending was not happy. My baby girl had too many problems. She lived only two weeks. . . . It has been four years and I have not conceived. I hope and pray each and every month that this will be the month. . . . My doctor said

that my uterus was not "sewn very well" (This was the OB who did the sewing, mind you.)—would this have any effect on what has been happening?" [Yes, the risk of placenta praevia, which increases the likelihood of "failed pregnancy," continues to rise with multiple cesareans.][51]

Bleeding Sweethearts

A woman who is having a repeat cesarean leaves behind her other child or children and becomes a hospitalized patient for a number of days. Her recovery time is extended; she cannot lift her two or three year old when she gets home. They cannot sit on her lap—it is too tender. Without saying a word, and even if the woman is "delighted" with her section, children begin to believe that having a baby makes you sick and weak. A generation of children with this notion can only beget another generation of sick, weak, debilitated mothers.

Our other "sweethearts"—our spouses—are also often left behind, always physically, sometimes bodily, and often emotionally.

"The doctor picked up a device that resembles a large, white garlic press with which he fired 15 stainless-steel staples into my wife's abdomen."

—Cesarean father[52]

He kissed her and took her hand. "A cesarean is a perfectly respectable way of being born," he said. "What about me?" she said. "What about getting all stuck up with tubes and cut up into little pieces?"

—Laurie Colwin, *Another Marvelous Thing*[53]

How can I explain it to her? Women are not raised to abort tears. For us, tears are a masculine demerit.

—Mark Gerzon[54]

Cesarean section affects fathers in many ways. Some are relieved that they don't have to "coach" the labor anymore and that the baby is finally being born. Others are angry about what happened. Some feel deflated or partially responsible and wish that they had been "better help." A number of dads have called me, far more upset about the situation than their wives. Once or twice, a woman has called who has said that she'd be just as happy having another c-section, but it's her husband who wants the VBAC.

Many labors present a catch-22 situation. If the father is an all-around nice guy, as most of them are, their wives often end up getting cut open. The doctor says, "Well, Bill, we've got a little problem here. Looks like Mary is going to need a section," and Bill sighs and shrugs his shoulders, and says, "Yes, I guess so. I see what you mean." Afterward, Mary says to Bill, "You let them cut me! Why didn't you fight them!" If, on the other hand, the husband is either strong-minded or hostile, the woman "gets it," too. John said, "I fought them all the way. I was angry with the staff and appeared rebellious: They were not going to hurt my wife anymore than they had! I threw one of the nurses out of the room, and told the doctor to go home. I helped my wife get up (they had wanted her lying in bed) and we walked around the room. . . . In the end, she got cut anyway."

One father said that he watched the operation and was amazed when the doctor took the uterus "right out of Kathy's body—he actually took it out! He wanted to show the residents his 'superior' suturing skills. It made me sick, and she had pain for months after the surgery. She said it felt as if someone had tried to close a drawer inside her, but couldn't because an article of clothing was sticking out." Another father said that he had been kept waiting in the credit department and came up to the OR floor to find that the cesarean had begun without him. When he finally was "released" and got upstairs, he was told that since the operation had started, he couldn't go in since nobody was allowed once the doors were closed, due to increased risk of infection. "So I stood outside the doors, not twenty feet away, but couldn't get in." Later, he found out that frequently various people enter the OR after an operation has begun.

A man's reaction to his wife's cesarean is not easily predicted. It is based on a number of factors and can, of course, be dependent on the woman's own reaction. "I couldn't touch her for weeks after the section. Her whole body hurt, from the IV, the epidural, the incision, her vagina from all the exams she had had, her thighs from the shots of pain medication—everywhere. It was not the tender and loving scene I had hoped for after the birth of our child." Tom said that his wife's section, for him, was "the worst encounter of the closest kind."

> He had been so brave and cheerful. He had held her hand while William was born. He had told her it was like watching a magician sawing his wife in half. He had taken photos. . . . He had bought her a book on breastfeeding. He had purloined his hospital greens to wear each year on William's birthday. Now he had broken down.[55]

As Barbara Katz Rothman states in her book on motherhood, "a birth management that routinely leaves psychological and social trauma in its wake for the members of families is measured as perfectly successful, unless the trauma is severe enough to be measured in appropriate 'medical' terms."[56]

I frequently meet young fathers who proudly announce they were present for the birth of their baby by section. Years ago, fathers were barred from cesarean deliveries. A number of us at C/SEC made it possible for fathers to be present at operative births. While I believe that father and mother should have complete decision-making power about the father's presence at any birth, emergency or not, I now believe that the incentive to avoid a cesarean is lessened with the "Oh, no sweat. He can be with me either way" mentality that many couples seem to have. Many fathers are unaware, however, how precarious their position in that operating room really is. At any time before or during the operation, if their presence is considered distracting in any way, they may be asked to leave. The father who objects or protests is labeled difficult, making reentry unlikely. Author Mark Gerzon writes that Congress ought to pass a bill allowing the father to attend the birth of his child if the woman consents, no matter what the circumstances.[57] In an emergency situation, when it seems to me vital that the husband be present, many doctors insist that the father be removed—either because "he won't be able to handle it" or because there should be no "witnesses" in this day of rampant malpractice suits.

In one hospital in Mississippi fathers attending cesareans must sign "disclaimer of liability," which says: "We understand and agree that the visitation of the father, unusual to the operative situation, places both the mother and infant at greater risk. . . . In other words, we accept the fact that our visitation into the OR places the lives of both wife and child at greater risk and accept that risk despite the fact that we have been counseled against it. . . . We release and waive any rights we may have against the doctors and hospital for any injury, either physical or psychological, which results as a direct or indirect result of the father being present during the procedure or any part thereof." By any standards this is a remarkable document.

Many of the same fathers who are proud to have been present at the c-section also boast that they were the first to hold the baby. But the mothers are supposed to hold them first! The father's role is to see that the mother gets that baby, not that he gets to hold it first. Since the beginning of time babies have been welcomed into the world by the mother's own efforts, from her body into her arms, feeling her skin, next to her breasts, next to her heart, hearing her voice, feeling her breath, smelling her, seeing her, being at one with her. It has nothing to do with loving them more; it has to do with so many other things, and if you don't understand it in your heart without my telling you, then there is really no point in my trying to explain it. Lynn Richards writes that father-centered cesareans ("cesareans where the father participates in the birth and bonds with the baby INSTEAD of the mother") have become "the rage" in operating rooms across the country. "Mothers are supposed to be grateful that their husbands are mothering their babies, while they lie like lumps of lard on their backs with their hands tied down as if they were being crucified."[58]

Just When You Thought it was Safe to go back in the Water

Even in the animal world, more and more cesareans are being performed. I recently read that Soviet scientists have begun performing sections on beluga whales, so as to harvest their eggs for caviar. Once sectioned, they are thrown back into the sea. Closer to home, a local veterinarian explained to me that certain animals are favored for being small. The prized females are so tiny they cannot birth normally. Many of you already know about the controversy surrounding "Babe," the elephant in a New York zoo, who died right along with her infant a few weeks after she was sectioned. Many felt her death was the result of the operation; others felt she should have been sectioned sooner. Babe's ordeal was one of the most touching and disturbing stories I have encountered in all my years in this field. Feminist thinking challenges exploitative hierarchies: "In the process of struggling for our own rights, we should not participate in the victimization of those even worse off than ourselves in the pecking order. We need to develop fresh ways of seeing the world if we are to get out of ignoring the realities of how other non-human animals are living."[59]

Ouch, a Breech?

Breech babies born by cesarean section don't necessarily do any better than those born vaginally. In fact, in several studies, breech-cesareans had a less favorable outcome.

Even breech premies do far better vaginally delivered than surgically removed. This makes so much sense when you remember that even full-term cesarean babies have much more difficulty breathing. They have a greatly increased incidence of hyaline membrane disease ("immature lungs"). Labor helps to ready the infant for survival outside the mother's body; it matures the lungs, so to speak. Tiny babies, so often delivered by c-section in this country "to insure a better outcome," do better when they can experience labor and be stimulated to breathe by the cyclical rhythms of the contractions and by the natural passage through their mother's bodies into the world.

And what about the big babies? Throughout this book you will find accounts of women who had wonderful full-term breech deliveries. Dr. Michele Odent tells us how: "With a breech, you *do nothing* [emphasis in the original] to interfere with the first stage of labor. If the first stage goes well, there is no reason to believe that the second stage won't. The only "intervention" is to insist that the woman be in a supported squatting position." Episiotomies are rarely even necessary! And twin births whether baby #1 is breech or not are "not a big effort for that breech expert."[60] Another doctor, who attends many breech deliveries, says that women are made to feel that they will "damage" their babies if they birth naturally, so they "choose" a c-section. He says that sections could be avoided if the doctors would get off their high horses and be willing to learn how to assist at a vaginal breech birth. Many times, a doctor has insisted on a cesarean because he was "certain" the breech baby was at least 9 or 10 pounds, only to discover that the baby was 7 1/2 or 8. Many women have delivered large breech babies—they either remained at home or came into the hospital pushing.

There are positions and exercises for turning breech babies, and many of them do work. Perhaps, though, we need a different orientation for breech deliveries: a certain percentage of babies presents breech, and this is normal. You'd never know that, seeing the way doctors react when the baby is breech. First of all, they tell you that the baby is "feet first" when you are thirty weeks pregnant (many babies are breech at this time) and make you nervous and uptight. Dr. Leo Sorger says that before the thirty-second week, breech position is not even

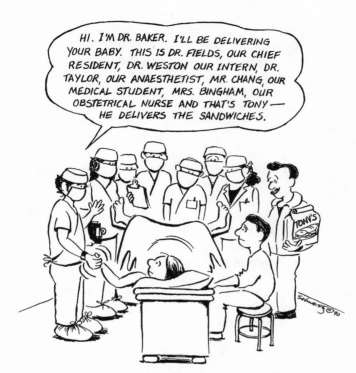

considered important.[61] Between the thirty-second and thirty-fifth week, he may "flip" a breech or transverse to vertex easily in just a few seconds. Even later, if it is easy, he doesn't hesitate to turn a breech. If this fails, exercises may be recommended. Occasionally, an external version is done, [one midwife recommends a sash after a breech baby is turned—a "belly binder"], or the decision is made to honor the babies' naturally chosen position, and birth breech. Doctors often panic because they don't have the slightest notion how to attend a breech birth; rather than admit it, they frighten you into a cesarean for which they have *plenty* of experience. Doctors could learn a great deal about breech deliveries from homebirth midwives; but they're rarely interested in learning from them since they are not university trained.

Some women have turned their babies by simply talking to them (or to the uterus), or by writing letters to them. Some have used acupuncture points, acupressure points, reflexology, healing touch, homeopathic remedies, and herbs. Each of these methods and a number of others, can positively affect the uterus and cause a change. One woman spent a few days swimming in a pool—she played like a child in the water, doing gentle turns and slow somersaults—and the baby turned. Other women have done absolutely nothing at all, and their babies have turned.

Chiropractors can help breech babies. Of the twelve women I have sent to a particular chiropractor, nine have turned—three within a few hours of the adjustment (called, I am told, the "Webster breech-turn technique"). Dr. Stephen Stern is currently preparing an article on chiropractic in pregnancy and has had a number of speaking engagements in the New England area. He explained to me that when the spinal column is in alignment and everything is "in place," we have the optimum chance that everything will go well within our bodies. If one or more of the bones of the spine are "subluxated," (out of proper alignment), the ability of the body to function normally, from a structural standpoint, may be impaired. One woman said that she felt as if her chiropractor had given her baby that extra little space that he'd needed to turn "bottoms up." Healer Shirley Luthman claims that chiropractic helps because it "unblocks"—and that blood and energy cannot flow through the body unless the spine is kept mobilized.[62]

More and more, I'm beginning to believe that flipping babies, external version (which often requires both ultrasound and muscle relaxants), upside-down exercises, and so on, are interventions into the pregnancy. I generally recommend starting out with uninvasive activities, like visualization. If they are not effective, it might be valuable to talk to your baby again. If the baby persists in a breech position, learn about breech delivery. As author-educator-healer Cathy Romeo says, "Our babies have energies of their own that cannot be discounted and they may be fulfilling their own need."[63]

One childbirth educator wrote,

> I am so incensed! One of my women just had an absolutely unnecessary cesarean! She got to the hospital at 5 a.m. very calm and peaceful, and doing beautifully. Her doctor confirmed his suspicion that the baby was breech by doing an ultrasound and then X-rays! I told him that most midwives know how to determine position without all that dangerous equipment. Anyway, Debbie said she wanted a healthy baby, and a vaginal birth. The doctor said they'd "give it a whirl." Meanwhile, he kept explaining what he considered to be the terrible risks involved about the head getting stuck in the bones and the cord getting pinched so there is no air— he was graphic!—He talked about fractures, dislocations, nerve damage, brain damage—and scared her half out of her mind. He hooked her to a monitor and confined her to the bed. Lo and behold, for some strange reason, her contractions slowed. Two hours later he told her she hadn't made any progress. Then he checked her again, and said she had gone down to 3 centimeters. She had a cesarean with general anesthesia—she was told that she wouldn't be allowed to bond with her baby even if she was awake because all breech babies are sent to be observed in the special nursery, so it didn't matter if she was put to sleep. This doctor rarely diagnoses a breech prior to labor—I have some questions about that.

The policy of one doctor in my area is never to deliver a breech baby vaginally. I have some questions about him, too, as well as about the doctor who was incensed when his patient came into the hospital already in the pushing phase of her labor with her breech baby. "He yelled at me, put me on a delivery table, tried to yank the baby out with forceps, but he couldn't quite get it, so he did an emergency cesarean. My son had horrible bruises on his little buttocks and was cut on the cheek during the section."

Frequently, there are surprises: a baby thought to be vertex may be breech. Michele Odent reminds us that we must be prepared—we cannot only "know" cesareans! A number of breech babies have been born at home; the women have chosen to stay there so they can have a calm, uninterfered-with delivery. Traditional midwives are well versed in the breech technique. One midwife wrote that she was quite certain all along that the baby was breech. "But the doctor's ultrasound 'confirmed' a vertex presentation. The woman returned home and continued laboring. Well, a few hours later, out blurps this wonderful, not so little, breech!"

Vice versa, the breech may actually be vertex. Many letters echoed Laurie's: "They cut me open to do the c-section and I heard someone exclaim, 'It's not a breech!' I didn't need that operation at all, *not at all!*" In one case, the woman heard the doctor say, "Forget it. It's not important."

Martha writes,

> My child was in a breech position. Immediately the doctor wanted to put me on an IV in case I needed a section. . . . then he took a needle and punctured a tiny hole in the water bag, thinking he could bring the baby down slowly but it didn't help. . . . Then he broke my water completely and reached way in so he could be sure nothing bad happened to the cord. When he did that, my labor stopped completely. That's right, my labor stopped completely. I didn't have another contraction. I begged him to let me get up and start walking to try and get this labor started again. By 2:30 a.m. I was so-o-o tired from walking the halls and still no labor except for every so often I would get a sensation like a contraction was trying to start but couldn't. They told me to lay down and rest. That felt so good, but I couldn't sleep because as soon as I did, I felt alot of movement . . . the doctor came to check me and said that the baby had come down and had turned, but the cord had prolapsed. (He had broken my water to prevent that, and now it was happening!) [Note: Amniotomy increases chances of cord prolapse.] There was no heartbeat. They did an emergency section. By 7:36 a.m. our stillborn baby boy was born, or "taken from me" might be a better way to put it. The doctor told me that he thinks it is the way my pelvis is shaped that caused the prolapsed cord. . . . Another question is this, was this cord prolapse Dr. created? If you can only spare me a few minutes and answer my questions, I would appreciate it from the bottom of my heart!

One woman with a breech baby writes that she was one day short of a month past her due date when her water broke. There was some meconium staining in the fluid, but the heartbeat was good and strong, so she went to sleep for a while. The next morning, she went to the hospital to "evaluate the suitability for a vaginal delivery." By most standards in this country, this woman was already four times a section—one for overdue, two for breech, three for meconium, and four because she had had a previous section. Labor started in the hospital.

> I was 4 cm dilated at my first exam, around noon. It occurred to me gratifyingly that labor had started (relatively) spontaneously. This had been my concern as I

never got into labor with my first birth. . . . The threat of a cesarean was constantly present to me. Deadlines were mentioned. I was encouraged and then discouraged. Labor deepened. When I heard, at 10 p.m. talk of being "deliverable," my spirits were buoyed. Felt a few pushing urges though not fully dilated. At eleven, the doctor strode in and said, "Time to get the baby out." I didn't ask what expediting techniques were to be—I was still worried about an unnecessary cesarean. . . . Episiotomy was the first of the obstetrical devices used. I later learned that they were routine at this hospital. Then I got the vacuum extractor. Finally forceps were introduced. In spite of all this, the baby emerged, and only then did I believe it! Our son was 9 lbs. 9 oz. The pediatrician grabbed him ["grabbing" is a new technique, used widely in hospitals all over the United States], and for the next few days, he was tested frequently. Throughout it all, my baby was healthy. [Not all babies get through this lucky with all those interventions. But more on that later.], and I was overjoyed at not having to have another section.

In "Baby Came Breech" Gloria Eng-Enorvac writes that at thirty-six weeks,

baby decided that head-up was preferable to head-down. Attempts to turn baby through massage, exercise, and the herb Pulsatilla were unsuccessful this go-round. My dream of a homebirth shattered, Jane [the midwife] advised me to see a doctor several miles away. . . . She had a reputation for non-intervention and was comfortable with vaginal delivery of breech infants.

Labor began and the contractions got strong very quickly. They knew they wouldn't make it to the hospital. There was a doctor's strike at the hospital closer by,

but that hospital wasn't midwife-friendly. I had wanted this baby at home. Jane's home the next best thing. . . . In 15 minutes I was 8 cm. dilated. . . . I knew I shouldn't push too soon. I tensed, trying not to push, and Theo and the midwife encouraged me to let my body do the work. I relaxed, and soon enough the little bum appeared. Katrina's meconium preceded her! . . . The rest of her slid right out into my hands and onto my chest. It was wonderful. The rest of a beautiful, warm June morning lay ahead of us.[64]

Charlotte, a woman from California, canceled the appointment for a cesarean-for-breech and had a joyful, safe homebirth delivery. She writes that, although there may be a slight increase in risk, the bad outcomes for breech births may be a result of drugged labors and the use of forceps. "What are the statistical results of [natural] labors in upright positions?" she asks. She says that it appears that the breech issue will have to be helped in the same way that the VBAC issue was helped in the beginning: "with birthing moms and midwives willing to face the risks and develop their own statistics" that will influence others that vaginal breech deliveries are safe.

R.N. = C/S?

As we learned in *Silent Knife* a high percentage of nurses end up with cesarean sections and difficult vaginal deliveries. This should come as no surprise when you consider who trains them and where they are "indoctrinated." Lynn Richards says that most of us as little girls grew up to trust the doctor. "Nursing intensifies this belief. Nurses are trained to obey the orders of the doctor. Therefore, perhaps for more than any other sociologic group within our culture, it is most difficult for nurses as mothers to question the authority of a doctor, and place trust in themselves and in their own intuition."[65] I continue to get a cartload of mail from sectioned mothers who are nurses. (Doctors' wives get sectioned even more.)

Judy, an RN in Florida who had had a cesarean with her first baby, wrote,

> It became obvious after I had been at the hospital for twelve hours, that I had to change something in order to feel relaxed enough to start dilating again. My husband suggested leaving the hospital, walking around at a nearby mall. My doctor laughed. So we signed out AMA—against medical advice—and came home. As we were leaving, the nurse said "Wouldn't you rather rupture here than at home?" I predict that she'll have a section with her first baby like I did unless she wises up quick! I didn't return to the hospital until I was fully dilated and pushing. My 8 lb. 12 oz. daughter was pink, gorgeous, and 2 1/2 pounds bigger than my first. I felt GREAT!

An article in *Holistic Nursing Practice* reports that nurses don't refer to vaginal deliveries as "normal" because it infers that cesarean births are "abnormal" and may upset the cesarean parents. "While this may help the parents to respond more positively and quickly to their cesarean experience, it may also encourage the belief that abdominal delivery is just another (maybe a better way) to have a baby. Have nurses become so accustomed to cesarean birth as an alternative that they view cesareans to be as natural as a vaginal delivery? It might be more reasonable to foster an awareness of the cesarean section as a surgical birth, which if in fact it is, done for specific indications." The article goes on to say that repeat cesareans are mostly unnecessary surgery and that nurses have an excellent opportunity through client education, to "preserve the personal and physical integrity of many expectant women."[66] True, but how can they when they are so busy climbing up on the OR tables getting sectioned themselves?

Joyce, originally an RN, does not believe that her nursing experience was responsible for her cesarean. She writes,

> I loved working in labor and delivery because it was always such an exciting and happy place. I worked in a hospital where, initially, there were only two fetal monitors for twenty beds. Things were not yet "routine." As nurses, we used our sense of touch, healing, smelling and seeing to ascertain how women were doing in labor. I even "caught" quite a few babies myself when the doctor didn't make it or we were so busy that there simply weren't enough doctors around. C-sections were not yet commonplace. I gained a healthy respect for the beauty and miracle of childbirth. However, in 1973, I left that wonderful experience to attend medical school. All of a sudden, my perspective on childbirth began to change. I became a deliverer of babies instead of a childbirth advocate. I could no longer sit with mothers and sponge the perspiration from their brows, hold their hands, and talk to them. I had to concern myself with delivering Mrs. X, sewing her up, and

getting her off the table before Mrs. Y had to deliver. But I didn't realize how much my perspective had changed until I became pregnant. I was a lost soul. I had lost confidence in Mother Nature's complete ability to orchestrate the birth experience. More importantly, I had emotionally forgotten all those wonderful experiences during my nine year nursing career before the birth experience became the technological web of the 80's.

Joyce had a homebirth with her second child.

Nora writes,

> I am a nurse. Now that I have become a mother—a cesarean mother—I am not very proud of the way I handled my maternity patients. I said things like, "No complaining! After all, you've got a healthy baby, and you didn't have to go through labor and delivery!" I thought the c-section mothers were too pampered. Most of my other post-op patients were up and about pretty quick—I thought my sections should be, too. I forgot that sectioned mothers had often long labors before their operations, not to mention the nine months of pregnancy. In addition, they had to go home and care for a baby—my other patients didn't! . . . When I had my own baby, I was really upset, not so much because I had a section, that didn't bother me too much at first, but because I expected I'd be up and about quick, and I wasn't even able to move for the first few days. I thought about all the mothers that I had been insensitive to.

Cynthia reported that when she told members of the hospital staff that "I felt like I was having my appendix out and adopting a baby by not being able to birth normally, I was told that I was ridiculous and that I should be grateful that I didn't have to go through labor and delivery! I felt as if I had trained for the Olympics and was disqualified at the last minute. Would an athlete be grateful? I didn't feel grateful—I felt cheated. I got no understanding, sympathy or support from any of the nurses there."

Sandi said, "I wanted to spit on all the nurses who came in and said, 'Okay, Mrs. Brenner, up and at 'em. You aren't dead, you only had a c-section." Easy for them to say—they weren't the ones who were cut! But how could I spit on any of them—I am one of them!"

"Let Them Eat Jello!"

Let's talk a little bit about doctors here, and, then you'll get to read more about them in a future chapter. One woman wrote that when she went into the hospital in labor she had an argument with one of the doctors about interventions at birth. "He told me I was dead wrong about everything. I found out later that he wasn't even an OB—they were short staffed and had called in a few other people to help—he was a dermatologist!"

One father wrote that when the doctor demanded that a cesarean was necessary, he demanded a second opinion. The second doctor said he didn't think that a section was necessary at that moment, that they could wait and see. The two doctors started arguing. "Although it could have made us tense, we actually found it amusing," said Rob. My wife and I started to laugh. She had the baby, naturally, a while later. So much for needing a c-section. If we hadn't asked for a second opinion, we'd have been up a creek. And even if the other doctor had agreed with the first, we know now that their opinions are subjective and don't really have to count."

In Rhode Island, a commission was formed to study the section rate at a particular hospital (44 percent). Several of the women's groups in the area "expressed concern about the impartiality of the investigation, as all the investigators were male physicians paid by the hospital, who could not be expected to understand the quality of care from the perspective of a woman in labor. . . . Despite considerable community pressure, the suggestion to make the investigators more representative was rejected, and the community itself was excluded from the official process."[67]

Peer review boards to lower section rates don't often work. For the most part, everyone ends up agreeing that the operation was indeed necessary. After all, the same doctor who questions whether a cesarean was necessary on Monday might perform one on Tuesday, and then it'll be his turn to be roasted. If he lends support today, he'll get it back when he needs it. Attorney Mark Mandell says, "Peer review? No doctor is going to say his colleagues screwed up . . . and residents don't criticize chiefs."[68]

I learned that for a period of time last year, however, one hospital in the Midwest with a very high cesarean rate required that all sections be justified in front of a board of selected obstetricians. During that time, the cesarean rate dropped by one-third—to half the national average—and the infant mortality rate was lower, even though they served a predictably "high-risk" population.[69]

Karen writes, "I had two terrible c-sections. They were really hard on me. When I got pregnant with my third, my doctor said, 'You need a good experience.' Well, he promised me a good experience, and he gave me a good experience—a c-section with an epidural that I recovered from faster than the spinals. But he knew I didn't want a c-section. When I took him two books on VBAC, he said that since they weren't written by a doctor, they weren't true."

Ruth said, "My doctor told me, 'You are going to get cut because in this day and age it is too expensive to birth vaginally. I can't sit around all day.' He said that!"

Abby's doctor told her that if she didn't take the epidural at that moment (for the cesarean), "he'd make me suffer." I am reminded of a question that was asked in one of my classes: When and where does "natural aggression become raving violence?"[70] Abba Eban once said, "History shows that men . . . behave reasonably only when they have exhausted all other alternatives."

Sandra writes,

> I was placed in the little cubicle and asked to sit on the table and wait for the doctor. You talk about the steps that it takes to go from being a healthy, normal woman who is about to give birth into "patient." I felt not only reduced to patient,

but a better word is "prisoner." This mentality set me up, easy, for the section. Also, while I was waiting for the doctor, I picked up my medical records. The receptionist walked in and asked me not to look at them. She said that she could lose her job for letting me see them. "But they're mine!" I said. Then she told me, 'Sometimes doctors write things they don't want their patients to see and it could upset things.' The medical profession is more sneaky and underhanded than the CIA."

Jody McLaughlin, the American distributor for *Compleat Mother* magazine, sent me a poster she found hanging up on the wall in her local hospital: "Unauthorized disclosure of information could be hazardous to your health." You may, however, want to read the article on medical records entitled "Absolutely NOT Confidential"; evidently, everyone gets to read them—"and you—like an open book. . . ."[71]

"A Section Handicaps Us All"

Judging from the letters I receive and the things I've heard, the vast majority of special-needs moms in this culture get sectioned a high percentage of the time. In "A Long Overdue Feminist Issue: Disability and Motherhood," Anne Finger writes that "Disability in and of itself is much less a problem than the social structures and attitudes towards disability. . . . our particular needs and concerns are rarely addressed, much less fought for. . . . There is a pervasive stereotype of disabled women as being asexual: How did you get pregnant?" She says that disabled women are treated as children and that they are often exploited and ignored.[72]

Marsha Saxton says that disability triggers much fear in our culture. Despite media coverage and an attempt by many schools to implement "physical challenge day" or "handicap awareness" programs, old attitudes persist. "Perhaps from prehistoric times, disability must have appeared to humans as some mysterious force leaving many human beings with physical limitations, loss of bodily functions . . . it is no wonder we have feelings of powerlessness about disability. It forces us to confront our own vulnerability."[73] [I heard from a nurse that she saw one doctor 'snuf out' a baby—he prevented the child from breathing because it was deformed. I was appalled—she said this happens on occasion—". . . they say that the baby was stillborn and that it was 'for the best'."] Saxton says that pregnancy or parenthood in a disabled person triggers alarm, ridicule, or even disgust. It is often assumed that the child will be disabled too, even when the likelihood is nil. She says that having a body with physical limits is "a snap when compared to dealing with [patronizing, pitying and invalidating remarks from others]. The oppression . . . is what's disabling."[74]

In *Childbirth Wisdom*, Judith Goldstein says that many cultures exhibit compassion, hospitality, and respect for those with differences.[75] From a number of the letters I have received from women with different challenges, I am certain that we in the United States have a long way to go in order to meet those with special needs and to help them to birth well. So often, the extra time and sensitivity that would have helped a woman with special needs to have a natural birth are nonexistent. One hospital, for example, would not allow a woman who was deaf to bring in someone to sign for her. They would not bend the rules to allow an extra person in the room—they said that if they allowed her an extra person, everybody would want one.

Lisa Roush, a VBAC mother and childbirth educator from California writes,

> I want to tell you about the deaf situations with doctors and cesareans. My deaf friends and I attended hearing childbirth classes at the hospital with an interpreter, but we couldn't really catch what the instructor was saying and we really missed a lot. Most of the deaf women ended up with cesareans! Deaf women try to watch the doctor's body language and they bow and obey, same thing as I did. I am so glad that I kept reading and learning about natural birth—I had a beautiful natural birth—I am so glad I didn't have another cesarean! I tell everyone that if they use a pain-killer, they may hurt their baby and they will miss something inside that there is no way to describe.

Lisa goes on to say that in her area most of the special needs women end up being sectioned. The doctors have no understanding—or interest—in helping these women to birth naturally. The women are regarded as stupid simply because the doctors cannot understand them. Although different areas across the country have some programs for special needs mothers, there aren't nearly enough. One blind woman said that having a cesarean was like being "blinded from the neck down, too." She told me that she had a number of unsighted friends and that they were all c-sectioned, too. Why not? They can't see how ugly the scars are anyway. I can't begin to imagine having to undergo a cesarean without my ears or my eyes to assist me with the ordeal. My heart opens to any woman who endured the surgery without interpreters or familiar, trusted, and caring assistance.

When one woman heard I was writing another book, she asked that I include another prejudice in my special needs discussion—obesity. This woman had a cesarean because "they said they couldn't find the baby's heartbeat under all my fat. Everyone panicked and I was on the operating table faster than I could eat a bag of chips." Her next baby was VBAC: "I told them just to assume the baby was all right and leave me alone." Another woman said that on the operating table "everyone kept saying how hard it was to do a cesarean on an overweight woman. It was as if I had asked to be sectioned, and they were doing me a favor by performing the surgery." *Our Bodies, Our Selves* says that overweight people encounter daily hostility and discrimination and that the medical world blames a whole range of problems on the problem, even those that may not really be associated with it. Fat women are often ridiculed, judged weak-willed, and made to feel ashamed.[76] They often end up with problems at birth, but these should not occur just by virtue of their overweight. Their bodies conceived and grew a child, and they can birth one also.

Blood in the Classroom

Later in this book we have a separate chapter on childbirth classes. Many of these classes merely pave the road to a section. Noel writes that childbirth classes in this country are not natural childbirth classes at all. They do indeed "prepare" you: you come to the birth prepared, with your camera, your chosen outfit, cassette and tapes, picnic lunch, and so on. As many of us have been saying for years, the classes prepare you to listen to the doctors, behave nicely, and say "please" in the corridor on the way to the OR if you want a mirror to see the baby as it is removed from your uterus.

As for cesarean classes, with that mentality, why not just bring together a group of battered women and teach them how to get hit so that it doesn't hurt so bad? C/SEC co-director Beth Shearer thinks that information on cesareans should simply be given in any discussion about emergency situations, so that everyone will get the picture. She says that couples must know the risks (including, of course, anesthesia, and risks to the baby) benefits (no comment), indications (absolute and nonabsolute), and contraindications. They must have local and national VBAC information, and they should be familiar with pre-operative, operative, and post-operative procedures. I suggest that a couple who has had a purebirth VBAC be invited in to listen to the class and discuss the differences between a section and a natural birth. (See Chapter 12, which covers how a cesarean class should be taught.) (Hint: Bring tomato juice and a pairing knife. Napkins will be provided.) As father Dave Barry said, "I remember at one point our instructor cheerfully observed that there was 'surprisingly little blood, really' [at a section]. She evidently felt this was a real selling point."[77]

Craigin's Demise

I borrowed that subtitle from Chris Sternberg, a VBAC midwife. Dear Dr. Craigin. If he wasn't already dead, he probably would have had a heart attack when Gwen, who had had six cesareans, had her seventh baby right there in her very own home a few months ago. His dictum, "Once a cesarean, always a cesarean" has been demolished.

Most of the women who have had c-sections could/should be having VBACs! At the present time, only about 8 percent (up from 2) are. Repeat cesareans still account for an enormous chunk of the overall cesareans performed every year in this country.

From the headlines, you'd think that the doctors are really into cesarean prevention and VBAC. Even *Reader's Digest* had an article that mentioned VBAC. The problem, however, is that everyone is writing about the safety of VBACs, but few are doing them.

Women are getting every excuse in the book for not allowing a VBAC. Stephanie had the best one I've ever heard: hospital renovations. Her doctor told her that if she was due in April or May, she could have the baby vaginally, but since she is due in mid-March, she is out of luck. As Stephanie told me, "So because some construction workers decided to take an extended lunch hour delaying completion of the construction, I must undergo unnecessary surgery. The doctor said that right now, the delivery rooms are too far away from the operating rooms. My doctor did say that they will start allowing VBACs after the completion of the renovation."

Linda reported an almost equally unbelievable reason: "My OB said that the policy here is no VBAC's because the hospital has no resident anesthesiologist on the premises for twenty four hours." You don't need an anesthesiologist for a VBAC. And what, pray tell, will the hospital do if a woman has a placental abruption—tell her to drive to the next hospital where they have a whole bunch of anesthesiologists sitting around?

One article says that although VBAC has been shown to be safe in many circumstances, "scheduled cesareans are the most efficient for all concerned. A practical reason to continue the practice of elective repeat cesareans relates to the time requirements of allowing a patient a trial of labor, which affects the delivery room staff and interrupts the patient schedule."[78] Anne, from Tennessee, writes "I am unable to reconcile a healthy pregnancy as a valid indication for surgery . . . the lack of compassion and concern for the well-being of mother and child permeates the OB literature and is appalling."

It has been said many times: the best way to avoid the second cesarean is to avoid the first. And don't allow the first just because the doctor tells you that you can have the rest of your children vaginally if you want to. There's more on that later. Three new beauty shops opened up in my home town. They were named Snip n' Clip, Shear Madness, and The Cutting Edge. I thought they were OB offices.

Bleeding the System

According to Paul Starr, doctors and other professionals claim authority, not as individuals, but as members of a community that has "objectively" validated their competence. The professional offers advice as a representative of a community of shared standards, standards presumed to be rationally and empirically based.[79] However, the establishment of a medical monopoly, which emphasizes commonality of practice rather than diversity, "has been clouded by the fact that the M.D. degree does not suggest that those who possess it necessarily espouse similar treatment philosophies. There is wide diversity and much tension between practitioners based on scientific principles and clinical experience and judgment."[80]

In the nineteenth century, physicians advocated legislation that would penalize various kinds of sexual behavior. Starr says that "the medical" went hand in hand with the extension of state power into private life. "With evangelistic fervor, the medical profession made decisions, proclamations, and injunctions on subjects from child rearing to international affairs."[81]

Since then we have continued to give doctors an unbelievable amount of power. But they are no different from any other professional: they give advice and they offer suggestions; they sometimes help us and they sometimes screw us. Stanley Gross says that all professionals must mystify the public by making their services appear to be expert and altruistic.[82] Virginia Lubell says, "We need to decide what role we want doctors to play in our social fabric. They are a service profession and if they become judge and jury then that is a distinctly different relationship."[83]

According to Jay Katz, doctors believe that a better appreciation of the uncertainty of medical knowledge will only make patients anxious and nervous. Sharing the burdens of decisions with patients will create new tensions in the area of authority and autonomy. Insistence on the doctor's authority has "stifled any serious exploration as to whether physicians and patients can interact; patients are seen as children whose capacity for choice is fully impaired." Informed consent, Katz says, is a mirage: "Yet a mirage, since it not only deceives, but can also sustain hope, is better than no vision at all."[84] In the late 1950s, judges began to ask a revolutionary new question: Are patients entitled not only to know what the doctor proposes to do, but also to decide whether an intervention is acceptable in light of its risks and benefits and the available alternatives, including no treatment? Later in this book you will begin to see how important this question is.

Dr. Robert Howard says that we have entered an era of medicine and law in which patients are to be considered responsible and capable people—which means they have the primary responsibility for the physical and emotional care of their bodies.[85] Jay Katz again: "Every human being of adult years and sound mind has a right to determine what shall be done with his/her body; and a surgeon who performs an operation without consent commits an assault for which he is liable in damages."[86] READ THAT LAST QUOTE AGAIN. Keep it in mind for a little later in this chapter.

Malpractice

Birth is a government regulated business performed by state-licensed specialists in socially designated institutions.

—Judith Goldstein, *Childbirth Wisdom*[87]

Do you know what they call a medical student who graduates last in his class? Doctor.

And did you hear the one about the medical student who decided to go to law school in case he was a lousy doctor?[88]

One of the most frequent reasons cited for the rise in cesarean section in the United States is fear of malpractice. In spite of all evidence to the contrary, doctors still believe that you get a "better baby" by doing a cesarean. Nothing could be further from the truth. You get better babies by believing in the process of birth and by not interfering in it. When doctors interfere, the woman's body and baby get confused. Things begin to "fall apart," and then a cesarean that would not have been necessary is the only way out.

According to more than one obstetrician, insurance companies are essentially telling them how to practice. Insurance companies spell out the "standards of practice" so that they won't get sued as much, and if they do, their behavior will be defensible. If you don't use an electronic monitor, for example, how do you "prove" that the fetal heart tones were normal? No one believes the human ear anymore. So doctors hook us up because the insurance companies have decided that this is the way it has to be. One obstetrician who attends homebirths said that these days we might as well call pregnancy "intrapartum fetal surveillance" and the birth "interior-exterior squadron patrol." She says that as a doctor in our sue-conscious society, you cannot afford to make others angry. Doctors are scared and angry, too, and so there is much dishonesty and "politicking" in each physician-client relationship. "Consumers are getting obstetrical care that is bastardized by fear," she says.

Columnist Margery Eagan writes that "common sense tells you a woman is much more likely to sue the physician who has rushed around her for nine months—or the stranger she meets in the delivery room—than she is a caregiver she trusts and who stays with her whether the labor is one hour or fifteen." Eagan's appointments with her own doctor lasted "one and a half minutes. I switched to a midwife, whose walls were covered with pictures of newborn babies, glowing mothers, and thank you notes. My appointments lasted forty minutes."[89]

In *The Great Malpractice Scandal*, Richard Moskowitz, M.D., writes that he and a number of his colleagues who have refused to purchase malpractice insurance were dismissed from the medical staff at their local hospital. The hospital claimed that its own insurance premiums had gone up because of uninsured physicians, although they had never produced any evidence that this had happened, or that it ever would. "The truth is exactly the opposite: We have never been sued for malpractice, yet are being compelled to underwrite *their* [emphasis in the original] malpractice risk, which . . . is growing all the time." Moskowitz writes:

> We do not oppose malpractice insurance simply because it costs too much. It costs too much because of the kind of medical practice it creates, because of the extra diagnostic and treatment procedures that it requires, and because of the mutual fear and distrust that it engenders between doctors and patients. Malpractice insurance means high-cost, high-technology, high-risk medicine: that is why we want no part of it.[90]

In malpractice cases, Moskowitz observes, the doctor and the hospital are almost always acquitted, leaving the victim without any compensation whatsoever. According to Moskowitz, with the present system, doctors and hospitals never have to take responsibility for either their mistakes or for accidents. The patients who might sue them and win are generally the ones who died! The patient stands alone against the entire medical system, with good reason to be afraid of it, no effective protection against it. A malpractice suit after the fact is the only possible recourse open to her. "The present malpractice crisis is essentially an expression of the growing resentment of the patient against the doctors and hospitals upon whom [the patient] depends." The insurance company is a threat to us all, doctors as well as patients, because by deciding which doctors it will insure and how much it will charge them, which practices it will defend and which it will settle out of court, "the insurance company has come to exert a decisive and largely destructive influence over how medicine is actually practiced."[91]

Insurance companies sometimes create their own standards, based loosely on the record of their member clients in court and their own corporate motives, "and then enforce them by investigation and even intimidation and blackmail of applicant doctors seeking to sign on for the malpractice 'protection.' The malpractice risk factors of each applicant are assessed, which can be anything from 'an extramarital love affair or an unsubstantiated rumor of homosexuality . . . to a tendency to prefer unconventional medical techniques, such as . . . medication instead of conventional drugs and surgery."[92] The insurance companys' threats are quite persuasive, because the physician understands that what he is buying into is the probability that he will be acquitted of any malpractice charges, provided he adheres fairly strictly to the companies' standards and guidelines.

Moskowitz, whose practice is homeopathy, homebirth, and natural healing, wanted to find out if the insurance company would be willing to insure his somewhat unusual practice, which was based on education, advice, simple caring, and a minimum of high-risk intervention.

> This [insurance agent] could dismiss my entire career, my years as a healer and a student in the natural world, because he had arrogated to himself the authority to decide what Physician's Mutual believes, and what he and his companions do to their patients, is what passes for medicine, for the real thing, while everything they could not understand, including a lot of the real healing that goes on in the world, is not. This was my initiation into the fact that Physician's Mutual is not simply a financial institution, but above all a kind of medical FBI, designed primarily to enforce a certain Neanderthal conception of what health care is all about.[93]

According to Moskowitz, malpractice insurance arises out of the prevalent belief that "birth and death, health and disease are essentially technical or professional matters, for which physicians must take ultimate responsibility. . . . The incalculable risk to which malpractice insurance does in fact address itself is the added liability that the physician incurs by taking away the ultimate responsibility from the patient, and vesting it in our own person, our own ego." He and his colleagues believe that life and death, health, and disease are natural processes and that their role is simply to assist the natural healing effort in any way they can. "This is our insurance, and ultimately we believe that there need be and can be no other."[94]*

Obstetrician Gerald Bullock writes, "Fear of malpractice does not make physicians practice better medicine, it merely makes them practice more compulsive medicine . . . cookbook medicine. A specific physical complaint no longer prompts a rational pattern of evaluation and management based on experience and judgment. Rather, it prompts an exhaustive list of tests so that if something doesn't go right, nobody can claim that the doctor didn't do all he could. . . . Fear of lawsuit in fact produces a poorer quality of care and forces unnecessary, dangerous surgery . . . I teach 'informed refusal'."[95]

Esther Rome, representative of the Boston Women's Health Book Collective, writes, "Once you are in the hospital you have very little control over what happens. . . . You have the right to refuse medical procedures, but be aware that this may affect your insurance coverage."[96] One woman, upon choosing a VBAC, heard that she had been dropped from her insurance plan. Leslie Belay, co-editor of *The Midwife Advocate*, asks, "Who will determine if a woman is 'high-risk' and by what criteria? Women . . . must take responsibility for their own births. They must trust themselves and honor the natural, biological process, and must be in an atmosphere of informed choice rather than informed consent."[97]

The most effective way to reduce medical malpractice litigation is for the health provider to obtain the woman's informed consent to the proposed treatment, and to document, "in a manner that leaves no doubt," that the woman had enough information to make an informed choice. An adequate patient consent form will not only protect the physician from "lawsuits born out of misunderstanding and anger, but will also ensure that pregnant women are involved in the decision-making process involving their care."[98]

My stomach started to turn a few years ago when I learned that childbirth educators were receiving letters from insurance companies that they, too, should get on the bandwagon. I am delighted that many of the childbirth organizations are neither offering nor supporting this craziness. I recently read that there is talk about whether society should scrap its problem-plagued medical malpractice system in favor of a no-fault insurance scheme similar to workmen's compensation.[99] *Everyone is missing the point here, especially in birth. In fact, in countries where malpractice is not an issue, the cesarean rate is still rising.*

We are heading for Margaret Atwood's *Handmaid's Tale!* Hospitals can refuse admission if the couple refuses to sign a consent form. Do what I say or you get it right across the belly. Pretty scary, isn't it?

David and Lee Stewart, Executive Directors of NAPSAC, write that the solution to the malpractice problem may be found in "identifying, promoting,

*The Gesundheit! Institute in Massachusetts was founded in 1971. Patients are treated as friends and no malpractice is carried by physicians. "There has never been a lawsuit and the practitioners are the happiest group of doctors around," says Dr. Mark Warren, who practices there.

and implementing the safest alternatives in childbirth."[100] They state that obstetricians are ten times more likely to be sued for malpractice by their clients than midwives, and whereas doctors are losing more and more cases, midwives, even when sued, seldom lose. The majority of midwives practice in out-of-hospital settings: "Hence, from a purely litigational view, the statistics suggest that the number of malpractice actions, and thus the cost of malpractice insurance, could be reduced by greater utilization of midwives, both in and out of the hospital." The Stewarts report that every study ever done comparing doctors to midwives shows better pregnancy outcomes for midwives.

The Stewarts state that insurance companies should favor doctors who work with midwives and out-of-hospital programs and the practitioners who engage in them. They urge governmental agencies to encourage good nutrition in pregnancy, breastfeeding, natural childbirth, homebirth, birth centers, and midwifery: "These factors will not only produce the healthiest babies and the lowest rates of mortality and morbidity, but are also the least costly and the least likely to result in malpractice insurance. . . . Thus, by the same set of actions, we could optimize pregnancy outcomes and solve the malpractice crisis at the same time."[101]

So the doctors are blaming the insurance companies, and the insurance companies are blaming the doctors. And we are blamed by both of them. The only good positive outcome of the high cost of malpractice insurance is the number of obstetricians who are leaving the field. The stress of wondering if "this will be the time that I'm going to be sued" has led more than one to teach rather than practice obstetrics. You can't teach what you don't understand.

I don't believe that obstetricians belong in childbirth. Even so, I don't want them to leave the profession in anger or in fear. I want them either to become midwives, to become surgeons (making themselves available in the rare instances that a section is necessary), or to leave obstetrics because their hearts are open and they realize this is not where they belong.

Court-Ordered Cesarean Sections: Cut it Out!

- In Missouri, two judges ordered a woman to undergo a cesarean section because the woman had had three previous sections. She preferred a natural birth. The doctors went to court and obtained an order. The judge said that the right of the child to a healthy birth took precedence over the mother's request not to have an operation. This was in 1987, long after the safety of VBAC was known and long after many women with multiple cesareans had birthed vaginally.[102]

- A nineteen-year-old in Washington, D.C., was ordered to have a cesarean section. She was in labor, and she was given one hour to find a lawyer to "prepare her case." The judge ruled against her.[103]

- A twenty-seven-year-old woman who was dying of cancer was twenty-six weeks pregnant. Her baby had a 50 to 60 percent chance of survival. The woman did not feel that the baby had enough of a chance to warrant the operation, and she did not feel that she was in any condition to withstand surgery. The court ordered a cesarean: the baby died within two hours, and the mother died two days later.[104]

- In Georgia, a physician determined that a woman had a complete placenta praevia. The woman had notified the hospital that her religious beliefs precluded surgery and that whatever happened was God's will. The doctor testified that there was a 99 percent certainty that the baby would not survive vaginal delivery and a 50 percent chance that the mother would not survive. The next day the court order was issued requiring the mother to submit to a cesarean section. The woman petitioned the court to stay the order: the court denied the motion. However, the woman delivered a healthy baby a few days later vaginally.[105]

- In Colorado, a woman was forced to undergo a cesarean for a baby that was supposedly in distress. Nine hours elapsed from the time the monitor tracings indicated distress and the delivery. The physician was "surprised that the outcome was not poor. He indicated that the case simply underscores the limitations of continuous monitoring as a means of predicting neonatal outcome."[106]

- In New York, a woman was told that if she didn't deliver her child by 11 A.M., the hospital would have a court order to deliver her by cesarean section. The woman broke down and said, "I knew I couldn't fight it. . . . My husband didn't know what to do either. They brought me the forms, and at 11:33 A.M. . . . my son was born. . . . My unborn child was a ward of the state."

- In Michigan, a woman was ordered to have a cesarean section. She had a placenta praevia. She went into hiding and when her minister was questioned he said that he didn't know where she was but he was praying for her. She had a healthy baby vaginally at a different hospital.[107]

- Several women have birthed vaginally while their doctors have been in the process of locating lawyers or getting court orders. Others have gone into hiding and had their babies at home.

The cases from Georgia and Colorado were decided within hours after they were argued. The courts made no attempt to analyze the rights of the pregnant woman. They decided that in each case the unborn child "merited legal protection," and they authorized administration of all procedures deemed necessary by the attending physician. Judges are not terribly good at making emergency decisions, and they don't belong in delivery rooms anyway. In both the Georgia and Colorado cases, serious errors were made. "In the first, a 99% certainty turned out to be wrong: the supposed 1% reality occurred. And in the Colorado case, the fetal heart monitor significantly overstated the amount of damage. . . . So permitting physicians to judge when fetuses are in danger may simply be giving them license to perform cesarean sections whenever they want to, without regard to the pregnant woman's desires."[108]

George Annas, Professor of Law and Medicine, asks: Do we really want to restrain, forcibly medicate, and operate on a competent, refusing adult? "Such a procedure may be 'legal' . . . from a judicial viewpoint; but it is brutish and not what one generally associates with medical care." It encourages an adversarial relationship between the doctor and the mother, and it gives the obstetrician a weapon to bully women he views as irrational into submission. When fetal surgery becomes accepted, will women be forced to consent to it as well? "And if one can lawfully force surgery, one should certainly be able to restrain the liberty of a woman for the sake of her fetus, e.g. by confining her during all or part of her pregnancy. . . . It seems wrong to say that patients have the right to be wrong in all cases except pregnancy—in that case, why should only the doctor have the right to be wrong?"[109]

The view that women who refuse cesarean sections are in some way willfully abusing their infants seems prevalent and deeply held by some obstetricians and judges. We must honor the rare case of a woman's refusal. "The choice between fetal health and maternal liberty is laced with moral and ethical dilemmas. The force of law will not make them go away."[110] Boston lawyer Alan Dershowitz says that "some mature mothers reject medical advice that it would be advantageous for the fetus if they were to give birth by cesarean section. They fear the surgery or worry about its disfiguring effects." Others, he says, refuse to stop smoking or drinking or "other things that are pleasurable to them, but harmful to their babies."[111] Where do we draw the line?

Women don't generally sue a doctor who has delivered a healthy baby by cesarean, even if the operation was unnecessary. Those who do find it difficult to get cooperation. Bonnie, a woman who took her doctor to court, told me, "I am a nurse, but I will never go back to teaching. How can I tell my students about the ethics of the medical profession when I know doctors who won't even help me out by testifying against someone else. When I decided to go to court, I couldn't even get counsel in my own state—they didn't want to be involved in suing the large hospital medical center here."

Medical researchers Dr. Nancy Milliken of the University of California and Lawrence Nelson of the University of California at Berkeley urge physicians not to turn to the courts to force women to undergo c-sections. Such a use of the system, they say, is unethical and could open the door to interference in such personal decisions as whether a pregnant woman continues to work. "Judicial involvement inevitably invades a woman's privacy [and] entails the disclosure of confidential and personal information." Once in that system, the woman must defend her choices on a highly personal matter at an extremely sensitive time. They say that a significant number of gynecology heads believed that court intervention is acceptable to force women to accept treatment on behalf of the fetus.[112] Bridgett Jordan, medical anthropologist, remarks that "it frequently happens that the first set of new procedures is tried out on people who are powerless," and mentions the irony that "a women's voice is not there, is not heard, is not a part of the proceedings."[113]

At a lecture I attended on court-ordered cesareans,[114] a number of interesting points were raised: With an elective cesarean section, we do not find out if the doctor was wrong. The legal system supports the present medical paradigm by making those who refuse to comply examples (allegiance between law and medicine). There is rarely time for due process; the doctor simply gives up trying to communicate with the woman and takes his "request" to a judge. The woman must then find a lawyer quickly, one who sees her under adverse circumstances and represents her to a judge who is fearful that if he doesn't act quickly he'll have the dead baby the doctor is predicting. These forced sections are just a symptom; we must understand the disease and its etiology. Court-ordered sections are plainly and simply a misapplication of the law and a travesty of justice.

Cold Sores

It's hard to imagine what it would be like to be forced into a c-section. Yet, in a sense we are all "forced": we wouldn't allow ourselves to be cut open unless we believed it was necessary or unless our internal fear prevented us from birthing normally. We are all forced to comply—it's a form of "forced consent."

Many people think that a woman who undergoes a section recovers and gets on with her life. Sadly, this is not always the case. The physical and psychological repercussions of cesarean sections are numerous and grim. The women who have written me, whose letters I have quoted throughout this book, were not trying to scare anyone when they wrote to me. They themselves were scared, and they were simply telling their stories.

The view of birth as emergency is reflected in the number of complicated pregnancies and difficult births. Pregnant women are in an opening state; they receive negative input from the medical system, and their fate is all but sealed. We have come to believe that postpartum depression is a "given" after birth, and while hormonal changes and other factors (exhaustion, poor diet, etc.) can indeed contribute to a need for a period of adjustment after birth, we must look at why American women are more susceptible to this phenomenon than many of their sisters world-wide. One woman went to her doctor several months after her section. She sobbed about her experience and asked him for help. He ordered blood tests, but they revealed no abnormality. He finally told her to "wait it out," that it was "normal" for women to feel depressed for a year or two post-partum and that it was foolish to feel that not pushing out a baby—or being separated from it for a few hours—was such a "big deal." Other doctors prescribe anti-depressants. The real issue, once again, is denied.

Writer Gregory Lay remarks that there occurs a phenomenon of "distanced observation by which we avoid looking directly at the issue—which we do not presently know how to improve—and spend energy instead on matters which are really not about the issue at all. This (superficially) absolves us of any responsibility."

In any society, the way women birth, and the care given to them "point as sharply as an arrowhead to the key values in the culture."[115] Robbie Davis-Floyd says that by making "the naturally transformative process of birth into a cultural rite of passage, a society can ensure that its basic values will be transmitted to [those] born [and re-born] out of the process. . . . Society must make certain that the new mother is clear about these values and the belief system that underlies them, as she is . . . the one most responsible for instilling this belief system in the minds of her children—society's new members and the guarantors of its future."[116] With a cesarean section rate climbing to the 50 percent mark in many areas, our children may learn that you do not participate; rather, you "get taken." Unless we shake the "knives of apathy and indifference slashing at our souls," unless we reach first-time mothers as well as VBAC women, the hands that rock the cradle will either be tied down or will belong to those whose chromosomes contain a Y. In addition, we will all remain "birth-colicky."

Cesarean section is not a failure on the part of each individual woman; it is a sadness. For many, it is a deadening instead of an enlivening. For some, like labor for a baby, it is a "wake-up call." In the end, it is a failure on the part of our entire culture as a whole.

Any process is marked by stages, but we seem to be stuck in hurt and hate. Sister Teresa has said that the moment you start thinking about other people as opponents it becomes impossible to find a solution. "There are no opponents in a disagreement; there are simply two [sides] facing a common problem. In other words, they are not in opposite camps, they are in the same camp. The real opponent is the problem."[117] Until we can proceed to other stages—those of healing and coming together—everyone should have a stomachache. As childbirth activist Patricia Barki has said, at the present time cesarean section in this country is the growth of an enormous abdominal social canker.

5 *Voices, Lowered*

More letters to add to those you've already read. I have received so many thousands that after a while I had to begin putting them in cartons and bringing them up to my attic to store them. When I go up there to get the winter boots or the summer clothes, I can almost *hear* the tears. As always, I read them and weep.

LYNN (California)
They say to be thankful. Your baby could have been (a) dead; (b) brain damaged; (c) etc. etc. So you feel like a crumb for saying you hated your cesarean.

PAT (Louisiana)
I want my scar to go away. How I would love to feel normal. Sex is terrible when as a woman you feel ugly. As a child, I wanted thirteen babies. One scar is enough. Here is hoping alcholo [spelling hers] doesn't make this letter too hard for you to read.

PHYLISS (Montana)
Now I found out (at a meeting where there were many women) that my doctor tells all the women who come to him that they have perfect bodies for delivering a baby and then he sections them all nine months down the road.

MARY (Michigan)
On my predelivery tour of the Labor and Delivery Unit, I was told that if the baby is healthy it is always brought to the mother, even if she is in the recovery room after a c-section because of the importance of that early bonding period. Nobody brought me my baby. Nobody asked me if I wanted him. Nobody told me I had a little boy. Nobody even told me if he was alive, dead, normal, or deformed or maybe brain damaged . . . I was in too much shock to ask, and I was too sick to hear bad news, so I couldn't ask. It would have been so healing to have him brought to me in the recovery room like they had promised if the baby was okay.

MARCIA (Washington)

I finally dilated. I was pushing but they said no good, so they called the doctor. He never came until after the fourth call. By that time I was so worn out he said he couldn't get forceps on the head, but he did manage to bruise my son's forehead. It was like he waited till I was worn out so he could come in and say c-section time. They gave me a shot in the back and said push. How could I push? I couldn't feel anything. I was then hauled to the operating room, given another shot in the back, and they pulled out a baby boy. The doctor also cut him by his eye. I can't even remember when the first time I held him was and that hurts.

KAREN (California)

I should have known it'd end up bad. My doctor chain-smoked his way through all of my prenatals. The hospital treated me like trash.

MARY (California)

Reading your information confirmed what I have known by instinct for many years and brought me to a place of sorrow and regret because I have had five completely unnecessary cesareans. My first was performed as an abortion in the second trimester of my pregnancy and was forced upon me by my parents when I was 15 years old. It was very traumatic; I wanted to be a mother and very much wanted my baby. I will never forget that initial nightmare.

I was told that since my uterus was incised vertically, a natural birth was completely out of the question. I numbly acquiesced to two more cesareans. I was 19 years old and I had had three cesarean sections!

When I was 27 years old, I developed a strong longing for another baby and decided even before I became pregnant that I wouldn't allow myself any more perverted birth experiences. I was told during labor, however, that since my water had broken two days earlier, there was a possibility of infection to my unborn baby. Shaking and in tears, fearful that my decision to birth normally would harm my child, I regretfully agreed to another painful invasion.

Some months later, a surprise pregnancy became apparent to me, and I once again began to plan for a natural birth. I signed up with a "progressive" hospital that boasted an 80% VBAC rate. I overlooked the fine print, which stated that women with a vertical incision was high risk and a definite health threat to herself and her baby. I again succumbed to a cesarean, not knowing what else to do.

During my fifth cesarean, I had a tubal ligation to insure I would never have to go repeat these experiences again. I am deeply disappointed about my five birth experiences and am also quite sorry that I have ended my fertility. I am 31 years old and have longed for a "real" birth experience all of my adult life. I love motherhood and have a strong trust in nature and my body. This trust, of course, didn't survive in the midst of AMA scare tactics. If I had had your material earlier, I believe I could have been more trusting through labor. I feel very empty and a deep despair and wish that my opportunities were still intact.

CHRIS (New Jersey)

The doctor assumed the cord was wrapped around the baby's neck. They did a c-section—the cord wasn't wrapped. I didn't get to see the baby—they took her to the nursery immediately, even though she was ok.

Later, a nurse came in and said, "We've got a problem." My baby had been cut on her right cheek. They called in a specialist and at 12 noon that day—at five-and-one-half hours old, my husband watched as they stitched her—six stitches. She will need plastic surgery. The doctor said this couldn't have been prevented—but he was talking all during the section—not even about the surgery.

ROSE (New York)
For two days afterwards my stomach blew up and they couldn't figure out why. They got pus and gas out of a tube inserted through my nose. It was HORRIBLE.

SUSAN (Missouri)
Since I am large boned, 5' 11" tall and very healthy, I never even seriously considered a cesarean. My membranes ruptured and I didn't go into labor. I felt my body betrayed me and I was a complete failure.

For my second baby, labor began on its own. My body could produce a contraction! However, when I got to the hospital, the contractions stopped. Two hours later, the doctor broke my water. He must have used ten different wires before he got one to stick in the baby's head and register on the monitor. At the same time, nurses were trying to insert an IV in my arm, also with great difficulty. I felt like a human pin cushion. I stayed like that for a few hours. My body was failing again. Another cesarean. Oh well, we tried.

We also tried to get hospital policy changed so that fathers could be present during cesareans, but no luck. I did receive a letter and basket of fruit from the hospital president—some consolation. I begged the anesthesiologist for a spinal or epidural, but as with our first child, "It is not our policy to use regional anesthesia for "emergency cesareans." (Emergency = unplanned.) I argued with him long enough that he suggested I ask for another anesthesiology group. Forget being awake! This whole thing is a nightmare! However, I was almost awake because the stupid doctor started cutting before I was asleep.

PEG (Maryland)
Now I understand that a nine-month crash course in natural childbirth isn't enough to uproot what is embedded in our minds for 20 plus years . . . By the time I was able to hold her, everyone had held her already but me—even the grandparents. I kept crying and saying, "I'm your mommy."—I was sure she wouldn't know. I wonder if this has affected my relationship with her. If she had been born vaginally would we feel differently or more towards each other?

DEBORAH (Mexico)
They're coming south, those blankety-blank cesareans of yours. In Mexico City they're all over the place—like a fungus.

VICKI (Oregon)
What scares me is that I felt I was an intelligent, motivated, and enthusiastic Lamaze "birther." But I was not prepared—the books I read helped me more than the classes. I received absolutely no support from the hospital staff: as compassionate human beings giving help over the rough spots, they failed miserably. I'm sure they'd be shocked to hear this from me; they probably think I was a perfect patient. After 15 hours of labor with no food or water, and then a cesarean, I was too physically and emotionally drained to be my usual complaining, questioning self.

Looking back, I cannot believe that not one nurse or my doctor even bothered to ask me if I was depressed or wanted to talk about my birth.

EILEEN (Arizona)

In my eighth month I was diagnosed with herpes. Besides feeling dirty and talked about, I was terribly frightened. The only information I could find talked about brain damage. I had a daughter after I was conned into a c-section. I say conned because I have since met several women who had herpes and had a healthy baby and safe, vaginal births.

LAUREN (Alaska)

Something has to be done to stop this atrocious butchery of women! Here in Anchorage nearly one-third of all births are cesarean! I am learning that there are some hot politics involved in childbirth policy. Yes, indeedy, it can get very cold up here, very, very cold.

MICHELLE (Louisiana)

Last month we did a section for a supposed cpd and fetal distress. The baby had no molding and weighed just a little over six pounds. She had an Apgar score of ten, no meconium, no nothing. As a labor and delivery nurse, I asked the doctor why the cesarean was performed. He said: "She wanted a tubal anyway."

MALINA (California)

I think a labor support person would have helped me avoid a cesarean, but no hospital here permits them in.

KARLA (Illinois)

About three months ago I had a repeat cesarean which left me feeling very depressed. I love my baby, but the c-section really took something out of me, I'm not as happy as I used to be, there is no zest. Here at the Air Force base I saw seven doctors during the course of my pregnancy and I didn't meet the surgeon until the day before the surgery. The reason I met him was that I didn't show up for my cesarean the first time around . . . So two days later he asked me to come to his office. Well he broke me in two. He gave me a choice of the 12th or the 15th, I picked the 12th, to this day I don't know why. He told me if I didn't schedule a cesarean he would drop me as a patient and we didn't have medical insurance. I deeply regret that I didn't wait until the 15th, I've thought about it every day since my child was born.

RENA (Mississippi)

I'd like to tell my story but I don't know if anyone has the time to read it. I need to tell someone desperately. I dilated to eight centimeters with my first baby. I had three doctors I had never seen and they all examined me, one after the other, and they all said I was different. One said I was six centimeters, one said nine. One said I was at zero station and another said I definitely wasn't. They didn't tell me he was posterior but they broke my water. I am absolutely certain I was more than they said, I was wanting to push and they kept saying no. I keep wondering about all of this. Please forgive the manner in which I wrote this letter.

SANDRA (Nevada)

I need help. I am a registered nurse with all my experience in ICU and OR. OB has always been my weak spot. I found that when the obstetrician finds you're a nurse, they explain less and less and are less help to you. My doctor is a lovely man, we had a good relationship, but when I went to see him with questions, I never really understood the answers. So each month I came back with the same questions and he became very impatient with me. Sometimes he almost acted like he didn't know any answers so he just covered up by acting impatient. I know some questions don't have concrete answers, but even the basic support seemed to dwindle. Come to think of it, I saw my doctor close the fascia on a section and to tell you the truth, I wasn't impressed.

BARBARA (Canada)

I have been afraid of the rage I would feel if I began to believe that my cesarean wasn't really necessary or could have been avoided. So I have justified it, over and over again, in my mind. I can't kid myself anymore.

JOHN (Ohio)

Dear friends, here is a humble letter of our experience.

Our first baby was born just fine—a healthy baby boy. I felt so unworthy of being a Daddy, our whole lives would be changed now, it was a change we looked forward to, so when I stood there, looking at our sweet little baby, secret tears of joy stole to my eyes. Two years later, on Friday the 13th, which turned out to be the unlucky day for us, our doctor was on vacation and the other doctor said they had to do a c-section because one hand wanted to come out first. I had to wait in the waiting room until they were ready for me. My wife so hated the spinal. One and a half years later we were very disappointed when our doctor told us we'd have to have another c-section because my wife's incision was made the wrong way. We had another baby girl, she wasn't really "born" to us or was she. I think she was stolen out through that ugly cut. My wife thought the spinal was worse than labor would have been. One year later, my wife started in labor so we rushed to the hospital as the doctor had been warning us that it's very dangerous to be in labor after a c-section. But at the hospital, nobody seemed to be in a hurry, and we were put in the labor room to wait for hours and hours, and labor getting strong, if only we had a way of making this baby hurry and pop out, but a nurse warned me that it never could be done. Finally, after six hours of labor our surgeon was ready to perform our 4th c-section. In the meantime, some of our friends were having VBACS after 1 and 2 cesareans without having the doctor's consent. So we decided then and there that labor wasn't as serious as the doctors like to say it is. (Note: Please see a subsequent letter from John in the chapter entitled Voices, Raised.)

CYNTHIA (British Columbia)

I became a victim five years ago when I was pregnant with my first and only child. After all the things they did to me in the hospital, I was in such a mess they sectioned me. They told me so many lies they started to screw up their own stories. Finally I demanded my records. I found out they not only lied to me but to each other.

I have since questioned the doctors involved. Most sit in silence. One admitted that what happened shouldn't have, one even said I would have been safer in the woods with a stick between my teeth. I believe that the ones who sit in silence think it was mishandled, but even those who voice an opinion wouldn't stand up in court and say it. I believe that doctors use women for medical experiments and that is the number one reason for all these sections. Joseph Mengele could fit in any maternity ward in North America, as long as the sheets are clean and you don't get gassed at the end of the experiment.

I once thought I'd never have another child but I am not going to let them have that power over me. I'll never have another section. If need be, I'll throw myself on the electrical fence before I go back to that lab.

My feelings about doctors have turned to hate and mistrust which is poisoning me. I went and spoke to my priest about it. I felt better when he prayed for me but he wanted me to talk to a woman doctor who had been sectioned. I met her in a coffee shop and we had a chat that reinforced all my beliefs.

TRACEY (New York)

I wonder why hospitals keep records when doctors can write anything they want whether it is accurate or not. . . . I was given 14 hours to deliver, so I raced the clock. I suspect that the CNM [Certified Nurse Midwife] thought that telling me of my time limit would make me get the baby out faster. It only planted a horrifying thought in my mind: I admitted to myself to the hospital and now they were controlling my destiny. The CNM kept pulling my cervix toward where she thought the head was—excruciating. Who can dilate with someone pulling at you? By 9 P.M. she suggested demerol to relax me—this was a joke because I had fallen asleep to rest. She woke me up saying, "You have to get going—you're running out of time!" I later learned that demerol can slow labor and cause the baby to be distressed.

I ended up with a cesarean. I asked for a bikini cut. The doctor waved his hand condescendingly and said he didn't do them. So I have a classical incision. I was wheeled in for ten minutes of needle stabbing, while contracting. I was told, then screamed at, to be still. My husband was not allowed to stay.

I asked a number of questions during the operation. I didn't feel numb so they stopped several times to poke me. My punishment for wanting to know what was happening to me was the gas mask! I still cry when I think how close I was, probably a minute, from witnessing my son's birth. But the mighty anesthesiologist gassed me so my questions wouldn't bother anyone. The doctor told me there was a Bandl's ring in my uterus and that I'd have to have all my children by cesarean. I signed myself out on the third day.

When I received my records a year later there was no mention anywhere that I had a Bandl's ring. In the doctor's detailed report of my operation, there was no mention of this, or of my questions to him, or stopping to check if I was numb, or when and why I was gassed.

MAUREEN (New Hampshire)

They yelled at me because I had my baby sleep on my shoulder. Do you know any hospital that does not ever separate mother and baby, even at night? I am thankful to learn that other cesarean mothers have sex problems after a cesarean. My doctor says it's because I'm too busy.

DIANNE (Massachusetts)

I recently read an article about cesarean prevention and VBAC and relived the extreme anguish and pain that I still experience in recalling the c-section birth of my son 9 and 1/2 years ago.

After 18 hours of labor, hooked up to graph paper, fetal monitors, etc., the staff decided the baby was too large to fit through my pelvis. After he was delivered, they flashed his genitals at me to show he was a boy and took him away.

They claimed I couldn't nurse him with an IV in my arm. In desperation, on the third day after his birth, we begged them to bring him to me and my husband so that my husband could feed him. They brought sugar-water. As soon as the baby was alone with us, I nursed him. It was the first time I'd ever touched him. I had to stare at him and say to myself, "Yes, I think this is the same baby." The nurse came back before we were done and RIPPED him out of my arms and said, "If I had known you were going to do THAT to the baby, I would not have brought him to you and you can be sure I will not bring him to you again!"

The next day my temperature went up slightly so I was informed I would not be allowed any contact with my child. I was forcibly catheterized against my will (held down by four people) which made urination painful for weeks and which I remember as RAPE (which it psychologically was). When I finally got home and sat in the rocking chair to nurse my own son, he was so frustrated from a week of no food, no touching, NO NOTHING, that he nursed for eight hours straight. If I tried to stop he would get hysterical.

Now, 9 and 1/2 years later, I still turn into one big knot when I think about it; I still can't discuss it without crying, and I am 5 weeks pregnant. I am in a state of terror and I don't know what to do to release all of the horror that seems bound up in every cell of my body. The thought of the last experience paralyzes me with fear and anger.

LEAH (Idaho)

I just heard about VBAC and I want to hug you people! It has taken me so many years to integrate the pain and disappointment of my first birth. It still causes lumps in my throat and tears in my eyes. The quack of a doctor first tried forceps and damaged my cervix. My baby was taken away for six days after the cesarean because of an infection (from the unsterile tools). We live in the woods—4 and 3/4 miles up a bumpy dirt road that is sometimes washed out. I'm staying home for this next birth. (Note: You will find a subsequent letter from Leah in chapter 15.)

DONNA (Colorado)

I feel I was set up for my cesarean and I hurt for other women who are being set up and deceived into thinking that a section is the only way to produce a healthy baby. All the women around here think their doctors are right. Baloney. Those doctors aren't anywhere near us when we are home mending our hearts, bodies, and spirits from the hurts and disappointments of our births. Where are the doctors when the depression becomes almost overwhelming, when the only activity you do is basic care for your baby while the rest of you slowly deteriorates. We're Christians. This time we're putting our faith in the right place.

PAULA (Maryland)

I took classes at the hospital and we were led to place all our trust in the medical profession. About ten days past my due date the doctor tried to stimulate my cervix but to no avail. My baby just wasn't ready! That was very painful. At twenty days late, x-rays were taken to see why things were so slow and I was told I was much too small to deliver vaginally. Then I read how dangerous x-rays are, and how they don't tell you accurate information. But I didn't know that then, and a few hours after my x-rays, I was lying naked in front of six strangers—an anesthesiologist, a pediatrician, two nurses, and two doctors. I was extremely embarrassed. I felt helpless and bewildered. In recovery I shook violently inside. I couldn't open my eyes to see because of the medication I'd been given. I was freezing and sweating. I felt incomplete and inadequate. I pitied myself. It took over a year to begin to recover emotionally.

ROSA (Georgia)
It should have been the most rewarding experience in my life. Instead, it was like going to the electric chair. The so-called doctors who attended me shouldn't be allowed to treat a dog, let alone a human being. One in particular was rude and cruel and had the manners of Attila the Hun.

KAREN (Rhode Island)
I let them talk me into an induction of labor. I feel like such a fool. As I look back, I don't see any reason for it. The doctor said he wanted to get the whole thing going because the placenta could start to decay at any moment. But I felt fine and all the tests were fine. I should have trusted myself. When I was still having postpartum depression I used to hold my son and cry and apologize to him, telling him that I had done the best I could. I guess some of the feeling was guilt that maybe I hadn't done the best I could, that I should have been stronger.

LIZ (Vermont)
You get to the point where you want to flatten the next person who tells you to put it behind you because you and the baby are ok so why fuss. The baby is fine but I have eight inches of scar of my stomach and a lot more on my soul.

LISA (Virginia)
They just undermine your confidence and that keeps on and then you just get to believe them and throw in the towel.

CONNIE (California)
Five months ago, my wonderful life came crashing down around me. I had a cesarean section that has left me with overwhelming feelings of failure. I feel like a failure as a woman, and a fraud as a mother.

PAULA (New York)
My strong anti-cesarean feelings began on my first visit to a maternity ward in the Bronx. I went to look at babies, but all I could see were the cards attached to the bassinets. Nearly half read "c-section." Chills ran up and down my spine.

When I found out that my baby was breech, I was sorry to be pregnant. I no longer wanted to be. I spent the whole month falling apart. Of course, no one told me the things that can be done to help turn the baby. For the entire month, I cried my eyes out and was constantly nauseous. I could not believe that the simple act of making love with my husband had put me in a position to have major abdominal surgery. The joy I had felt turned to dread. I felt like a caged animal ready for slaughter. Could I simply stay at home and deliver alone? Would the baby come out? Who delivers animals?

. . . My ride to the hospital was like a ride to hell. . . . My doctor walked in, did a vaginal exam, and said, "I feel toes." I said I wanted to deliver. "You can't!" When I began to protest, she said, "This is an emergency!" She told me that footling breeches born vaginally usually weren't alive after the delivery—I knew this was a lie since my own father and husband were footlings delivered vaginally. She told me I would kill my own baby. After only an hour and a half in labor I was already four centimeters dilated. I knew I could do it. "You don't want to take the chance," I was told.

. . . My poor squeamish husband looked on as they began to torture his wife— jabbed, stuck, and "prepared" was I. Immediately and simultaneously I was jabbed with a catheter and IV which made me crawl up the back of the bed in pain . . . Once in the torture chamber, my body was covered with sheets, only my genitals were exposed. One arm was tied to a blood pressure machine. The other arm to the IV. I felt my left hip propped up. My mouth was muzzled with oxygen. I saw faces all around me, but not once did anyone look at me.

Inside I felt they were all laughing at me because I had lost the battle. My heart pounded. (My God, "Why hast Thou forsaken me?") I felt like an unwilling victim of sadism in a porno flick. Was this any different than the holocaust, operating on people who did not need surgery? It was exactly like being raped. The only difference was that I somehow had given my permission to have this done to me.

In the blackness I heard a baby crying as if it were in a tunnel. A woman's voice said, "Boy." I opened my eyes (I am still alive) and saw my husband's face. Then PAIN, PAIN, PAIN—it's been done. You've been sectioned. You've been mutilated. Your baby cut from your womb. You've been violated, tortured and the doctor made a bonus on you—fool.

. . . 2 A.M. I was given nothing to drink—I was choking. Nothing for pain—I was dying. I was refused an extra blanket—I was freezing. Then I was refused my baby. My buzzer didn't work either. So I banged on the bedrail. I told her I would not stop banging until I saw my baby, got some ice, and a warm blanket. Can you believe, I got all three. But it was awful. I was on my back and could not move a finger to hold him, could not turn my body and look at him. I could not cradle him in my arms the way I envisioned mother and child. I was a weakened creature.

. . . Everyone of us on that floor had cesareans. All week long we came and went—c-sections. My roomate developed a horrible complication. Her incision bled, the internal muscle wall ripped open, the bowels fell through and stopped functioning. She had to undergo major surgery again to repair the job. The sight was pitiful as I watched her kiss her baby goodbye as she was wheeled into an operating room for the second time. Two years later she was urged to immediately sign a sterility consent form before she underwent an emergency cesarean. She did, twenty-five years old.

I bore a child, I know he's mine, but I did not give birth to him. Forgive my anger, but I am pregnant again.

ANNE (North Dakota)
I was induced because I supposedly had diabetes. They said the baby was going

to be a giant. He was 7 lbs. even, and I never had diabetes but I'll always have a scar on my belly from now on.

DALE (Hawaii)

Aloha from another cesarean mother. It wasn't any luau, believe me. If they'd put an apple in my mouth, they could have sliced me and served me as the main course.

JANA (Nebraska)

I thought cesareans saved all babies! Mine died.

CAROLINE (Ontario, Canada)

Those bastards. They raped my first two babies out of me. So I labor slowly, but damn it, normally. Those damn bastards stole my birthright. They robbed me of my primal scream of triumph. They cheated me of my celebration of womanhood. Damn them all to hell.

6   Birthcrap!
Interfearences and Interveintions, Once More

Language—words—are not apart from thought. Our minds are literally streams of consciousness and of unconsciousness as well. We cannot hear a particular word without having some reaction to it on some level. If I were to say "doctor" right now, a series of feelings would begin to surface, depending on what your past experience with doctors has been. If your life had been saved by a physician at some point in your life, you might have feelings related to relief and gratitude and admiration. If you have never been to a doctor in your life, or if the only doctor you've seen in the recent past is Doogie Howser, then your reactions will be far different.

I listen to women very carefully when they speak to me. A few times, I have predicted a woman's cesarean based on just a few words. Lewis Mehl and Gayle Peterson did quite a bit of work years ago on predicting birth outcome. By asking a number of questions, we can often identify "a woman at risk" (for a cesarean, for example). It is then possible to help the woman refocus and redirect her thoughts and perhaps affect the outcome in a positive way. One woman, for example, kept using the words, "the upcoming delivery." There is only one way that I know of that babies "come *up*" and out of the mother's body, and we all know what that is. Another woman kept talking about the "impending" birth; I had a feeling she would be quite "overdue" (a word on that later on). Another must have told me three times in the course of a ten-minute conversation that she didn't want to fall apart during labor, that she wanted to "keep it together." There's a tension and a tightness in our bodies when we are working to "keep it all together." I asked her if she wanted some feedback about her conversation, and we spent the next hour "loosening up." There is a balance between telling someone something that may be of use to them, and planting a seed of doubt in their minds. Generally, I point out the "red flags" to women; as they change their language, a new concept develops.

The words we use are so important! Throughout this book you will find many examples of things that were said to women that influenced their births in either positive or negative ways. There must be a famous quote out there somewhere about words being swords or rose petals. It's true. Fran had back labor and was at six centimeters. The people she was with said, "It's going to get worse as the baby moves down. You're going to need to take something for the pain. You can take it now and get ahead of it, if you want to, or wait until later and hope that it'll do some good at that point." She ended up with a you-know-what. Heather also had back labor and was dilated to six. The first thing her LSP (labor assistant) said when she arrived at the birth was, "Open your back." "Open my back??" Heather said. "Yes, Sweetie, open your back." "Oh, okay." Heather wrote, "Thinking about opening my back really helped me as I opened and let the pain go. . . . I was checked. Seven? More like eight . . . (a contraction) oh, nine . . . ten centimeters, there you are! I knew I could start pushing and the back pains would go away."[1]

When a woman says that her doctor is going to "let" her do thus and so, that's a red flag. We stop right there and rework the whole concept of permission at birth. It's a wonderful opportunity to talk about responsibility and power and a multitude of other things. When she says she is going to "attempt" to get through labor without drugs, or "try" for a VBAC, we also have some things to discuss. Other word flags from just this week alone: I'm going to *beg* the hospital to let both of my friends be at my birth; I'll *fight* not to have a monitor; When my midwife said that, I practically *split a gut*. One woman who called me and said that she was "fine" with her c-section, kept referring to the baby as "it." When I asked her if she would be willing to use the baby's name, she said yes. When she did, the tears of healing began to fall.

Another woman called and said, "I'm a cesarean mom. I'd like to have a normal birth next time." During the course of the conversation, she referred to herself as a cesarean mom several times. She was, but that's not the point. If she continues to label herself that way, she imprints "cesarean mom consciousness" on her brain. This could make it more difficult for her to birth vaginally. How many times does the brain have to hear "I'm a cesarean mom" before it believes it as truth? If these words are inked indelibly onto the brain, it might be difficult to have a VBAC.

In *Silent Knife*, Lois and I talked about the many words used at birth that give us a headache. I think they bear (intentional use of the word) repeating. It's okay to "rupture" your membranes, but uterine "rupture"—now, that's a no-no. We labor in "stages"—three different stages: the "latent" phase, the phase of "dilation," and second stage, also known as, get this, "expulsion." Our babies are supposed to "drop" (many don't, and there is nothing wrong with that at all), and "engage." There is a birth "canal'" (a canal is artificially made and bordered on two sides by concrete or an embankment!), and we are "monitored."

We are measured in centimeters and by fingerwidths. Our babies' position is announced to us as "plus" or "minus" a "station" (and we wonder why it is hard to loosen up and open up and give birth?). The image of a train barreling into the next town doesn't exactly fit the feminine vision of birth, but then, we end up with "skid marks" (bruises in the vagina), so, why not? We are told that we make far too much "noise" in labor. We supposedly get an "urge" to push.

A few of the words that have become commonplace at birth really get to me. To tell you the truth, I don't care who Braxton was, nor Hicks. "EDC"— estimated date of confinement. LISTEN LOUD AND CLEAR! It is only an estimation. Yet women count on it (notice my carefully selected choice of words) and go bananas if they're "overdue." I know women who have been three and yes, even four weeks past what the doctors carefully determined was the date. Babies still can't tell time. And we aren't supposed to be "confined."

Bloody show. Now that's a good one for you. What woman who wants to feel the fullness of her sexuality and femininity wants to have a "bloody show"—or, better yet, a "mucous plug." A plug of snot. Makes you feel soft, and warm and open, and sexy, huh? I refuse to use that term. The whole birth scene in this country is a bloody show, and not a very bloody good one, at that.

Contraction. Nope. I won't use that one any more either. Birth is an opening, not a tightening. Every time we talk about contractions, our memory bank, the one that knows the definitions of words and creates physical reactions to those words brings "contraction" images: secure, fixed, taut, closed, inflexible. When people get angry they often contract; they roll up inside themselves into a little (or big) ball. I shuddered the time I heard a nurse saying to a laboring woman, "C'mon! I really want to see you contract good and hard with this next pain!" So many of us have been talking about how inappropriate and damaging this word is to laboring women; yet few have consistently avoided its use. Ina May Gaskin calls the rhythms of labor "rushes." I like that word in the sense that the sensations are, in fact, flows of energy, but I don't like the other connotation of the word "rush"—to hurry along. Labor must be allowed its own time.

The word "labor" itself no longer feels right to me, but I'll let that one go for a little bit.

Sometimes we think we are talking the same language, and we're not. For example, someone tells you they are going to call you "soon." A week later you get a call. "Soon," to you, was Tuesday, or maybe Wednesday. Words have different connotations to different people—which is why if a doctor tells you he'll "let" you labor for "a while" before performing a section, you'd better define "awhile."

Thomas Kuhn, author of *The Structure of Scientific Revolutions*, has found that the scientific community shares a common world view, a reality concept, called a paradigm. A dominant paradigm always exists during each scientific period and provides the basis structure within which all scientific thinking and experimenting are done. "Thus, all experiments tend to support and entrench the dominant paradigm of the moment. . . . When a new and better paradigm begins to emerge, scientists welcome the chance to verify it with rigorous and creative experimentation. Right? Wrong! Nothing, it turns out, is more threatening to the scientific community than the thought that the paradigm is failing."[2]

So, we are asked, how does a new paradigm break through the "logjam" of existing thoughts and beliefs, grimly held together by an unyielding leadership? In a surprising and exciting way: by the emergence of a new concept, "so large, so poetic, so stimulating, so above the battle, that defending the existing ideas becomes less important than exploring the ideas suggested by the emergent paradigm."[3] Kuhn says that new ideas are taken and tried in light of the new paradigm. Most of them fit, which indicates that in a paradigm shift, it is always more important to have a *change of vision* (italics his) than to have a series of small, new ideas. Without the statement of a new dominant paradigm, new insights will never gain hold: The ideas supporting a new paradigm cannot be explained or articulated in the language of the old paradigm.[4]

It may be time, Kuhn says, for a new social paradigm. "It is clear that our present institutions have not absorbed the flood of new knowledge now available to them. They cannot do so and still continue with their present forms and obsolete rituals. Thus, they daily grow more dinosaur-like, and lose the loyalty of their once-faithful True Believers." We now know, he says, that major new truths don't come from the drip-drip-drip of tiny new "truths" being added to old truths; rather, major changes occur with a leap to a new, more enlightened level of perception.[5]

Once we realize that we have bought somebody else's (the OB's) paradigm (Barbara Katz Rothman calls it the male medical model) lock, stock, and barrel, and once we decide it no longer fits and that we are going to create a new one, we're cookin'. The words that the doctors have given to me no longer fit in any way, shape, or form the view I hold of birth. I need all new words.

In *Growing Up Free*, we are made ever so much aware that the words we use reflect how our society sees women. A "man in the street" is Mr. Average; a "woman of the street" is a prostitute. The unmarried man is a "bachelor" or a "swinger" or a "free agent"; the unmarried woman is a "spinster" or an "old maid."[6] There will be more on attitudes about "male/female" in Chapter 7.

In my birth class we talk about language. We begin to change how we talk about pregnancy and birth. One woman called me and said that a doctor walked into the labor room and told her that she was making too much noise. "Noise?" I said to him. "That isn't noise! What's the matter with you?! This is my *birth music!*"

It may be the "field" of obstetrics, but to me, birth is better placed in a meadow. Women rarely want to see, let alone touch or smell, "bloody show," but they are delighted and interested in "baby gel." What an incredible, wonderful body we have that can create something like that! Our bottoms do not "tear" or "rip!" Sue, in Ohio, says they simply "unfold." I say they "smile." A "bag" of "water?" Cradle basket. Second stage? No. "Openhome," or "Babytime," but not "Rush hour!" Open. Expand. Melt. Float. Be.

We are blooming, blossoming, opening, unfolding. We are doing a lot of things. One woman in my classes calls contractions "babyhugs": when you get one, you just let it hug the baby. Soon, your baby will want another hug, and another. Other words in my classes are angeltaps, cuddlebunnies, pillowfluffs, sunflights, bellybounces. Hey, don't knock 'em; they all beat "contractions." In Lynn Richards' book, *The VBAC Experience*, one doctor said, "If the baby is, say 6 or 7 pounds, you could possibly pass it. "Pass it??" says Lynn. "We weren't talking about a kidney stone. People "pass" kidney stones. Women "give birth" to babies.[7]

Bruria Husarsky, a childbirth educator from New York, says that the term *cesarean birth* annoys her. She says that no one bats an eyelash these days at cesarean sections. She says that we should call it what is really is—open uterine surgery! How about calling it an ouch—open uterine cutting at the hospital.

Brian, a dad from Ohio, thought that LSP—labor support person—wasn't enough. He thinks PSS is more appropriate—your personal spiritual sister. I like that, too. The words come to you when the vision—the new paradigm—takes wing in your heart.

I needed a word to refer to the people in my classes and workshops. I was both tired of and uncomfortable with the words "spouse" or "mate" or "partner." These people are certainly not patients or clients. I call them "momdads." If it is a woman to whom I refer, it looks like this: Momdad. If it is a man, it's like this: momDad. I especially like this because it encompasses the male/female principle (which we'll talk about later) and for a number of other reasons as well.

There is so much power in one word: NO. Three are even nicer: *No, thank you. I love you.* I may have already mentioned that in *Sense and Sensibility*, Judy Herzfeld says that if the American pregnant woman could only learn a few words, she's be in good shape, such as: stop, wait, slow, take it off, take it away, go away, be quiet, when I'm ready, when it's time.[8]

Our names are words. It's time we all started calling our OBs and anesthesiologists by their first names. It will change things, I tell you.

Words can heal, destroy, empower, alarm, soothe. At some births, we talk a lot. At one birth, no one spoke for four hours. It was beautiful: "Language is so often more relevant in its absence. When a person's essence unfurls from her it silently vocalizes her own atmosphere."[9] Samuel Thomson reminds us that physicians have learned just enough to know how to deceive people, and keep them in ignorance, by "covering their doings under a language unknown to their patients."[10] In my opinion, this is where real "pig-Latin" originated.

Tests in Pregnancy

The height of the ridiculous came when a [medical student] asked me: "Have you had all those genetic tests? Like for sickle cell anemia?"

I looked at him. He is white. I am white. "I'm not in the risk group for sickle-cell," I said gently.

"Yeah, I know," he said, "but if there's even one in a zillion chance . . ."

—Perri Klass[11]

"Good prenatal care here means lots of tests."

Mary S., Florida

Grown-ups love figures. When you tell them that you have made a new friend, they never ask you any questions about essential matters. They never say to you, "What does his voice sound like? What game does he love best? Does he collect butterflies?" Instead, they demand: "How old is he? How many brothers has he? How much does he weigh? How much money does his father make?" Only from these figures do they think they have learned anything about him.

If you were to say to grown-ups: "I saw a beautiful house made of rosy brick, with geraniums in the windows and doves on the roof," they would not be able to get a picture of that house at all. You would have to say to them: "I saw a house that cost $130,000." Then they would exclaim, "Oh what a pretty house that is!"[12]

The above paragraphs are excerpted from one of my favorite books, *The Little Prince* by Antoine de Saint-Exupery. I took a little poetic license: the house the little prince was describing was $20,000 at the time. It's been a while. The answers to the questions, if you really want to know are: rhythm of the rain gently patting on a roof, softball, no, 45, 1, 153 (give or take), I don't know.

Thanks to people like Barbara Katz Rothman (*The Tentative Pregnancy*) and Robin Skynner (*Test-Tube Women*), as well as Anne Frye and Robin Blatt, who have written books on tests in pregnancy,[13] I have only to add a little of my own two cents and then be on my way. I won't be repeating much of the information on testing that was in *Silent Knife*, so if you are interested, you can also read the chapter entitled "Diagnostic Test Bombs?" in that book. The news today is that with the oversupply of doctors, the number of unnecessary tests and treatments is increasing.

In *Silent Knife* we talked about some of the tests that were available for your consideration during pregnancy. For your viewing pleasure, we have your basic ultrasound. For those of you who wouldn't mind going into labor a little early, we've got your basic stress test and for all the rest of you, we have your basic nonstress test, too. We even have a nipple stimulation test. But if it's a little baby juice (amniotic fluid) you want, no sweat. We'll just set you up for an "amnio" (along with the ultrasound, of course), and you'll find out what you want in no time. Or will you?

In *Childbirth Wisdom*, Judith Goldstein remarks that, unlike modern Western women who rush to doctors for lab tests to confirm pregnancy (although with the do-it-yourself home kits, this is ruining a whole segment of the doctor's role in life), tribal women know they are pregnant by the changes in their bodies: they are in tune with these changes.[14]

Recently, I received an article from a newspaper in a town not too far from me. Apparently, tests done in the eighth month of pregnancy indicated that the fetus was no longer alive. A few weeks later, the operating room was readied, a priest was called, and a cesarean was performed to remove the "dead" infant. The mother is quoted: "When I saw the baby, the color wasn't consistent with that of a child who had expired. I'm saying, 'Oh my God, maybe the baby isn't dead.' Before I could think of anything else . . . her little eyes opened and blinked and she started to scream!" The doctor in question was quoted as saying, "I think it was a mechanical error. The machine we used just didn't pick up the heartbeat."

More than two hundred "fetal conditions" (including "fetal sex determination") can now be determined prenatally, from the more well-known circumstances to "Maple syrup urine disease."[15] In an article entitled "The Promise and Problems of Prenatal Testing" by Barry Seigel, we are told that our ability to diagnose defects has far outpaced our ability to cure them, or even to describe accurately how they will affect the baby. "Their science has transformed the amorphous embryo into an unborn patient, but the chief therapy for most problems remains selective abortion. So with the wondrous new advances come anguish and uncertainty and hard choices. Advancing technology already on the horizon promises even greater complexities and moral dilemmas." Despite such difficulties, Seigel says, more and more couples are turning to prenatal diagnosis; for many women an introduction to it often comes unwittingly: "sometimes it's the result of a simple blood test taken in their doctor's office." The routine test shows "a little something" that isn't "quite right," perhaps, and the couple is on their way to the AFP (alphafetoprotein) test. It is highly inaccurate as tests go; "It's merely a screen, so it sometimes leads to more advanced procedures such as ultrasound and amniocentesis."[16]

Cheeriocentesis

We told you some of the dangers of ultrasound in *Silent Knife,* and you'll learn more in a little while. As for amniocentesis, the risks of the procedure are still horrendous and high: infection, hemorrhage, fetal damage (including puncturing the baby), miscarriage, embolism, premature labor, abortion, damage to uterine and placental vessels, and sudden deaths, to name a few. (Unexplained respiratory problems at birth may be another.) Yet women go in for their amnios as if there was nothing to it. (In *Silent Knife* we said they make the appointment as if they were having their hair done.) I've taken to calling them "cheerios" (Cheerio and all of that, everyone; I'll see you after my stomach gets punctured!").

Let Them Eat Worms

A procedure they've been working to perfect is called fetal endoscopy. A cut is made into the pregnant woman's uterus, and the endoscope is pushed into the baby cradle (amniotic sac). In this way, it is possible to "peer at the fetus through the telescopic lens in the instrument. Then the doctor will clip off a piece of the baby's skin and draw blood from it for what doctors call 'diagnostic purposes.' " The risks are frightening and numerous: spontaneous abortion (as if it happened on its own, right?), damage to the eyes of the fetus, uterine trauma, and psychiatric disturbance.[17] I don't know if the article means psychiatric disturbance for the mother or the baby or both—or maybe for the doctor when he finds out he's killed a kid?) The ability to perform fetal testing and surgery opens up a whole new can of ethical and moral worms.

Alphabet Soup

Another fairly new technique is percutaneous umbilical blood sampling (PUBS—sounds like a place to go for a beer). In this procedure, a "highly trained specialist" (you hope) guides a fine needle through the mother's uterine wall directly to the point where the umbilical cord joins the placenta. The "target point" (more war words) is a spot of vessels 3 millimeters (less than an eighth of an inch) in size. Do you wonder if this test brings with it an increase in the risk of problems with placentae and cords? I sure do. An article on PUBS tells us that this is sometimes difficult to administer: "When the fetus is moving around a lot, the sampling is possible but may take a little longer. . . . When the baby moves, the cord may shift and throw you off target,"[18] says the good doctor. Don't you mothers have any control over your children at all? Can't you get them to be still???

The test that gets to me the most is chorionic villi sampling. The test is no bargain, believe me. It is done to find chromosomal abnormalities. Villi form right at the beginning of the pregnancy (they are the tiny (microscopic!) "fingers" that reach into the uterine wall) and eventually form your placenta! In one article I read that the villi disappear as part of the chorion develops.[19] They don't disappear; they become a part of the placenta! Women are told that the sample that is being taken is not an anatomical part of the fetus (not to worry). What in the world do these ostriches think is going to happen when they take even one of the villi? Nothing? How can they think that they can remove something as precious as a villus without any consequences? Am I angry? You better believe it. How dare they. Current studies suggest that the test carries "about a five percent risk of fetal demise."[20]

We are told that the advantage of CVS over amniocentesis is that it can be done early in the pregnancy (the eighth week versus the sixteenth week for amniocentesis). "When defects are found, decisions about continuing the pregnancy can be made with less stress and anguish."[21] Have you noticed that we are always told the advantage of the newest test over the previous test. They won't tell us the problems associated with amniocentesis until CVS becomes "the way to go." Then they'll say something like, "Amniocentesis? Oh no, we don't do that any more. You see, it's far too dangerous. What we do nowadays is. . . . " And we won't be told all the risks associated with CVS until something newer gets discovered. For now, we are told that CVS is the "new alternative" to amniocentesis, that it may "rival" amniocentesis.[22] It'll be a contest to see which of the tests "wins out." How many babies will we have to lose in order to find out?

Correcting Tests

Barry Seigel says that doctors who work in the field of fetal diagnosis have little time for philosophy. "If they get too philosophical, they can't come to a decision and that their certainty diminishes each day. . . . They steel their minds and live with the complexity and gray areas. They say they accept their perpetual uncertainty." How well they live with it is a matter of opinion. In Chapter 8 Seigel presents a discussion by an OB who made an inaccurate diagnosis. Seigel says: "Whatever one finally thinks of prenatal diagnosis, this much can be agreed upon: once babies were either born or they were not. Now there are options. [Choices] provide opportunities and burdens."[23]

In my hometown recently, a couple was tested for Tay-Sachs disease, a rare but invariably fatal disease that affects mostly Jews. They waited for the test results and were told that their baby had the disease. They chose to abort the fetus. Several months later, a baby was born in town with Tay-Sachs. The test results had been mixed up: the "wrong" couple had been given the bad news. In an article entitled "Ethical Issues in Prenatal Diagnosis" we are asked whether or not doctors must tell a woman when (not if, mind you), by mistake, a normal fetus is aborted. "It might be extremely difficult for a physician to tell a woman who had been trying to conceive for years that such a mistake was made."[24] Yes, it might be, mightn't it. Because if we knew how often mistakes were made, we'd stop having tests, and after all, what is a doctor for if not to prescribe them, diagnose them, and analyze them? (In the same article the question was raised as to whether all women should "enjoy" equal access to testing programs. Then it states that, "Despite [several] unresolved ethical issues, the mass screening program will begin. . . . " In another article, we are informed that in spite of protests from the American Academy of Pediatrics and even ACOG, the FDA "signaled its approval of wider use of laboratory tests that detect neural tube defects in fetuses."[25] Now if you can't trust the FDA, who are you going to trust?

We all know that doctors order too many tests and that testing itself is a lucrative enterprise. Many articles state that hospitals waste millions of dollars on "unindicated tests"—tests ordered for people who are extremely unlikely to have the abnormalities the tests detect. Most often, malpractice is cited as the reason for failing to detect an abnormality might be grounds for a lawsuit. A research team at the University of California at San Francisco discovered that 60 percent of pre-op blood tests were unnecessary.[26]

Another article states that doctors favor the Pap test on an annual basis, partly because of concerns about their accuracy. "There are inherent inaccuracies in the whole process. . . . Errors can occur either because the doctor took an inadequate sample of cells. . . . or simply because the sample was not properly examined by the lab technician."[27] Yet another article confirms that the more tests you have, the greater your chances of receiving incorrect reports. The same sample, tested twice in one day, or sent to two different labs, may yield different results.[28]

Is the barrage of routine tests ordered for pregnant women really necessary? Pregnancy normally alters the body. "In a normal pregnancy, there is some doubt as to the need for frequent blood testing, or for ultrasound scans at all."[29] In a normal pregnancy, there needn't be any testing at all, as far as I am concerned. The problem is, most doctors convince us earlier on that our pregnancies are not normal. Then we are like putty in their hands.

In an article entitled "First Trimester Prenatal Diagnosis," I read that the problem of how to become skilled at some of the finer sampling procedures is being handled in a number of different ways. At two large well-known institutions, the Institutional Review Boards gave the researchers permission to biopsy women who were planning to have abortions anyway, as long as the women gave informed consent (but there really isn't any such animal, as we all know). Other institutions, finding that method unacceptable, gained their experience, instead, by practicing on women who had blighted ova—"a condition in which the embryo dies early in pregnancy—but in which the chorion is the last to go."[30]

One big concern about tests is, of course, accuracy. Often when the tests come back "iffy" everything is really perfectly fine. Many times in my eighteen years in this work, women have called me in tears because of a test. Do you think it is accurate, I ask them. Do you *feel* that it is? What do *you* think? Most of the time, they have a sense about what is going on—a far more accurate account, it turns out, than most of the tests.

This one hurts. I received a letter from a woman in West Virginia. "Mindy," an RN, had a routine mammogram done, and the results showed a lump in one breast. The lump was removed and found to be benign. Since she had cystic breasts, her doctor recommended that she have most of the breast tissue removed and have implants. "During the surgery," Mindy said, "they ran into bleeding problems—the plastic surgeon didn't have any blood available. I lost over half my blood volume. Three days later, the surgeon came into my room and said that he had bad news. The pathologist's report had come back—'You have cancer in both breasts.' I was told that I had three types of cancer and one was an invasive type—the rapid-growing type. It was suggested that I have a modified radical mastectomy and all the lymph nodes be removed. The surgeon told me that I had between six months and a year to live. This happened on Mother's Day, and I had the surgery to remove my breasts a few days later."

In the weeks following, Mindy had time to think: "How could I have had a benign report one month, and then 72 days later—three cancers?. . . . So I picked up my slides at the hospital and brought them to one of the top pathology labs in the nation. The doctors did not know that I had my records. Four days later, one of the leading pathologists at the lab called me. He said that there was absolutely no sign of any breast cancer in any of the 112 slides. He said, 'I advise you to get an attorney.' "

Mindy got an attorney, and she "won" the case a few years later. She said that there was a coverup in the hospital, that the trial was delayed, and that the pathologist who diagnosed her "cancer" is still practicing. He is 85 years old. "It scares me to death that he is still out there doing lab work," she says. Mindy is alive and angry, ten years after both breasts were removed for three kinds of cancer that she did not have. She wants everyone to know how inaccurate test results can be—and the devastating consequences "trusting" them sometimes has.

"Skipping Exams"

Not one of fifty women who have called me in the last few years with a question about gestational diabetes has had it. It is testimony to their strong, healthy bodies that they didn't end up with eczema or heart palpitations from the grief they had in removing the label. Insisting a woman fast when she is pregnant is tantamount to child abuse.

Leslie had tests done when she was six days "overdue." The signs were worrisome, but it was not yet time for panic. Five days later, she was told it was time for panic. If things "deteriorated" any more, her baby would die. She didn't want a dead baby, did she? To make a long story short, two weeks after "panic-time" Leslie had a beautiful ten-and-a-half pound baby (a VBAC). She had "checked-in" with her baby, with her own intuitive wisdom, and had decided to trust in her body and in the process of birth. Another woman, Terri, was twenty-three days "past term"—and decided not to have any testing at all. She had a beautiful little girl after two cesareans. Lynn's fundal height did NOT change for six weeks; she decided not to have any tests and delivered a healthy baby at term.

Pop Quizzes

Monika wrote that the results of her AFP test indicated that her baby might have Down's Syndrome. "After participating in a genetic studies program at [a university medical center], two ultrasounds, and amniocentesis," she was thrilled to learn that her baby was okay. She said that the stress of waiting for the results was insurmountable. (And we all know what stress can do to a body.) "I would surely not wish the red flag nightmare on anyone. Even with the 'assurance' that things were fine, I held my breath in the delivery room. And then, when the results are back, you have to wonder if the tests themselves did any damage." I often wonder how women who have had an experience like Monika's can continue to put their faith and trust in "the system" and subject themselves to modern obstetrics at the actual birth as well.

When a woman who swims at my Y heard that I was writing a book on pregnancy, she asked me if I had planned to include any material on prenatal testing. She said that when she was pregnant, she had had a routine AFP test done. The test showed that she was carrying an anencephalic baby. She insisted that the test be done again. This time the test came back with different results: the baby had Down's Syndrome. The third test? "Not completely normal," said the doctor, "but close enough." (whatever that meant). Judy said once you get the results, and there's any question at all, you are no longer waiting for a baby. You are waiting in the delivery room for the doctors to tell you if they were right or wrong. She said that her husband was great throughout the pregnancy: he said to her, "Don't worry, honey. If the baby is this or that we'll deal with it." But he fell apart afterwards (the baby was perfectly fine). Judy said, "He never played with the baby. He just kept *testing* him." Her relatives, concerned that the initial diagnosis might be right, continually asked, "Do you think he looks alright? Don't you think his eyes are funny?" Clearly, they had been prejudiced by the results of the test.

Judy observes that once you are pregnant, there just isn't enough time to learn all the things you might need to know about tests. And when you are pregnant, you are so involved emotionally that it is sometimes hard to make decisions. She recommends that women inform themselves ahead of time as to whether or not they want to get involved in the testing scene. Her neighbor had an AFP test and was told that everything was "A-OK." A few months later she had a baby with Down's Syndrome. Judy says, "Her doctors kept shoving the test results in front of her nose to show her that it wasn't possible for this baby to have Down's. Even though you could tell that there was a problem, the doctors kept insisting that the baby 'looked normal,' and they wanted to do some tests to prove that they were right."

Another woman I met at the Y was told that her baby was severely deformed. She decided to continue the pregnancy and prepared herself for the worst. She gained an inordinate amount of weight: "The stress!" she said, really got to her. The baby was born; it was fine. The doctor showed her five times on the sonogram photograph where the "problems" were.

I know there are people out there who are going to stamp their feet and tell me how testing saved their baby's life. In Chapter 7 we learn that there is room for more than one reality in the Female System: tests are not okay sometimes and at other times they are clearly needed. As one article suggests, the testing can be a "marvel or a menace"[31] depending on what side of the fence you're on. In a number of articles I read that eventually, all our tests will be handled by computer. I love my computer, but I wouldn't want it to tell me everything everyone else thinks I'm supposed to know about a pregnancy or a birth.

They're All Boobs, Anyway

Breastfeeding and breastplay (during love making) stimulates the release of oxytocin. Oxytocin helps to strengthen labor contractions. The nipple stimulation test that I referred to earlier, however, is called the nipple contraction stress test. According to one source, it offers "significant advantages over nonstress testing for antepartum surveillance." A quote from the same article, same doctor: "The nipple stimulation test must be performed in the hospital area for safety. . . . It offers a remarkable savings in time, convenience, and cost over the oxytocin stress test."[32] Twiddle my nipples and you're a dead man, doc. He recommends that the nipple test be done in the hospital because "there are half a dozen cases on file at this hospital in which nipple stimulation led to a seriously abnormal heart rate pattern that made immediate intervention, including cesarean section, necessary." Dr. Nippleman's article in an obstetrical journal cautions against home use of nipple stimulation to ripen the cervix. (I wonder how he plans to monitor that.) He also discusses the "hyperstimulated patient."[33] Next, we'll have machines that do it for us. I clutch my chest in total disbelief.

I read an article entitled "A Test About Just Who We Are" by "a former defective fetus who was not aborted."[34] So many issues are raised in such articles! Amniocentesis can sometimes uncover defects but cannot always predict the severity of the problem. Barbara Katz Rothman asks, "What does it do to motherhood when we make parental acceptance conditional, pending further testing?"[35] Columnist Margery Eagan writes, "This testing lets women say, 'This is not the child I want, I want a different one, a better one.' Some women hold off telling people they are pregnant until they 'know' [quotes mine] the health of the baby—or whether or not they will keep the child. Then the decision is made on the quality of the fetus."[36] Barbara Katz Rothman tells us "No matter how hard we try, we cannot know what kind of a child we will have, whether it will be healthy and able-bodied and remain so, or what sort of [person it] will grow up to be. No amount of prenatal testing can guarantee any of that.[37]

These days, you can get tested for everything from A to Z (literally). The choices you make may depend in large part on the "system" you choose (medical or nonmedical), on the paradigm you adopt, and on the beliefs you carry in your heart about birth. The choices you make for yourself during your pregnancy will influence those you make during your labor. Please remember that at most hospitals the tests are not over when the birth is over: our sweet little babies also become "pin cushions," too.

William Roper, chief of the federal Health Care Financing Administration, says: "It's time to get serious in limiting unnecessary testing. . . . As long as doctors are paid to do tests, and not to think, they will do tests and minimize thinking.

... In too many instances ... tests turn out to be worthless—or even dangerous."[38]

Let Them Eat Sprouts (and Fruits, and Veggies, and Whole Grains. . . .): Nutrition

The number of U.S. medical schools with a required course in nutrition: 30. The training received by average U.S. physicians during four years of medical school: 2.5 hours.

—John Robbins[39]

Maybe our grandmothers didn't know it because they were misled, but our great-grandmothers knew it. They would eat for two—chickens, eggs, meat. They didn't go to the hospital to be weighed, their salt wasn't restricted and they weren't given drugs. Yet they had strong, healthy babies. . . . Now if a woman has a 9-pound baby, they think that's abnormal. The common sense of people is an idea that needs to be dug up, resurrected and . . . brought to prenatal care. Common sense is suspect, however, because it's not electronic.

—Dr. Tom Brewer[40]

Dr. Brewer goes on: In the well-fed mother you can see that her hair has a nice texture, her skin is smooth, and her gums don't bleed. The well-fed mother hardly ever gets stretch marks, her liver functions well, the placenta's working, and the baby's growing. When the babies are born, they are a good size, not premature. He says that when a mother eats well and salts her food to taste, she will usually go ten to twenty days past her traditional due date, but the babies aren't overdue. Well-fed mothers have an abundant milk supply, recover quickly from birth, and have the energy they need to begin mothering. "An adequate diet must be provided all through gestation—for each and every pregnant human being! No civilization can afford less!" As always, he tells us that the role of malnutrition during pregnancy in causing reproductive pathology is the "best kept secret" in this country. The survival of our oncoming generations hangs in doubt, he says, in every mismanaged pregnancy, labor, and birth.

A lot of excellent information is available on diet for pregnancy. You can read things by Dr. Tom Brewer, Gail Sforza Brewer, Nan Ullricke Koehler, Phyllis Williams, and many others. Taking care of yourself nutritionally isn't an "option," it is a must. I'm just going to add a little to what we said in *Silent Knife* and then assume that you will read the material from the experts.

Tom shared a letter with me from a woman, Susan, who after giving birth was in a coma for over two days. Her 2 pound 11 ounce baby was in the hospital for six weeks. Twenty-eight years earlier Susan's own mother had died of eclampsia when Susan was one day old. Susan had followed the 1,000 calorie a day diet her OB had given her. "She had the diet sheet taped to the refrigerator and was weighing her food on scales! My God, we're back in the Dark Ages! They told her that eclampsia was a 'genetic disease.' " Susan sued her doctor for malpractice. In the court proceeding when Dr. Brewer criticized Susan's doctor for making no notes whatsoever on her prenatal record about diet and nutritional counseling—"not even the 1,000 calorie diet was recorded"—the doctor's lawyer asked, "You don't expect a busy ob/gyn to write down notes about the pregnant woman's diet, do you?" "That's why we're here!" Brewer responded. "If her doctor had given her even ten minutes of proper education and stopped the 1,000 calorie reducing diet, we would not be here suing for malpractice!"[41] Tom says that one-third to one-half of the cesareans seem to be for pregnancy-induced hypertension when, in fact, doctors don't understand that the women don't have it (and it's "curable")! They're just pregnant, and that changes blood volume and blood pressure.

I received a letter from a woman in Alabama. Her doctor had delivered her baby by cesarean ten days early because of IUGR (intrauterine growth retardation). He had tried to induce her twice, but the inductions didn't "take" well. Her water broke during an exam to check for dilation (will wonders never cease?), and the baby's heart rate dropped to 60 during each contraction induced by the pit. The baby weighed 5 pounds, and the doctor said it was the "driest birth" he had ever performed. The placenta was sent to the lab. "There was nothing wrong with it, except it was half the size it should have been." I wrote back to the woman and asked her about her nutrition. Sadly, no one had bothered to ask her before. I referred her to Tom, and I am sure her next baby will weigh a lot more than 5 pounds.

Contrast the above story with that of another woman who learned that she had IUGR at thirty-seven weeks. When she called me, I advised her to talk to Dr. Brewer. It wasn't that she was eating poorly, but she was definitely not eating enough. Instead of inducing labor, she started feeding herself differently from that moment on. She ate every two hours, almost around the clock. Six weeks later she delivered an 8 pound 3 ounce son. This is no excuse to eat poorly at first, but it does show that with proper information and nutrition the label high risk can be removed.

Childbirth Wisdom states that six of the ten leading causes of death in the United States are linked to our poor national diet. We have so many riches, and we eat such junk! "Rather than concentrating on new pieces of hardware for the operating room, doctors should have a much stricter insistence on a better diet, and an overall healthier lifestyle. All the substances that we use that interfere with pregnancy and birth (alcohol, drugs, caffeine, sugars, fats and milk) are absent from tribal diets, and the health of those mothers and their babies is, for the most part, excellent."[42] It is perhaps unrealistic to ask doctors to counsel us in nutrition; have you ever seen the way most of them eat?? One doctor said that diet is very important after surgery. "In fact," he said, "many of us eat a chocolate sundae after we operate."

Childbirth educator Nancy Hatch Woodward says, "It is one of the primary responsibilities of the obstetrician to work with each woman nutritionally so her baby has the best chance of being born healthy. . . . Unfortunately, they often know very little themselves . . . and [therefore] give diet guidelines that are harm-ful to mother and infant."[43] Nancy says that it is tragic to note that many women do not receive any prenatal care and equally disturbing to find that those women who are seen by doctors privately or in a clinic have the same nutritional deficiencies as those who have gotten no care. As Dr. Brewer says, "We feed our nation's pregnant dogs and cats and hogs and cows better than we feed our pregnant mothers; animals are rarely nutritionally mistreated the way women are." But then, "How can the blind lead the blind?" Besides, there is no money in "safe motherhood."[44] Poor outcomes are big business.

In a number of areas, if you have high blood pressure, the doctors assume you have toxemia, put you in the hospital, and give you drugs. Apart from all the other problems that drugs can cause during pregnancy, they can interfere with your appetite, and so compound any problem. Brewer says that pregnancy-induced hypertension is *not a disease of pregnancy*. It is not even a clinical syndrome, but only one clinical sign.[45] He says that it is a mistake to focus all the attention on the pregnant woman's blood pressure while ignoring her nu-tritional status, blood volume, liver function, and her emotional state. Most PIH as presently defined by U.S. obstetricians is benign physiologically and has no connection with MTLP (metabolic toxemia of late pregnancy) in the doctors' minds. "Most babies would be better off if they grew to term in a cabbage patch, tended of course by an organic farmer. Is know-nothingism forever in this field? Only if the AMA-ACOG's Stone Age three N's for prenatal care is forever: Nutritional Nonchalance and Neglect. . . . There is no true prevention of pre-maturity and low birth weight in the United States without a program of primary prevention of maternal malnutrition and legal drug abuse.[46] Bed rest and drugs are not the answer to problems in pregnancy.

One woman wrote to Dr. Brewer that she had seen an advertisement in a nursing journal that touted aspirin as protection from PIH. "I wonder how many stillbirths or IGUR babies will result from premature closure of the ductus arteriosis that aspirin is implicated in? Why are drugs being promoted for pregnant women when a superior diet will prevent problems? Too simple a concept I suppose. . . . I want you to know that some of us are 'believers!' We are listening! I am an RN and I have worked three years in labor and delivery and three years in the NICU. I am a convert—I now truly believe that superior nutrition is the key to prenatal care and healthy babies and moms. Fifteen months ago, I gave birth at home to a 10 pound 2 ounce baby. I went twenty days 'over,' which we all know is what well-nourished women often do. . . . Many doctors still teach that after the first 24 pounds, 'all it is is fat.' No wonder weight-conscious young women in our 'skinny is beautiful' culture stop eating . . . and as a result end up with MTLP, other problems, and damaged babies."[47] You can't get a "blue ribbon baby" dieting, smoking, and/or eating unconsciously.

Penny goes on: "I also thought you might be interested to know that of the five nurses who were pregnant with me, I was the only one who didn't have any problems and the only one who followed your diet (despite my urgings). Two of the nurses had severe hyperemisis, one of who, went on to develop MTLP, premature labor on Ritadrine, etc.—the whole nine yards. She ate candy bars all day long. One nurse had second trimester bleeding and a small (?) abruption. And another had IUGR [intrauterine growth retardation]—no weight gain after thirty weeks and no uterine growth after 32 weeks with reduced amniotic fluid. She ate very little protein. . . . After delivering her IUGR baby she bragged that she only had six pounds to lose to return to her prepregnancy weight! The last nurse, who worked on the postpartum floor, bragged to me she only ate a bowl of Cheerios all day. This was while she was eating candy out of the vending machines. At fifteen weeks she had already developed severe preeclampsia and told me the doctors had put her on a low salt diet. When I asked her, 'Didn't you know that salt was essential for a pregnant woman?' she looked at me as if I were crazy. These are not stupid women, but their ignorance in the area of nutrition is appalling."

We know now that even moderate amounts of alcohol affect the fetus. Fetal Alcohol Syndrome is a cluster of several physical and mental defects caused by alcohol damage during pregnancy. These include growth retardation, with no "catching up" later even if the baby is well nourished; facial malformations; brain damage; and abnormal development of various body organs, among others. Alcohol can also affect infant development after birth. [48]

Excellent nutrition helps every aspect of pregnancy and birth. It lowers the rate of everything—low birth weight, prematurity, eclampsia, and cesarean sections. Tom Rush, a pediatric epidemiologist, remarks that increased awareness and implementation of nutrition programs in pregnancy result in fewer stillbirths, better brain development, fewer learning disabilities, and healthier children. [49] We also know that exercise helps. Women are stronger and healthier. They are better prepared for labor and delivery. Take a walk—now's as good a time as any—and don't forget to bring along a really good snack.

One of my cousins brought me a paper that her doctor gave her during her pregnancy. Every woman in that medical practice (she switched) was required to be tested for gestational diabetes. Pregnancy as pathology, once again! The form reads: "As pregnancy progresses, it becomes increasingly difficult for the body to maintain a normal blood sugar level. [Wrong—it maintains a level that is normal for pregnancy.] Some patients will actually develop a type of pregnancy-induced diabetes. Since we cannot always predict in advance which patients are likely to do so, we are strongly urging you to have a simple test." Among the instructions given is No. 5 which says: "As a general rule, avoid concentrated sweets, i.e., pies, cakes, candy bars, etc. prior to any prenatal visit." Is it okay to eat them at any other times???

Some foods, herbs, and teas actually help tone the uterus and build our bodies in more than twelve ways. You can gather that information; it is all out there for you to own, cheap. [50] One point of interest: a number of midwives recommend that women go easy on milk products. Milk is intended for calves, who start out their lives much bigger than we do and must stand minutes after they are born.

Cow milk grows cow bones. The instruction by many doctors to go home and drink three glasses of milk a day (that's about all the nutritional instruction many of them give) may be ill-advised.

In *Artemis Speaks*, midwife-healer Nan Koehler gives great advice on nutrition. Mix her information with that of the Brewers et al and voila! You have a great recipe for a great pregnancy.

Doohickies and Thingamabobs: The Power of Paraphernalia

The French Revolution gave birth to the myth that physicians could replace the clergy. Until the late eighteenth century, the trip to the hospital was considered a last resort. Typically, it was taken with no hope of return.[51] Today, most people believe that hospitals increase one's chances of surviving a crisis. With some clear cut exceptions, more often than not, they are wrong. Intensive care, Ivan Illich says, is merely the culmination of a public worship organized around a medical priesthood struggling against death.[52]

Susanne Arms states that women are confused as to what constitutes a genuine crisis in childbirth requiring intervention and what is actually within their own strength and capacity to handle.[53] In *Childbirth Wisdom* we are told that there are far fewer complications of childbirth than the man-made troubles that emerge when we fail to understand the process of birth and its "demands."[54]

In cultures where birth is understood, that is, respected and allowed to unfold naturally, there are seldom any difficulties and rarely any accidents. Among one tribe of North American Indians, there was no placenta praevia, no infections, no toxemia, and no phlebitis until the women "started living like the whites."[55] Yet, the vast majority of births in the United States are considered high-risk situations: all birth must be "risky"—why else would we be in a hospital while it is taking place? Contemporary women find it impossible to imagine how they could live without the technologies that past women lacked, never missed, and were often better off without.[56] "These days, a woman in labor is considered to be in an intensive-care situation," says an assistant professor of obstetrics and gynecology at Cornell University and Medical College, speaking for ACOG.[57]

So many of you work in hospitals, you say, where things are changing. "Your" women stand in labor! They even have a little yogurt! They don't get monitored for the whole labor; they just get hooked up for "strips." You don't even have "delivery rooms" any more: all your rooms are "birthing rooms!" Please!: Don't let your little world view cloud you from reality. There isn't a whole lot of natural childbirth going on out there yet, you know. Not yet. Each normal birth is still a victory rather than an "of course!" One nurse wrote to me and said, "Keep writing. I'm sending you lots and lots of good vibes. I just finished working another horrible shift at an area maternity unit. Add together a few sections, some mid-forceps (they still do them, you know), some vacuum extractions, and virtually one-hundred percent medication of mothers and one-hundred percent monitors, and watch this nurse and mother finally go to pieces." Another RN wrote, "I always thought that I could make a difference at my hospital. But I seem to be spinning my wheels."

Ruth Holland and Jill McKenna observe that birth technology has never been properly evaluated, but its availability has been used to pressure women into acceptance "on the false assumption that they make pregnancy and childbirth safer."[58] They go on to tell us that all this undermines a woman's confidence in her ability to give birth—and that even midwives, once the skilled and trusted companions of the pregnant and laboring woman, too often have become mere handmaidens to doctors and machinery. Jay Katz, M.D., remarks that the controlled studies that are being done now "may very well sacrifice a generation of women, but scientifically it does have merit: the altars of science are presided over by gods who at times demand human sacrifice."[59]

Maureen Ritchie, tells us that, from bitter experience, many of us know that we will not "be given" a good birth, that we have to "take it." In other words, she says, "to retain control over our bodies and our babies in pregnancy and childbirth, we have to resume more responsibility for ourselves than we are usually expected to."[60] In an article on feminine ethics, Janice Raymond tells us that the medicalization of women's lives brought about by technology produces continued debilitation to our bodies and spirits. "Woman adapts to a self and a world she never created," Raymond says. "In the midst of a man-made environment, it is important to persist in asking woman-centered questions. Why, for example, does technology reinforce the biomedical 'fact' that a woman's reproductive system is pathological and requires an enormous amount of intervention? Why do these technologies reduce the totality of a woman's being to that which is medically measurable?"[61]

Some of the letters that arrive at my house, and at C/SEC and CPM's doors as well, could melt stone. Many of them are pages long, with details from the very first sign of labor to the bitter end. One woman sent me a single-spaced typewritten letter that was thirty-one pages long. Another sent me a handwritten letter; it was forty-four sides of a large yellow legal pad. Another woman, who wrote a quick little "note" (eighteen pages), apologized and said she hadn't really meant to "go on" for so long: she's actually just sat down to write for information. So many of the letters start out, "I hope you aren't too busy to read my story. . . ." Surely every woman who has endured hour upon hour of labor, hooked up to every machine and gadget known to the field of obstetrics, deserves a listening ear. One of the most touching letters I have ever received was from a woman whose labor was one of the most gruesome I had ever encountered; there wasn't an orifice in her body that wasn't poked or "inserted into." Her baby died. She sent me a copy of her child's little footprints.

Space-age analogies are frequently used to describe birth nowadays and doctors even make references to exploring "inner space."[62] Those of you who have heard

When I Play with My Child

Sometimes we wrestle
I get him locked
between my legs
and start to tickle

He fights to be free
All the while laughing
And I find myself imagining
I'm birthing him
I'm finally birthing him.
                    Colleen Redman-Copus

me speak have seen me dress up into my version of modern-day woman's "birth outfit." I start with my hospital jonnie and then put a "catheter" (garden hose) into my jeans. Then I take a small-size plastic Pepsi bottle, and suspend it upside down from a wire coat hanger. There is usually a blackboard or something tall that I can hang the hanger from. Attached to the mouth of the Pepsi bottle is a long telephone wire, which has a letter opener on the end. This is my "IV," of course. I usually ask if there are any nurses in the audience who would volunteer to "hook up" my IV (via masking tape). Once they do, I tell them I hope that this is the very last IV they ever hook up to a birthing woman. Fortunately, it often is.

I then continue my "labor." I have an extra-large shoe box with buttons drawn on it—my external fetal monitor—and I wrap two wires around my belly: one to monitor me, of course, and one for the baby. Since everybody knows how important it is for a woman to be upright in labor these days, instead of lying down with all this apparatus, I put my monitor onto a wagon (or a set of luggage wheels). Most hospitals boast the new portable fetal monitor units! I can also put my IV on a mobile pole and stroll down the promenade at my leisure. I shouldn't go too far; after all, they have to do "a check" every little while to see if I am progressing. So out come a dozen or so rubber gloves.

I now attach a second bottle to the IV—it is a baby bottle turned upside down. They now come in a new shape so the baby can hold them sooner. (Soon we won't have to feed our babies at all; computers will do it.) Into this bottle will go some pitocin, because my labor isn't going fast enough. Then, since the baby is going into a little distress, we will break the water. Out comes the longest knitting needle I own, and voila! we have ruptured the membranes. Now for the internal fetal monitor. A sharp little thumb tack will do, or better yet, a screw, attached to a tube. Look out vagina, here it comes. Sorry, baby, but this is for your own good. . . .

I'm hungry! No, not more juice, although you have been most generous with that, thank you. But I'm hungry, not thirsty. Oh, I'm not allowed to eat? Okay. So I hang a big sign around my neck that says "DO NOT FEED." I can barely move from all the tubes and wires. I can't do this labor any more—someone give me drugs! And, of course, I pull out a big glass jar with "pills" in it (marshmallows!).

Okay, I have managed, somehow, to get this body to the "pushing" stage. I puff out my cheeks and grunt and groan a while. But, no, it isn't going right. So I guess I'll have to have a forceps delivery. Out come my salad tongs. Ah, but wait! Why not use the latest in modern technology—a vacuum extractor— a "baby-sucker-outer!" I lay down on the floor and get out either a dust buster, or, better, a vacuum cleaner with a nozzle. First, I do an episiotomy—that goes without saying. I turn on the vacuum and sssllllluuuuurrrrppppppp!—the baby is sucked out of my body.

I have forgotten the little details: I also have shoe covers and hats and masks, just in case I am in a location where hospitals still use those things. I also have a razor for shaving pubic hair—or beyond ("From stem to stern!" one woman called out. "That's what they did to me!"). Someone once suggested that I make chocolate pudding for the places that still do enemas.

I stand up with the baby that I "delivered." I put on a party hat. After all, it's my baby's birthday! I look ridiculous, as you can perhaps imagine, and the audience is usually quite amused by now. I must say, it is rather nutsy. But then, I say stop. Stop laughing, please, stop talking . . . just stop. The room gets quiet. Take a breath, I say. A big breath. Take another. And we all realize that we have all pretty much stopped breathing all the time I was doing this scene, because the truth is that it isn't funny at all. It is real, and it is awful.

The room generally stays pretty quiet. It's pretty sobering: More than 90 some-odd percent of American women birth their babies in a scene not too far off from the one I have just portrayed. When we breathe deeply, we feel the pain in our hearts.

A poem entitled "Long Memory"[63] reads:

> We are exalted to think back before machines which think
> like the men who think like them.
> You will find a long memory there—
> Now listen.
> now remember.
> To keep the long memory
> is the hardest, most dangerous thing that we can do.
> Yet it is all that keeps us human,
> saves this earth for our grandchildren.

Anesthesia

It's still dangerous.
I almost burst a blood vessel a year ago when Hal Linden had a thirty-second

spot on TV that aired a few times in which he said that women should not be martyrs in childbirth. He said that childbirth anesthesia was safe and that each of us should talk to our doctors about the anesthesia that would be best for us, personally. I couldn't believe it. All these young impressionable women out there, watching "soaps" after school, and this "expert" filling their heads with garbage. Hal, go back to "Barney Miller"!

Do you know that more than 80 percent of women "choose" epidurals? An article in one of those magazines that gets passed out in childbirth classes and through diaper services said so. The woman who wrote it also said, "The last four hours of my labor breezed by, and my baby was born no worse from wear from the drug."[64] (Note sarcasm.) In its favor, the article does point out some of the problems associated with epidurals. In another article, we learn that nausea, vomiting, and shivering are frequent side effects; however, "With re-assurance, most women accept the shivering as an unimportant side effect."[65] Epidurals increase the need for forceps (the woman loses the ability to bear down at the time of delivery) and episiotomy. In addition, the woman's mobility is restricted, so labor is often prolonged; hypotension occurs in almost 30 percent of the women who have epidurals; there is an increase in fetal distress, an increase in fetal malpresentation, and an increase in cesarean sections. "Depending on the anesthesiologist's skill, there's a slight risk (up to 1 percent) that the needle may puncture the fluid-filled spinal dura, which could result in dangerous overmedication of the patient."[66] Also health costs are increased, owing to the need for an anesthesiologist, IV fluids, and constant use of a fetal monitor. (If it is so safe, why do they have to keep monitoring you?) Many women wrote to tell me that they were charged for anesthesia even though they didn't use any.

Oh, and cardiac arrest, that's another "disadvantage." When we wrote *Silent Knife*, bupivicaine was used in epidural anesthesia. The following year, the FDA cautioned that its use was associated with at least sixteen deaths.[67]

And what effects do epidurals have on babies? Epidurals cross the placental barrier and affect the baby in both short- and long-term ways (drowsiness, poor sucking reflex, suspected hyperactivity up to seven years of age). One group of researchers found effects on the muscle strength and tone of newborns, "but these effects wore off rapidly as the drugs were eliminated from each baby's bloodstream."[68] Compared with babies in an unmedicated group, epidural babies "performed poorly on the motor, state control, and physiological response clus-ters, as well as their total score. . . . Mothers of [epidural] babies reported that they were less adaptable, more intense, and more bothersome in their behavior. . . . Mothers of [epidural] babies seemed to view them less favorably and in general found them more difficult to care for compared with mothers of unmedicated babies."[69] The final conclusions of this last article state that a "drugged" and disorganized baby can interfere with the development of a "positive, reciprocal relationship at home."[70]

Judy, a nurse from Florida, wrote: "I just attended a birth that I have to write about. I was nauseated and appalled by the experience. This woman's birth turned into a nightmare. She had an epidural at seven centimeters, after which 'everything' stopped. The nursing staff gave no support to Donna—come on, Donna, don't be so macho, everybody gets an epidural here. . . . The nurse-anesthetist that came in shortly after the initial dose of the epidural was administered and saw that Donna still felt the 'peak' of the contraction, said, 'Now honey, the point of the epidural is not to feel any pain,' and proceeded to give her a bolus of the epidural, after which Donna was 'paralyzed' like a bedridden sick old lady, couldn't feel her legs, her contractions, couldn't urinate, but of course promptly got the diagnosis of cpd and had a cesarean. I stormed out of the hospital, wishing never to return."

People still get spinal headaches and all the other things we said about anesthesia in *Silent Knife* still stick. In *Entering the World—The Demedicalization of Childbirth*, Michele Odent says that we live unconsciously; we use anesthesia from "the cradle to the grave."[71]

Drugs

Ivan Illich says that, increasingly, pain-killing turns people into unfeeling spectators in their own personal living experiences. He remarks that each culture "provides its own psychoactive pharmacopeia, with customs that designate the circumstances in which drugs may be taken and the accompanying ritual."[72] Childbirth educator Jane Szczepaniak reports that childbearing women have a virtual "pharmaceutical candy-counter" of drugs to choose from. In fact, women want their "sweets": "More and more women are asking for some kind of pain medication during labor."[73] Although Illich remarks that it has been rendered either incomprehensible or shocking that skill in the art of suffering may be the most effective and universally acceptable way of dealing with pain. He says that medicalization deprives any culture of the integration of any program for dealing with pain.[74]

In one article, we are told that "long before your due date, you should learn all you can about labor and delivery and the drugs that may be used. In an uncomplicated labor and vaginal delivery, the decision to medicate or not—and which type of medication to use—may be left, at least in part, to you."[75] If it is "uncomplicated," why complicate it with drugs? How about learning about labor and delivery and the things that can help you birth *naturally*? How about this is *all* your decision? The article states that when used judiciously, most obstetrical pain-relieving drugs do not adversely affect the health of the baby. But in the very next sentence we get a clear contradiction: "The babies of medicated mothers may, however, appear sluggish and drowsy for a short time after birth, as all of these drugs cross the placenta."

Dolores Krieger has developed the technique of therapeutic touch, which is based on the principle that the human body has an energy field that is responsive to healing. Those who have used her technique report less pain in labor, easier

Pregnant with Peace

I am pregnant with Peace,
  aching to give birth
    to the child of tomorrow.
My fear of labor
  gives way to the urge . . .
    an urge to push.

Part of me wishes for drugs,
  a numbing injection
    of unconsciousness
  to block the nerves
    to my feeling center . . .
Or to be able to sleep,
  and awaken with the baby
    already born.

But I know too much
  to allow myself to be drugged.
The birth of this baby is to be
  a conscious act.

Like a birthing ward, I see around me
  many pregnant beings . . .
    each of us becoming ready
    in our own way.
I pray for guidance,
  the courage to push at the right time
  the wisdom to rest
    between these contractions,
  the love to bear the pressure
    of this birth
    with the joy of knowing . . .
  not that I have no choice
    and must endure
But that I choose freely!

Dorothy Fadiman

births, and peaceful babies. Criticism about this natural healing process is, of course, still widespread; one nursing journal reported that therapeutic touch could never gain professional credibility without "clear, objective evidence to support it."[76] It is hard to document healings that include energy fields, visualization, and the like. As a result, the medical model will continue to label these methods quackery and tomfoolery. But they do work—as do crystals and gemstones and shells from the ocean and eagle feathers and herbs and songs and laughter and a variety of other "pain-killers."

I read that more than two hundred and fifty women in Chicago may have unknowingly taken a drug as part of a study to see if it could reduce fetal stress in cases of cesarean section. Only 5 of the women signed consent forms. For more information on drugs in labor, you should consult the works of Doris Haire, the founder and president of the American Foundation of Maternal and Child Care in New York.[77] I'm quite certain that Doris would disagree with a nurse who said, "After six centimeters, a woman's labor has progressed sufficiently enough so that she can take pain medication without the danger of slowing her labor." Medication taken at any point in labor affects that labor and the baby as well.

The Greek word for drug—pharmakon—does not distinguish between the power to cure and the power to kill.[78] Drugs in childbirth still cause placental malfunction, fetal distress, and jaundice, among other things. Harriet wrote, "I asked my doctor what I was being given and he told me the name of a drug. I asked what it was and all he would say is, 'It's fairly new.'" Liz said her doctor *promised* (emphasis hers) that the drug would not affect her babies (twins). *No doctor can promise that!* Brenda said that her doctor convinced her to take some demerol, and later morphine, and then wondered why her labor slowed down. Birth psychotherapist Stanislav Grof says that it is more scary for the newborn when the mother is not conscious. He says we may be programming a drug-dependent society by giving newborns a cellular memory of countering stress with drugs.[79] Susanne Arms says that when the mother is drugged, the tissue around the baby feels dead.[80]

A recent study in North Carolina showed that women who self-administered painkillers used less of it than women given the same drug by a doctor or nurse. The research says that "fetal exposure to drugs is reduced when the mother in labor takes less."[81]

The news on drugs isn't all bad. Since *Silent Knife* was written, Bendectin, a drug given to pregnant women from the 1960s through the 1980s, was taken off the market.[82] (Supposedly it prevented morning sickness, but it rarely did; instead, it had the potential to cause limb deformities, gastrointestinal birth defects, and a "possible three-fold incidence in the risk of defective heart valves" in the children of women who took it.) I was more than delighted. It was prescribed for me in my first pregnancy with the assurance that it was perfectly safe. Somewhere inside of me, I just knew it wasn't: I took two pills and threw the rest away. In an article about the Bendectin problem, Doris Haire stated that the FDA, "by its own admission, lacks an effective system for gathering and utilizing data on [a] drug's safety and that FDA officers have admitted that there is significant underreporting by physicians of adverse drug reactions.[83] Great. A front-page article in the *Boston Globe* says that the "FDA admits delay in seizing devices." On the eve of congressional hearings, "at which the FDA is expected to be accused of laxity, a top agency official has admitted that the agency was slow to seize a medical company's supply products that were implicated in the death and injury of patients."[84] The FDA was to have confiscated catheters over a year and a half earlier but apparently didn't get around to it.

The minute you take a drug, any drug, in labor, says Judy Herzfeld, "you automatically convert a low-risk pregnancy into a high-risk pregnancy."[85] Yet, when you ask questions about a drug and its effect on your labor and on the baby, you seldom get a straight answer. According to Maureen Ritchie, whatever decision is made should be based on full information, and not on whatever scraps have stuck in the ob's mind.[86] One woman wrote, "It's almost as if they can't hear you [when you ask a question]. They go on with the same sentence that they've been saying. And you say something new, and they somehow manage to evade it as if you hadn't said it. They somehow manage to sidetrack you so that you forget that you've asked it, and you only remember later."[87]

Electronic Fetal Monitor

Childbirth author Carl Jones calls electronic fetal monitors (EFM) "electronic fatal monitors" because they so often seal a woman's childbearing fate.[88] One woman in my class calls them "ground-level automatic pilots." Remember that the external monitor utilizes ultrasound, so check the information on the risks and problems associated with that, too.

Gena Corea remarks that the EFM, originally slated for only high-risk pregnancy, rapidly became routine for all labors, despite findings that half the tracings of fetal heart rate and uterine contractions cannot be interpreted, that 25 percent of the women describe fear and pain associated with the monitoring catheters (distressed mothers equals distressed babies) and that all the same problems that have been cited over and over again are still present with EFMs.[89] The *British Medical Journal* states that improved sensitivity of the ultrasound detection increases the likelihood of the maternal pulse being detected from uterine or iliac artery blood flow. "The resulting rate may be misinterpreted as the fetal heart rate, particularly if the maternal rate is raised." (Three cases were noted in which maternal heart rate tracings were mistaken for fetal tracings when the fetus was dead; two of these cases led to cesareans, which "might have been avoided if fetal death had been appreciated.") Dr. E. Hon remarks that doctors perform many more sections than are necessary because they do not understand the EFM tracings and they "panic unnecessarily."[90] It has been noted time and time again that fetal distress begins as obstetrician distress.

Emanuel Friedman, developer of the overused and grossly abused Friedman curve for labor, notes that, despite their technological promise and value in detecting fetal hypoxia, EFM and fetal scalp sampling "have only proved to be of limited use" and have "serious shortcomings."[91]

Joan said she arrived at the hospital and was asked by the nurse, "Are you planning to use the monitor?" Joan said, "No." The nurse said, "Has anyone

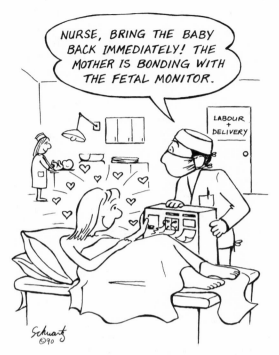

told you what you miss by not using it? Are you willing to take those risks?" Chris's doctor told her, "We always do a few hours on the machine, here. We get to see what position the baby likes so you get a better baby." Barb's doctor told her that the monitor would only be on for a few minutes. When she got to the hospital, the nurses told her that they would only put it on until the doctor got there; he was driving over shortly from his house. Barbara asked where the doctor lived, and found out that his hometown was a very long distance from the hospital. Marsha's doctor came in and ordered "a strip." Her husband thought she was supposed to get naked.

Remember the paradigm I mentioned in the section on language? Perhaps there's a new one on the horizon. In an article in the *New England Journal of Medicine*, we are told that not all pregnancies need continuous electronic fetal monitoring during labor.[92] Another article tells us that researchers have determined that electronic monitoring appears to be no better at picking up problems during the delivery of premature infants than the stethoscope and may be linked to a greater incidence of cerebral palsy.[93] An article in the *ICEA* (International Childbirth Education Association) *News* reports that, "Given the arguably questionable benefits of routine EFM, respect for women's informed choices is both legally and logically required."[94] "Internal monitors may cause infections in the newborn ranging from scalp infections in 80–95% of the cases, to scalp abscesses where the electrode is screwed into the baby's scalp in 5% of monitorings, to neonatal deaths from infections in scalp wounds."[95] Furthermore, continuous EFM is not helpful in "detecting infants who will show evidence of asphixia or hypoxia at birth."[96] A survey entitled "Fetal Heart Rate Monitoring During Labour—Too Frequent Intervention, Too Little Benefit" states that there is no justification for routine monitoring for all women during labor.

We now know that even ACOG admits that listening to the baby's heart rate is "as effective" as monitoring;[97] that there is a threefold increase in cerebral palsy in infants who are electronically monitored as compared to those whose heart rates were monitored with stethescopes; internal monitors are linked to an increase in endometritis.[98] Twenty-nine thousand (plus) women each year may undergo unnecessary cesareans as a result of electronic monitoring. (Two-thirds to three quarters of all women are monitored).[99]

I have four letters from women who were told that their babies were dead when in fact, it was a malfunctioning monitor that was the problem. One of the women, whose monitor started malfunctioning ("They thought the baby was dying, but it was the monitor that was pooping out"), said that "Everyone starts avoiding you like the plague when something is going wrong. The nurses and doctors would walk in and check the monitor without even looking at me. I knew he was alive, but they wouldn't listen to me!" Another woman sardonically said, "Well, at least with a dead baby, you don't have to worry any more about fetal distress." Another said, "I was so grateful that the baby was alive, that I didn't get angry for a long time. When I did, the — really hit the fan. I went through hell, all because of their stupid machines."

This might be a good time to mention a new "advancement" in birth technology. It is called the accelerometer. A spiral electrode is used for measuring fetal head rotation. "When the fetal head starts rotating, the output voltage increases proportionally to the amount of rotation. . . . Descent, flexion and rotation . . . can be easily measured with this element." There's one problem: maternal movements upset the device. "These possible disturbances can be detected and/or excluded by another measuring element attached to the mother. A ninety-degree combination of two or even three of these cheap measuring elements may give more detailed information about the rotation of the fetal head."[100] Only two or three? Why not an even dozen.

This might also be a good time to mention another device that is being used to control pain in labor. A transcutaneous electrical nerve stimulation (TENS) units sends electrical impulses through lead wires to electrode pads placed on the skin. These impulses are said to interrupt pain by overriding the pain messages that travel along the nerve pathways to the brain and also "stimulated the nervous system to release its own natural pain control substances in the body." (These are called endorphins; see *Silent Knife*.) We are told that results of studies in Europe show that women using TENS requested less pain medication in stage one of labor; there was no significant difference in second stage. One disadvantage of the TENS unit is that the unit causes mechanical interference of the fetal monitor—but never fear, a filter is presently being developed to eliminate this problem. In addition, the unit does not offer total analgesia, and "in most cases minimal amounts of other analgesics are required."[101]

One of the so-called advantages of the TENS unit is that the patient (sick person) is in charge of the unit and decides the amount and length of stimulation received. How about the amount of support and hugs she receives, instead?! This, the article says, gives the woman a feeling of control. Over what? A machine? I don't know. I know that a few women have found the TENS unit to be helpful. To me, it's just more paraphernalia. An extra support person would be better to me than ten TENS units, or even eleven.

There is also growing concern over the safety of video display terminals, which shouldn't surprise you, I'm sure. Dr. Louis Slesin, publisher of the VDT News (a bimonthly consumer report), says that "If these were chemicals, they'd be regulated pretty fast." Aside from headaches and eyestrain, other serious problems are associated with their use. He cited studies where the incidence of miscarriage was greater among VDT users. Another study done in Sweden documents that the weak pulsed magnetic fields emitted by VDTs harm the development of mouse embryos and increase fetal death among pregnant mice.[102]

Episiotomy

A New York obstetrician remarks that an episiotomy is simply an incision made to prevent tearing and that without it, the pelvic floor could fall out in later years.[103] I thought we debunked that one a long time ago. Another women's magazine tells us that whether you have had a cesarean section or an episiotomy, "You can expect sex to be as good as ever."[104] We all know that both a cesarean and a birth with an episiotomy can affect a woman's sex life for a very long time. In another magazine, a woman tells us that, although an episiotomy is painful, the pain of the operation (it *is* a surgical procedure) and the tenderness while healing were outweighed by a sensitive doctor who "gave me a choice."[105] Women do not "choose" to have their vaginas cut. They are given erroneous information that makes them believe that it is the best alternative. Nowhere in any of these articles is it mentioned that women's bodies were designed to birth and that many, many women (the ones at home births mostly) become mothers with an intact perineum. In other parts of the world, women *never* have them and they fare far better than we in the long run. Nancy S.'s doctor told her that if he didn't give her an episiotomy, her bottom was going to explode. Doctors who do episiotomies have no regard for the female body and no understanding of how to assist at a birth without mutilating the mother. Episiotomy has nothing to do with the adequacy of the perineum—only with that of the care provider. *Providing care* does not include cutting our genitals.

The National Center for Health Studies says that 60 percent of women have episiotomies. Far more than that are cut; the missing 40 percent are out there *getting sectioned!*[106] One article states that "review of the literature on episiotomy indicates the likelihood that it is overused."[107] From the CENMASAC News-letter, we read:

> "Come on now, Mrs. Smith. Hold your breath and push down as hard as you can. Hey, close your mouth. No noise now. That only wastes the energy you can use for pushing. Come on and get three good hard pushes out of each contraction. No! No! You're not doing it right. Close your mouth and hold your breath. Come on. It burns, you say? Well, keep pushing and push right past the burn. Well, Mrs. Smith, you've been pushing real hard but your bottom looks like it won't stretch enough, we'll just snip it a little bit. Whoops!" The onlooker sees the baby fly out and the new mother is left with an episiotomy extended into the rectum.[108]

Lidocaine, the local anesthetic given before the cut is made, may be hazardous to the newborn. Within one minute of injection it appears in large amounts in a woman's bloodstream, quickly passes through the placenta, and is detected in the urine of mothers and babies for at least forty-eight hours.[109] An article in the *British Medical Journal*[110] questions the current practice of carrying out episiotomies routinely in first-time "patients." The article says that the question of long-term prolapse "must await further study."

Ellie told her doctor that she didn't want an episiotomy. "He got insulted! He said, 'Well, there's nothing for me to do around here then. You handle it on your own,' and he walked out! In other words, if he couldn't cut me, he wanted nothing to do with me!"

Pam said her doctor was in a rush. He started stitching her before the novocaine had taken effect. The pain! He told her husband to just kiss her neck and whisper sweet nothings in her ear.

Here's one for you. I got a letter from a woman who had an episiotomy AFTER her baby was born. Her baby was born soon after she had arrived at a teaching hospital in New York; there was no doctor in the room at the time. The resident who came into the room told her he had to do one or his superior would be furious.

What still amazes me after all these years is the mentality of most women regarding episiotomies. One woman wrote that she did have a small episiotomy, "but only what was necessary; not a great big 'man's cut.' " Tears are usually surface and do not extend through muscle as episiotomies do. I can only begin to imagine what men would say if we constantly told them that their penises weren't big enough to get out the sperm. As we said in *Silent Knife*, they'd all be halfway across the world before they'd allow us to take just a teensy, tiny little "snip" in order to enlarge the opening.

There is hope for us. The paradigm is changing. Increasingly, episiotomy is being called "the unkindest cut"[111] (along with circumcision, and court-ordered cesarean sections). If we call routine episiotomy "crotch slicing," perhaps it will stop sooner.

Forceps

In the early 1600s, the Chamberlen brothers became England's most famous obstetricians. They were not even physicians, but members of the barber-surgeons guild: "surgery was a natural extension of the barber's art, for both occupations required skill in using sharp instruments." Behind the brothers' success, we are told, lay a secret invention: forceps. We learn that the Chamberlens went to great lengths to guard their invention. When they were called to help in a difficult situation, they arrived in a special carriage carrying a huge box. Others assumed that the secret was a huge machine. Only the brothers were allowed to attend the birth, and even the laboring woman was blindfolded! Several generations later, another Chamberlen allowed the secret to slip out, and "obstetrical forceps came into general use. Subsequently, the forceps were misused, enlisted in even normal births."[112]

"The child is seized by two steel tongs. His head is pulled forward at a force equal to forty pounds of tension on his neck. The slightest slip or too much pressure can leave his head permanently damaged."[113] And this is how so many of the babies in our culture are born! "There is no place for forceps in normal delivery," says Gregory White, M.D., president of the American College of Home Obstetricians.[114] Forceps delivery was based on the outmoded idea that the baby's head pounded on the perineum like it was made of concrete, he says; the perineum is, of course, soft and pliable. One doctor said, "Forceps are best taught in an uncomplicated delivery."

Babies still get brain damaged and die from the use of forceps. They often hemorrhage internally. Susan wrote that her son went into severe fetal distress just as the forceps were being used. An emergency cesarean was performed, her baby was resuscitated three times, suffered multiple seizures, and almost died." Hers is the only one in a series of letters I have received about forceps damage. If there is room to get the forceps in, there is room for the baby to come out, without forceps. Michele Odent says forceps have yet to be designed that are safe in any hands. "Women whose babies are extracted by forceps never forget it [he's right about that] . . . they should never be used—they belong in museums."[115] Forceps turn births into "vaginal cesareans."

IVs

They are still as unnecessary and dangerous as they were when *Silent Knife* was written. The whole rhythm of birth is "open, down, and out." IVs are just one more of the things that go on at birth in this culture that go completely against that energy. IVs are up and in.

Fairly soon after a woman arrives at the hospital, IVs are put into her veins. Everyone wants to be ready, "just in case." Life itself is pretty unpredictable: why not just stick an IV in everyone's arm and let them all go through life "prepared" for whatever dangers might come their way. We can all walk around with IVs on poles, ready to meet life head on.

Eileen wrote that "This is a teaching hospital, so all of the routine 'prep' stuff is done here by the residents on duty. One doctor wanted to start an IV on me, and I told him quite firmly there was to be none. He started explaining how it might be difficult to find a vein later in case of an emergency, but we read that chapter, buddy, and thanks is essentially what we said. So he quietly slipped away. The second doctor, however, was more insistent, but we held our own." Mara wrote that her birth was a "crashing medical success—and a horror for me. For example, during the epidural, they banished my husband, but even after the procedure they wouldn't let him back in. When I got upset, they ran a tranquilizer through the IV without telling me!! I realized a few minutes later what was going on, and I got even more upset—they simply upped the dosage! Although I was 'conscious,' I have virtually no recollection of her birth."

IVs cause a laboring woman's body to become exhausted. In normal labors all over the world, when a woman is hungry or thirsty, she has something to eat or drink. Her body begins to work; it digests what she has eaten and then it "rests." Later, when she is hungry or thirsty again, this process begins again— work, rest, work, rest. When an IV is inserted, and fluid is being drained into the woman's body every single minute, the body has no rest. The placenta has to work hard, too. Everything is taxed.

Professor-Doctor P. E. Treffers notes that a woman fatigued by hunger and thirst will be exhausted earlier, "with concomitant complications in labor."[116] IVs are not "food" and they do not nourish a laboring woman. They increase risk of infection, reduce mobility, and are associated with poor muscle tone and color in the newborn. Michalene Bratton, LSP, remarks that the hairier the arms, the more tape everyone uses to hold the IV in place.

Heparin ("Keep Her In") Locks

Many people see heparin, an anticoagulant, as a compromise. One compromise almost always leads to another at birth. If you are with people who insist upon a lock, you are with people who do not see birth as a normal process. They believe that something may go wrong; otherwise they wouldn't even be thinking "lock."

I wouldn't be surprised if heparin were associated at some point with placental abruption—a very serious circumstance—and with maternal hemorrhage. (After the baby is born, the placenta separates from the uterine wall and delivers.) There are many blood vessels at the point of attachment, and these must begin to coagulate or the mother will hemorrhage. If an anticoagulant is in the mother's system, clotting may be delayed or impossible. Certainly, they tell you that the heparin only stays near the needle in your arm. But they also told us that X-rays were safe and that fetal monitors were accurate, too.

An advertisement from a manufacturer of heparin mentions that it is *not known* (emphasis mine) whether the drug can cause fetal harm when administered to a pregnant woman or can affect reproduction capacity. Although it says that it does not cross the placental "barrier" (the placenta is *not* a barrier), it also recommends that it be given to a pregnant woman only "if clearly needed," and that hemorrhage is "the chief complaint that may result from heparin 'therapy.' "[117] It says: "Heparin should be used with extreme caution in disease states in which there is an increased danger of hemorrhage." Many women who have had heparin locks end up with cesarean sections, for any one of a dozen reasons. Major surgery certainly puts them in a state of dis-ease and at risk for hemorrhage. Mark my words, in years to come, we will hear that, although research had assumed that heparin did not cross the placenta, new findings indicate. . . .

Inquacktion of Labor

"Nice veins," said the nurse. "You would have made a lovely junkie. Now we're going to start the pitocin."[118]

"My doctor tried to induce labor three times," said Rona. "My water broke during an exam to check for any dilation" [Rona! It didn't "break" just like that! *He broke it!!*]

Jan wrote: My doctor told me my baby had to be born because it had IUGR [intrauterine growth retardation—talk to Dr. Tom Brewer about that, everyone. He's the expert! See the section on nutrition.] He said it was 'time' for the baby to be on its own—that I was, in effect, killing it if I kept it inside. He said my placenta wasn't functioning any more. Well, I was induced, it didn't take, I had a c-section, and my placenta was fine. My baby was only six pounds, but then, she was still three weeks early by my calculations."

Betty said: "I live on an island. A week before my due date, the doctor roughly dilated my cervix and told me to go over to the mainland hospital. A storm may come on the island, he said, and I wouldn't want to be stranded there. At the hospital my mucous plug [we call that baby gel, now, remember?] fell out and I thought that meant I would have the baby immediately [the gel fell out, not on its own, but because of what the doctor had done to your cervix. Vaginal exams can also affect the baby gel. It probably wouldn't have come out on its own just then. Even when it does come out on its own, it does not necessarily mean that labor is imminent. It can be weeks before labor begins. It just means that the hormones are beginning to change and things are going according to the natural process.] The doctor said that if I went into labor and delivered by the next afternoon, fine, otherwise he'd give me a c-section. They put me on a monitor and told me that if your pelvis was too small, your poor baby would be subject to a harsh labor, banging against my bones and could die of a cerebral hemorrhage if not delivered 'safely' by c-section. Nothing happened, so I had to have surgery. The operation was a shock! All my illusions were shattered, it was the worst experience of my life. . . . Not until I got home six days later, did I realize that the weather had been beautiful the entire time."

Valerie wrote: "My labor began six weeks early. After five hours, it stopped! I was only three centimeters dilated, but they wouldn't let me go home because "infection was sure to set in." My doctor routinely induces all laboring mothers with pitocin to help their contractions. My cervix was high and out of reach, so I quickly became quite bruised from the repeated exams. . . . I am certain that I would not have had my baby within a short time—shouldn't the location of my cervix have told them something? [YES!!] Thirty-nine drugged hours later and an episiotomy the size of Wyoming, all 5 lbs. 1 oz. of my son was born— with typical hyaline membrane problems as well as a heart murmur."

Valerie went on to say that with her next child, "The doctor wanted to do some tests to get a better idea of the due date. I went to the hospital for the 'tests.' I started having contractions and called a nurse. She placed her hands on her hips and declared, 'Of course you are! You are in here being induced, dummy!' If I had been smart, I would have removed the IV and left the hospital. But I was enough of a dummy to go through the doctor's evil-minded scheme. Twelve hours later, no progress was made, so he created an emergency c-section. My pediatrician said the baby was almost two weeks early and the problems our son had could have been avoided."

Oxytocin, which is used to induce labor, is associated with all kinds of problems, including uterine rupture. I've heard from several first-time moms who ended up with a uterine rupture and a hysterectomy as a result of "pit."

In *Childbirth Wisdom*, we are told that in the days before our cycles were confused by city lighting and indoor electricity, women, menstruation, and ovulation coincided with the moon cycles, and our bodies followed an established pattern. "The full moon is still the busiest time in modern obstetrical wards, yet many Western women are threatened with having their births induced if the baby has not come when the doctor predicted it would. . . . In many cases, a span of ten complete moon cycles from the mother's last period seems to more predictably indicate the time of birth."[119] Elaine, an LSP from Alabama, recommends that if your doctor is average, which means moderately anxious, add one week to ten days to your last menstrual cycle. If he is very anxious, "add two to three weeks!"

Jane is forty-one years old, and expecting her first baby any day now. In fact, her "due date" was eight days ago. When she went to see her doctor three days ago, he said her blood pressure was too high for his liking, and he wanted to do an ultrasound "to see if everything was okay" and then induce her. He's nervous—it took Jane eight years to become pregnant; this is a "premium baby." She's already had one ultrasound and decided that was enough. She went home, meditated, and talked to the baby. The next day her blood pressure was down. We all know that women who are well nourished often carry more than forty weeks and that our blood pressure often rises on our way to the doctor's office. Another woman wrote, "My due date came—and went. My obstetrician changed from a 'don't worry about it' flippant fellow to a very worried father figure. According to my calendar, I wasn't 'late'—according to his, I was—and we all know which calendar he wanted to go by."

Induced labors invariably end up in hot water—or on operating tables. It is the lucky woman who is induced and is able to deliver vaginally—and the rare woman who is then able to deliver naturally. The amount of dilation means nothing. One woman was six centimeters dilated and did not go into labor for three weeks. Another was two centimeters dilated—and had her baby twenty-five minutes later.

One way that doctors induce labor is by breaking your water (a no-no in almost all situations—it can even turn the baby into a posterior presentation). However, if your water breaks on its own, it breaks. Perhaps it will reseal. If you have Sharon's doctor, you'll immediately be whisked to the hospital. If you have Diane's doctor, you'll stay at home and wait for labor to begin, since, "as fate would have it, his wife also had premature rupture of the membranes and managed to stay four whole weeks before delivering healthy twins vaginally!" The male medical model labels it premature; it is not premature, it is on time in its own time. Again, vaginal exams are associated with PROM and should not be performed if your water breaks, so take heed. Numerous articles note that vaginals should not be performed in the third trimester unless a specific reason for examining the cervix exists. Rarely are there specific reasons. Pelvic exams are not a very good indicator of when labor will occur, which is the reason usually given to do them.[120] Moreover, they increase the risk of infection and may have an adverse affect on labor.

I've been told that one Miami hospital has a 55 percent rate of inductions. Lest we pick mercilessly on one place, please remember that most hospitals have high rates of induced labors. The truth of the matter is that every labor that is not natural—including cesarean sections—is an induced labor. The baby comes out not on his or her own time, but by someone else's timepiece. Nowadays, it's fashionable to induce with prostaglandins. Remember, there are prostaglandins in semen. Maybe you can "induce yourself"—*naturally*.

Meconium

Still mostly iatrogenic, meconium is secondary to fetal distress (and what baby in our country isn't stressed thinkin' about vacuum extractions and the rest?). It depends on how much meconium there is, when it was passed, how thick it is, and a variety of other factors. As we said in *Silent Knife*, some babies are "knee deep," and none the worse for wear.

Placenta and Cord

I thought I had held up pretty well when the doctor, who up to then had behaved like a perfectly rational person, said, "Would you like to see the placenta?" Now let's face it: Nobody would like to see a placenta. If anything, it would be a form of punishment.

Jury: We find the defendant guilty. . . .

Judge: I sentence [him] to look at three placentas.

—Dave Barry[121]

Pulling on the umbilical cord is practiced almost nowhere in the tribal world.[122] Many midwives from other areas of the world are known to have "patience without limit . . . and this has prevented many distasters. It is known that few deliveries will end unhappily if one has the patience to wait."[123]

The kind of tool used in traditional societies to cut the cord—a knife whittled out of plant stalk, usually bamboo—was superior to those used today. It prevented bleeding, and it negated the need to tie or seal off the end. Goldsmith says that Casablanca may have the wisest attitude of all: a cord that no one touches falls off in three days, while one that is carefully dressed takes four times as long. She notes that colostrum and mother's milk aid the healing because of their antibacterial qualities.[124]

Waiting to clamp the cord has many advantages. As early as 1893, some sound advice was given as to the care of the cord.

> Sever the cord when pulsation has entirely ceased in it. Use a dull pair of scissors, cutting about two inches from the child's navel. Following these directions, no tying is essential. This method has its advantages. By tying, a small amount of fetal blood is retained in vessels peculiar to fetal life. This blood, by pressure of irritation, may prevent perfect closure of the foramen ovale and can be a cause of hemorrhage. Besides, it must be absorbed into the system, causing jaundice, so common in young babies. Prejudices exist against adopting this treatment, as it is contrary to that which is usually adopted. I tested it and proved to my own satisfaction that it is the best method. One has only to recollect to wait until the pulsation in the cord cases entirely, then sever as before stated. [When in doubt, Shay states, wait. The last place to feel a pulse will be right up next to the baby.][125]

In the article, Shay goes on to say that the logic of this seemed quite obvious to her. "I live in a very rural area and each spring many new lambs, calves, and other baby critters are born without . . . someone on hand to tie a string around the umbilical cord. In fact, many books caution against clamping the newborn animal's cord in any way. . . . One comment that I have heard from various professionals . . . is, "Well, you've never seen the horror of an umbilical hemorrhage." Yet this complication that they spoke of with such dread must have occurred in newborns with clamped cords. Perhaps the clamping of the cord contributed to this problem, since it obviously did not prevent it."[126]

In several other cultures, women stand up immediately after the birth and walk. This helps deliver the placenta. Soon after, they often bathe in streams and lakes, even when it is cold. In one culture, women have intercourse immediately after the delivery. It is thought to be of value in aiding the internal organs to return to their pre-pregnancy state.[127] In many cultures, women rest in an upright position for several days and avoid a reclining position. If you leave the cord and placenta attached until they fall off on their own, this is called a Lotus birth.

All species of mammals practice placentophagy; the eating of the placenta. One British midwife researched this practice after suffering severe depression following the birth of her first child. She learned that eating the placenta could protect her from hormone imbalance that is associated with postnatal depression. "My theory was that if I ate this tissue, female hormones, which are types of steroids, would be absorbed and make the blood level drop more gradually." She tried it raw, "as steroids are destroyed by temperatures over 100 C." She reported some remarkable physiological effects. Her hair was silky and shiny instead of dry and brittle following the first birth. Postnatal euphoria set in: she felt so strong, as if she could do anything! She ate the placenta gradually over the next five days and it was an instant antidepressant. Her lochia (blood flow) lasted only ten days, as opposed to the five weeks following her first birth. The midwife who ate her placenta said that she felt she had to be secretive about what she was doing because "the practice verges on cannibalism."[128]

One woman wrote to me, "I held the placenta in my hands. It was big and dense and rubbery and wet. This was my third child and the first time I had even seen a placenta! I felt a little like an animal—I wanted to look at it closely, to smell it, to put it near my face. It was a very primal experience. If I had been in the hospital, I wouldn't have been able to get in touch with those deep basic reactions. My other two placentas were dumped into a steel basin and sent to a pathologist. I asked what they did to them after they were checked and the nurse said, 'chucked.' "

Ultrasound

There's some mighty good information in *Silent Knife* on ultrasound. Here's my update.

A woman from Texas writes, "When I questioned the practice of repeated, routine ultrasound scans, an indignant nurse said, 'All our ladies have ultrasound!' They had a machine in the doctor's office, and it was the doctor's pride and joy. He operated the scanner like a new toy and his practice had a special 'Scan Day' once a month when all that was done was ultrasound scans on all the ladies 'needing' it."

According to an article, "available data on the biological effects of ultrasound do not permit unequivocal statements regarding its safety. On the one hand, there is no doubt that ultrasound at certain intensities can be destructive. . . .

There are no definitive, replicated studies. . . . Many of the studies show defects in their experimental design. . . . Consequently, an undetected hazard may still exist despite negative studies."[129] The article says that there is good evidence that synergistic effects with other procedures may cause problems: "the biological damage caused by X-rays . . . is enhanced or reduced depending on the level of ultrasound and the sequence of application (i.e. before or after exposure to radiation." Another study reports that "When considering possible links between ultrasound and childhood cancers or developmental defects, risk levels cannot be assessed until a large adequately designed, randomized controlled trial with sufficient follow-up is conducted."[130]

Doris Haire is a veritable encyclopedia on the subject of ultrasound. She says that it is "essential that the National Institutes of Health and the FDA not permit pregnant women to be misled by obstetricians (or midwives) into assuming that ultrasound is without risk for the mother and child."[131] We know that exposure has been associated with hearing loss and dyslexia and may have an effect on maternal red blood cells. It may retard cell growth and interfere with maturation. Doris says that it is "frivolously overused! Even if twenty percent were high risk (and they are not), that still leaves millions who are getting it that don't need it!"

Exposure to ultrasound causes the amniotic fluid to bubble: The risk of acoustic cavitation "would be small, unless something as sensitive as an embryo is involved," and at that point, the effects would be "difficult to detect."[132] All the mothers undergoing ultrasound have "embryos" in them!!!

Laurence Crum has commented on the abuse of ultrasound: "People who use ultrasound are not careful enough, especially in regulating the intensity and the duration of exposures. There is potential here for causing severe damage that you probably wouldn't see immediately. It is incredible how unrestricted the use of ultrasound is."[133] Just like X-rays, it'll take them twenty or thirty years to find out—and by that time, the damage will have been done. Senator Kennedy (D.–Mass.) has said that "the time to find out is before millions of children have been exposed. Otherwise, we are playing an unjustifiable game of Russian roulette with the health of our children." He's right, of course, but it may already be too late. The wheel has already been turning for some time now. The saddest thing for me was learning that Maria on "Sesame Street" had told all the viewers about her ultrasound[134] and the picture she had of the baby inside of her. We aren't supposed to have photographs of our unborn; the pictures in our heads and our hearts should suffice.

Vacuum Extractors

This new gift to American women leaves bruises on the fetal scalp (and like forceps increases the incidence of jaundice) which "may be distressing to the parents if their transient nature is not explained." It may cause interventricular hemorrhage—bleeding of the brain.[135] It hasn't been around long enough, and so there haven't been enough studies. You know the story by now.

Talk about copout. A study done to determine whether vacuum extractors were better than forceps concluded that their trial was of insufficient size to rule out major adverse effects on the neonate of one instrument or the other. "Another larger trial is required to address this still open question more rigorously."[136] Any volunteers?

One article said that "these newest little patients exhibit the bruises and swelled head of a prizefighter after doctors employ the ominously named 'vacuum extractor' to deliver them. 'You're boxer-babies,' the pediatricians coo to these newborns."[137]

Why not vacuum extractors? After all, they cut them out of us and pull them out of us so why not suck them out of us, too? One of the momDads in my class said, "The next thing on ACOG's list of things to do to get a baby out (if vacuum extractions don't seem to do the trick) is: Blast the thing out with a keg of dynamite."

Vaginal Exams: "Let the Fingers Do the Talkin' "

Vaginal exams are absolutely unnecessary at most births (as are doctors). The rarity of puerperal fever in tribal cultures following birth is due to the fact that it was considered "abhorrent" to insert hands into a woman's vagina at this time.[138]

One of the "pioneers of gynecological surgery," J. Marion Sims, who is honored by a statue in Central Park—I hope there are lots of pigeons there this afternoon—practiced his technique of vaginal exams and suturing by using slave women given to him because they could no longer work or produce children.[139]

One doctor recommends that "mothers stop having intercourse after the eighth month of pregnancy."[140] (He didn't say anything about fathers.) He says that the cervix begins to open and that bacteria could enter the uterus. If this is so, then why does he do vaginal exams beginning in the ninth month?

Many nurses do additional vaginal exams as the labor progresses so that they will know when to call the doctor. No one who is opening to birth her baby should have to endure someone's hands up their bottom. Why we allow this is beyond me. If we allowed our womanplace to be really alive, we would know in a moment that this was a violation of our limits and boundaries. Most of us would just say no.

One of the momDads in my class said that he got a pain in his gut every time someone went to do a vaginal exam on his wife. Since he was at a teaching hospital, he had one major stomachache the whole time. At one point, three residents came in to check his wife. "If I had wanted a gang rape and a sloshing for her, I could have driven her to a nearby [rough part of town] and just let her out of the car."

Born (Stress) Free

In spite of surface appearances to the contrary, normal delivery is not harmful: "It is actually important to undergo the events eliciting the production of stress hormones." In fact, labor prepares the infant to survive outside the womb. It clears the lungs, regulates heat, nourishes cells, and ensures that there is a rich blood supply to the heart and brain (preventing asphyxia), among other vital functions.[141] Vaginally delivered infants produce a far higher level of these stress hormones, called catecholamines.

The fetus is better able to withstand asphyxia than an adult. A catecholemine surge in the fetus serves as a highly effective protection system. The advent of fetal monitoring made it possible to detect subtle changes in the fetal heart rate during uterine contractions. When complex changes were found, "the infant was often judged to be suffering from life-threatening asphyxia and was delivered surgically. Upon delivery, however, more than fifty percent of the infants were found to have few clinical signs of asphyxia."[142]

Concerned that many cesareans might be unnecessary, Lagercrantz and Slotkin decided to find out whether a normal catecholamine release in response to labor could account for the complex heartbeats in the fetus. "We found that catecholamine surges elicited by the normal birth process can indeed cause alterations in heart rate that might well be misinterpreted as signs of fetal distress . . . unless the monitoring is supplemented by biochemical tests."[143] Only when the pH level in the blood from the fetal scalp falls below 7.25 did the heart rate actually indicate a problem. The normal birth process, they say, gives rise to a surprisingly large increase in catecholamines in the human infant. Even early in labor, when a mother's cervix is barely dilated, catecholamine concentrations are extremely high.

This "stress hormone surge" not only protects the infant during delivery, but also enhances the newborn's ability to function effectively by facilitating normal breathing. It is well known that infants delivered by cesarean section are predisposed to breathing difficulties, especially when there has been little or no labor prior to the operation: no labor, fewer catecholamines. Fewer catecholamines, less respiration. Less respiration, more problems. Some researchers have advocated administering catecholamines to surgically delivered infants. These have proven neither safe nor effective. Others simply recommend a cesarean not be performed at all or, whenever possible, delaying surgery until the mother has at least gone into labor. Labor is not a cosmic scheme to harm babies; it is a beneficial experience that *alives* them.

Baby Interventions

Hopefully, the days of picking babies up by the feet, spanking them on the bottom, and tossing them around is behind us. But we are still a long way from giving infants the love and honor they deserve from the very beginning.

In other cultures, babies are born and introduced to the sun, to the gods, and to the community. There are naming ceremonies, and cord/placenta burials, feasts and welcomings—all within hours of the arrival. In our country, we are still measuring, weighing, and needling our little ones—right through the first week of his or her life. You can read about all the interventions to baby in *Silent Knife*.

Judith Goldsmith remarks that the alien environment of a hospital exposes the newborn baby to many contaminants it would not have encountered at home. Those institutions that still insist on wiping off the vernix remove its protective grease from the baby's skin permitting germs to settle on the skin, grow and cause infections.[144] She also says that other cultures are much more careful about the sensitivity of the newborn's eyes to light. (Some cultures, for example, fashioned "umbrella hats" out of leaves)[145]: our newborns are observed under bright lights in nurseries. As to their ability to observe their new world—after they've had all that unnecessary goop put into their eyes, how can they? Babies in other cultures are kept with the mother and not "put upon a shelf" [the bassinet].[146] One hospital issues a form that says, "Because of neonatal problems, which can develop right at the time of delivery—or soon thereafter—the first person to get the baby will be the pediatrician; and it is not until he feels comfortable that everything is going OK with the baby that parental bonding should begin."

The process for testing for PKU requires stabbing a baby's heel with a sharp, pointed lancet. . . . "Sometimes repeated stabs to the heel are necessary to obtain the quantity of blood needed."[147] (Ya, first they insist upon Vitamin K so the blood will coagulate, and then they have to keep squeezing to get out the blood they want for the PKU test. Talk about conflict of interest here. . . .) Williams remarks that her work required that she draw blood samples, and leave the nursery . . . full of crying babies. This experience caused her to seek an alternative solution to the "bloodletting" for her own child.

Barbara reminds us that the optimum time for performing the test for PKU is uncertain. Generally, it is done when the baby is discharged from the hospital, usually on the third day of life. However, since many babies leave the hospital before this time, there is no uniformity in testing. Some hospitals send parents home with a PKU packet: the parents are asked to dip a specially treated stick in the baby's urine. We are told that ketones in the urine may cause a false positive test and that brain damage may have already occurred by the time phenyalanine appears in the urine (four to six weeks).

Several risk factors can help determine the statistical chances for PKU. In Barbara's state, she was able to waive the test. She recommends that if you believe the test is necessary, you might be better off to take the baby to a laboratory, and to hold and nurse the baby while they do the prick. She also reminds us that it is best to postpone any Vitamin K shot after birth—if you think the vitamin is "necessary"—until after the PKU test is done. In my own case with our homebirth baby, a visiting nurse came to our home. I nursed Andrea as her heel was being pricked. She hadn't had any Vitamin K, of course, and her blood was coagulating very nicely—so well, in fact, that the nurse could not get enough blood. She went to stab Andrea again and I said, "NO!" She said she would come back again another day, and I told her not to bother.

For Crying out Loud, Leave the Kid Alone!: Circumcision

Circumcision is a crime. It is a crime against life. . . . It is a crime inflicted on innocent male babies by parents and medical professionals too hardened to see what they are doing. It is a needless and mindless act of violence that must be stopped if we are to raise boys and men more able to affirm life.[148] Thank goodness Blue Cross coverage has changed: Circumcision is no longer covered as part of the birth package. "You want your son's skin removed, you pay for the dubious privilege."[149]

I have an advertisement for a "Circumstraint." It is a small padded table designed for newborn baby boys. The "new improved design" features "better exposure" and is "ideal" for circumcisions. The velcro straps encircle the infant's elbows and knees, "depriving him of leverage. He is held safely and securely without danger of escape. Its comfortable . . . shape positions the infant, hips elevated, perfectly presenting the genitalia. . . . It is cost effective. It permits a nurse to quickly immobilize an infant . . . speeding procedures and saving valuable time for doctors."[150] At first, I honestly thought this ad was a spoof, but it's for real. We are surely a barbaric lot.

Anyone who has any question about whether or not to circumcise their son, consider whether you might do a clitorectomy on your little girl. Before you make a decision, read Ann Brigg's wonderful book on circumcision. Rosemary Romberg and Ed Wallerstein also have books on the subject.[151] I have been getting more and more letters from couples—including Jewish couples—who are making the decision not to circumcise. My own womanplace would never allow another child of mine to be circumcised: How can I teach nonviolence at birth and the perfection of our bodies, and then let babies get cut instead of women?

Bev writes: "I wrote to you a few years ago. At the time, the only voices of understanding for my anger, disappointment, and self-doubt were the writers of radical stuff. My families' attitudes were to be glad for a healthy baby. I am writing now to tell you that I had a home VBAC! We experienced the joy and the power—and for me, the tremendous boost in self-esteem and feeling grown-up and womanly. Between the cesarean and the VBAC, I had a miscarriage, a sad happening for a much wanted second baby. However, even then, I could feel pride in having it at home. And afterward, although devastated, I found the strength to refuse a vaginal exam, medications, and a D&C that the on-call doctor who examined the 'remains' recommended, and we had a simple burial at home. So we felt entirely comfortable with an attitude of being responsible for ourselves. It is such a growing and strong feeling, far different than when I went off to the hospital the first time and put everything in other people's hands. It has helped me to not circumcise this baby boy—unheard of in our Jewish families. We did a blessing ceremony on the day he would have been cut. He smiled through it all—and so did I. We don't make decisions just to be different. Now we think and talk about things we used to just conform to."

Hi Tech?—No!—Goodbye, Tech!

When the doctor has pulled out "all of his stops"—the monitors and the catheters and the IV and the pitocin, etc. and he's done all his little deeds— hooked you up, stuck it in, broken your water, etc.—and things still aren't "progressing," he generally says, "Well, we have done everything that we can. There is nothing left to do [except a c-section]." What he really ought to be admitting is this: "There is nothing else in my repertoire—nothing that I am aware of—that can assist you." His knowledge is *limited*! Chances are, he's never even had a baby before! There is a vast array of "other things" that can be done, including unhooking everything and letting labor progress on its own. We all know the best thing to do even in most "high-risk" situations is to trust the process and *not* intervene.

Michel Odent writes, "I used to ask the midwives, for example, 'Why did you break the membranes?' or 'Why did you cut the cord that way?' They always answered, 'It's what we learned at school'. . . . So together we tried to have another view of obstetrics. . . . To control is always to disturb. To control is always to interfere . . . I tell doctors, you should study less, study less and feel more."[152]

Daniel Grossman reports that Americans generally give an exuberant "Why not!" when they are invited to try something new. "Yet in the face of ever-more sophisticated technologies—with greater potential for disrupting our lives." The newly emerging neo-Luddite movement does not rigidly oppose all technologies, but believes that we should carefully consider which of them actually improve our lives instead of "passively accepting each scientific 'breakthrough,' " no matter what the cost.[153] The deeply passionate attachment our society has to technological advance is not entirely rational. "Rooted in colorful dreams, myths, and fantasies, expressed in recurring rituals that contain enormous spiritual energy" for those invested, the nation's commitment to and involvement with technology is, "among other things, clearly a matter of religious zeal."[154] Neo-Luddites believe that there are unwanted social consequences that accompany the technology that far outweigh any benefits. Shirley Luthman says that in the evolution of the race, the United States' contribution has been in the development of technology. "We have carried that development to the point of our own destruction. In order to prevent that destruction we are now forced back

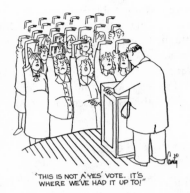

"THIS IS NOT A 'YES' VOTE. IT'S
WHERE WE'VE HAD IT UP TO!"

into the exploration and development of ourselves so that technology does not control or threaten us, but can be balanced with a sense of oneness with each other."[155]

Commentary: Common Territory?

There is a signature of wisdom and power impressed upon the works of God which distinguishes them from the feeble imitations of man.

—John Newton

Like a chain reaction, one intervention leads to another. If you allow your water to be broken (I call it "robbing the cradle"), then you increase your risk of infection—and so they'll want to get the baby out quicker and they'll speed up your labor. This causes fetal distress so you'll end up with a c-section. Or since your body isn't really ready to have to the baby—it is only tricked into thinking it is—your hormones won't be the way they would be if you let things unfold on their own, and so your perineum won't stretch as far as it is capable and you'll most undoubtedly have an episiotomy. If you are given an epidural, you will require forceps and an episiotomy. If you take drugs—which you'll probably need if you're on pit—your labor may slow down (so they'll give you more pit so you'll need more drugs). Your placenta will be compromised, and the baby will go into distress. If you are on a monitor and you are lying on your back, the baby will go into distress. External monitors aren't accurate anyway, so they'll rob your cradle and insert an internal monitor which causes distress and so on and on and on.

Most women do not feel calm or "safe" after they have been attached to all the interventions. Barb said, "I felt like at any minute, one of the machines was going to clang, jump, boogie, and gong: YOU'VE HIT THE JACKPOT! and I'd get a new car, a new washing machine, and an all-expenses paid trip to the Poconos right along with a new baby." Liza said, "I felt like a dog on a leash." And Anita said, "I was hooked up to everything in sight. I looked like the first monkey that was going to be sent up into space. I felt like they might as well just put me on 'automatic pilot' and leave the room. They could direct this whole thing from 'central control.' I should have known I was headed for an automatic—cesarean."

THIS IS IT FOLKS: YOU EITHER BELIEVE IN THE PROCESS OF BIRTH OR YOU DON'T. WHAT'S IT GOING TO BE? ANYTHING THAT YOU DO TO YOUR BODY DURING LABOR WILL AFFECT IT AND ADVERSELY AFFECT THE OUTCOME. We now have two generations of women's bodies who were either confused or blackmailed into thinking that they didn't know the blueprints! When each of those bodies became pregnant, it said, "I know what to do! I know how to birth this baby growing inside of me!"—But then someone decided that it didn't know how, and that there was a better way. What arrogance to believe that we can improve on, or change, the gift of bringing forth life.

Did I say that strong enough? It's hard for me to even do labor support in a hospital any more. All those interventions, just waiting for the "right" pregnant body; all those IVs just waiting for a vein; all those gloves, eager for a check; all those monitors, waiting for a fetal scalp. I walk into even the nicer ones and my heart says, "No, this isn't how it is supposed to be." This isn't where woman's sacred act of creation is supposed to take place. Outside perhaps. Near a lake or a pine grove or a mountain or the ocean. In your home, your friend's home, your grandmother's home; in an apartment, in a cottage, a cabin, a tree-house. With your partner, your children, your friends, your mother, or your best aunt. I do not see this as a romantic vision of birth: I know as well as anyone that the hours and minutes preceding a baby's entrance onto this planet are a time of reverence and awe. But to surround oneself with scared, dictatorial, uniformed, physically and/or psychologically vagina-less automatons in a steel and concrete medical/surgical warehouse makes absolutely no sense to me whatsoever anymore. Yet, women who birth in hospitals need the support so much!

Sonia Johnson says that the belief that one must have fear to have good judgment is wrong. Fear undermines our judgment. It prevents us from thinking clearly. It is the "supereminent weapon of men to keep women in their place."[156]

On Wings of Birds

Test Tube Women states, "Here is man's control of the awesome power of women; the last stronghold of [her] Nature which he can fully dominate."[157] In *Childbirth Wisdom* we are told that it is very rare to have problems at birth: the problems that do arise do so as a result of simple (and not so simple) mistreatment of the mother—not from "failures" within the bodily process itself.[158] There are few "faults" with the process of birth, but there are thousands of flies in the obstetrical ointment. This salve is spread all over the birthing women of North America; it oozes down to Mexico and seeps into South America. It becomes a flammable elixir and spreads like wildfire. It grabs on to gusts of wind, sticks to the wings of birds, drops on distant shores and begins to cover us all, smother us all, one IV, one monitor, one trickle of pit at a time.

I once heard it said that in the United States birth is "obstetrical self-defense: kung fu for the pregnant." And the battle is still raging. What are our options? To wait in the trenches (i.e., at home?) until we are attacked; to arm ourselves with ammunition (information, research articles)?; to catch them by surprise (arrive at the hospital fully dilated and ready to push—so why bother going in at all?); or to defend ourselves (by writing books, giving speeches)? Do we really want/need to fight? Do we need to struggle with this problem for the next umpteen years just to win a victory (such as, say, the "right" to birth without an IV)? We do not need to fight. We just need to do. One woman after the other doing her birth. Not being delivered by, or having someone "do" her birth for her, just doing what her body knew how to do from the moment it agreed to conception.

Almost every woman who walks into a hospital today is faced with acquiescing to hospital policies—or suffering the contempt and fear that accompanies her refusal to "comply." Women get any number of excuses why they ask (rather than demand or simply decide) to birth naturally: We've never done it that way; we're not ready for that yet; we're doing all right this way (or without it); we tried it once and it didn't work out; it costs too much; that's not our responsibility.[159]

In a presentation called "Being Born" we read, "Everything matters! Absolutely everything matters! . . . Every single thing matters, you know, the light in the room, the warmth, the blankets that may be around the mother, how cold she is, how warm she is, what people are saying. To really understand that everything matters . . . and to be aware of that. Yet tension can enter when we get too over careful. So we have to have a certain relaxation within ourselves, all of us."[160]

A certain relaxation . . . all of us. A belief in birth. We don't want fancy gadgets and machines! We do not need expensive birthing chairs that tilt up and back and sideways and spin around in midair—that look like a cross between Darth Vader's control room and Queen Victoria's throne. We do not want to be poked, prodded, pitted, placated, pummeled, or psychoanalyzed. We don't want to listen to scare tactics or old OB tales from the land of testosterone. We just want to have our babies. We must have our babies. We will have our babies. The world NEEDS for us to have our babies. We will not fight you or blame you or debate you. We will simply birth.

According to Harriet Goldhor Lerner, we are responsible for our own behavior, but we are not responsible for other people's reactions, nor are they responsible for ours. She says that guilt and self-blame are a "woman's problem" of epidemic proportion and that fighting (as in labor rooms) is a way to maintain the status quo. A colleague of hers tells the story of pausing on a ski slope to admire the view only to be knocked down by a careless skier who apparently didn't notice her. "I'm sorry!" she yelled out after him from her prone position as he whizzed on by."[161] It is not our responsibility to deal with the rage or the upset that our reclaiming our births causes the obstetrical world: it is theirs. We can empathize, sympathize, care, and offer our understanding—as human beings to each other—but it is not our problem to finally resolve.

Our Bodies Our Selves states that violence against women is any violation of a woman's personhood, mental or physical integrity or freedom of movement, and includes all the ways our society objectifies and oppresses them. "Violence against us occurs on a massive scale, no woman is immune,"—and the vast majority of individuals and public institutions are insensitive to it.[162] Mary Daly says that the mutilation that has become an accepted part of birth in the United States is no worse than the mutilation of women's bodies in Africa (or Chinese footbinding; see Chapter 7). But since it appears more "scientific," we allow it. Judith Herzfeld remarks that the physicians' motto of *primum non nocere* (above all, do no harm) has come to mean that it is acceptable to do anything at all that has not been demonstrated to be clearly harmful.[163] Medical intervention into birth is a vulgarity; in the United States birth is an act of violence that defies human understanding. I recently learned about a number of babies who were stolen from a hospital nursery in our country; baby abductors, posing in white coats as lab technicians, kidnapped the infants. That we live in a society where people could do this is almost incomprehensible and unbearably depressing. Our obstetrical system is one big semisolid mass of baby abductors; those who recover our infants do so one pure birth at a time.

When people are connected to their intuitive process and their aliveness, they do not need to control someone else. They can open themselves to whatever experience occurs and feel that experience to the fullest.[164] Instead of fearing birth (which arises from our fear of death), we could be supporting life. In this culture, however, we seem unwilling to merely observe and enjoy birth; we must control it. "We see 'progress' not in terms of our ability to work with the natural process, but in our power to 'improve' it, surmount it, or even eliminate it." Instead of being genuinely glad that a woman had a purebirth—instead of seeing that as one more affirmation of a process that works—most obstetricians feel that the woman was "lucky" this time. The fear is that when women discover their own personal power, and relearn that they can have their babies without doctors and interventions, then who will need/want an obstetrician? So they continue to make us believe that they are vitally important, and we continue to believe them. It's one of those co-dependent relationships everyone is talking about. It's time for us to tell our OBs, "Don't call us, we'll call you—if we need you." It's time to say "Get outta my face," (or wherever). It's time to realize that most intervention at birth is about as necessary or as beneficial as dog hair in an omelet.

Courage, we are told, comes from the heart, "and since the heart is where courage is generated and since what we need from these men is courage—we have to touch their hearts."[165] One of the men who allowed the women in his practice to teach him and open his heart (he's one of the reformed OBs who gets a "Tootsie Award"; see Chapter 8) writes "Are you keeping up with all the comments in the current literature regarding mandatory intervention on unwilling mothers? Appalling! Perhaps there is a place somewhere in all of this for "gentle coercion"—in the rare case of the woman whose baby is truly in jeopardy. But I am afraid we are in for a treacherous time from the standpoint of patients' rights. Can you imagine 'home monitors' that are required for rental [during pregnancy] or mandatory hospitalization for all third-trimester lovemaking? In my own case, my conservative colleagues would rather prove me incompetent rather than say they do not share my approach. If I ever accused them of not supporting natural childbirth, the criticism I would have to endure would be unbearable. Not one of them even knows what a real natural childbirth is like. How dearly I would love to help them know."

Hands Across the Sea

We have a distorted picture of non-Western childbirth: most eyewitness information concerns rare, difficult cases during which a Western doctor is called in as a last resort. Most births occur without much warning, a private affair, restricted to family and friends. "Pregnancy flowed easily into the act of childbirth, childbirth proceeds directly into the recovery time, recovery meshes neatly into the nursing period. . . . A pregnant woman becomes a mother easily and gradually."[166]

Sadly, our devious and destructive birthing practices are becoming popular in many other countries which look to us as exemplars of the way things should be. They emulate us. God help us all! As I see it, together with all our sisters in the world, we have a responsibility to preserve the natural process of birth. Unless we begin to say no, the cesarean epidemic will continue to sweep across both the Atlantic and Pacific and soon all the women of the world will show their great esteem for us by having identical scars on their bellies.

We all know by now that the emulation notwithstanding, American women are far more likely to undergo radical mastectomies, deliver their babies by cesarean, and undergo routine hysterectomies than anyone else in the world. "Americans would best be served by learning lessons from those abroad, among them: to rely less on radical surgery, prescribe lower doses of drugs, and put more faith in the ability of the body to heal."[167] Are we drawn, like magnets, to the knife? Have we given enough blood? Our foreign sisters are beginning to "donate" theirs as well.

The rate of cesareans is increasing in the west generally. Our Canadian sisters are being cut like crazy, as are women in England. Nina (Israel) writes: "There is only one hospital—one!—in the entire southern half of the country. Options are severely limited here and many women are sectioned. There is a love affair with things American." In New Zealand, an appalling article says that childbirth is no longer for women and their babies, but a "commercial venture for doctors on their own terms and at their own convenience."[168] In some South American countries, women choose to be sectioned. They regard this type of delivery as a sign of upward mobility. Nothing could be further from the truth.

We must relearn birth from the women that can still teach us. We must make certain that our negative influence is quickly nipped in the bud. As other countries become "civilized," we can only guess what will happen to their birthing practices. One country full of "obstetrical cripples' is enough.

Judith Goldstein states: "Unless foreign influences slow down, or change their emphasis, easy birth may become a thing of the past. . . . It is incredible that American women stand for [the] treatment [that they do], but to foist it on women whose traditional practices have for so long prevented many of the problems of Western childbirth is truly absurd."[169] "Although customs vary from one culture to another, there are certain constants: the maintenance of active life right until the moment of birth, the use of massage before, during and after birth, instant recovery (1/4 hour!), and prolonged breastfeeding—these are universal customs all over the world in cultures quite different from one another."[170] "It is time to take a fresh look at what the ancient world of traditional cultures may have to teach us. By ignoring traditional practices and denying them a place in our body of knowledge, we cut ourselves off from the rest of the world."[171] Hopefully, none of us is so ethno/egocentric as to believe that the American way is the only way, or that when it comes to birth, we are the 'best' at it. If we lose connection with the women who know how to give birth, we will lose our lives.

7 My Aching Feet

A group of childbirth educators, labor assistants and midwives in Ohio go out to a local restaurant for a light meal after each of their monthly meetings. While they are eating, they discuss (what else?) birth. The waitresses at the restaurant affectionately call this group "the vagina people."

Who are "vagina people"? Are they always viewed with respect and affection? And who are the doctors without vaginas, the ones whom I refer to less than affectionately on occasion as the "creeps"? I knew that I would have to begin to have some understanding of the two sexes in order to understand the birth problem in this country. I'd like to share with you some of what I have learned thus far. (As we might expect, we will be talking about women much more in the chapter on birth.)

Andrea Szmyt and Herb Pearce teach workshops together on male/female relationships,[1] and have emphasized the following basic similarities between the two genders: we all want to be loved; we all want to be valued and to be secure; we all want to be accepted and respected. They point out the importance of remembering the fact that we are both similar and different. In order to heal ourselves with members of the opposite sex, we need to heal relationships with members of our own sex. (In so doing, we forgive and heal the separation within us to our own femaleness or maleness as well.) We must remember, too, that the healing of male/female differences is a basic and profound principle for the healing of the planet at large. Communication, admiration, and appreciation between the sexes is not only possible but vital: for we share the earth. We must be willing to become true companions, for our mutual home may not be able to survive the abuse of our bickerings. No longer is there any room for karmic or cosmic sibling rivalry.

The *I Ching* (the Chinese Tao Book of Wisdom) tells us that there are two principles: the masculine and the feminine.[2] When they are in harmony, growth, energy, and spirit are possible; when they are in discord, chaos and destruction are the result. When the two are balanced, the earth revolves perfectly on its axis. When they are not, the planet tips ever so slightly; this change is imperceptible to humankind and immeasurable by our technology—but the earth knows, it "feels" it. It has been suggested that the earth's response to imbalance is manifested in part on a physical level—volcanos or earthquakes, for example.

Ilya Prigogine, a Belgian chemist, won a Nobel Prize many years ago for his theory that everything alive is *surprisingly* (his emphasis) alive and on a searching, upward journey. Such living systems, he said, periodically break into "severe twitchiness" and appear to fall apart. In fact, it is at such vibrating times that living systems—humans, whole societies—are shaking themselves to a higher ground. Transition to a higher order, Prigogine says, is universally accompanied by turbulence, and the disorder and harmony are a *necessary* (his emphasis) activation of growth to a higher level. The apparent upset is the way that things are "jiggled" into higher levels of development. The greater the turbulence, the greater the jump into a higher place.[3]

"Hi, Mom"

Our earth is a living planet, a female planet: "She" needs the right amount of "the feminine" in order to live and to grow, and in order to nourish—all of us. For a number of reasons, not the least of which is the massive problems with childbirth in this country—and in the world at large—there is a tremendous absence of the female in the atmosphere right now.[4] We are told that women always have the capacity to bring the light of consciousness to life and to others: men depend largely on women for light. The "touch of light" that we bring to the world is often very bright. It may "sting a man into awareness,"[5] which is one reason why he may fear the feminine so greatly.

(Pale) Pink

The lack of female energy on the planet has a number of consequences. Neuropsychologist James Prescott contends that the greatest threat to world peace, for example, comes from those nations whose children are most deprived and whose women are most repressed. Prescott observes that societies that provide their infants with a great deal of physical affection—touching, holding, carrying—are less physically violent than societies that give very little. When such countries acquire the technology for modern warfare, we are in trouble.[6]

When female sexuality is repressed, birth is affected. In our culture, women aren't simply "repressed" at birth: they are knocked out. Drugs and anesthesia are the norm here, reducing/eliminating the pleasurable sensations of human touch at that time. Babies, drugged themselves, are quickly wrapped in blankets and sent for footprinting, weighing and measuring—and then to nurseries for a number of hours each day. We allow babies to cry themselves to sleep, prop bottles, and fill up day care centers, teaching "distrust at a very basic emotional level, and also establishing patterns of neglect which harm the child's social and emotional health."[7] Modern hospitals, Prescott says, start us on the road to other harmful child-rearing practices.

Prescott interprets rape as man's revenge against woman for the early loss of physical affection: "A man can express hostility toward his mother for not giving him enough physical attention by sexually violating another woman," he says.[8] Whether or not this is one truism in a complex issue is a matter of conjecture; what is true is that hundreds of women over the years have described their cesarean sections and vaginal deliveries as well as terrifying moments of rape and violation. Dr. Lewis West, a psychiatrist from UCLA, remarks that violence toward children, including cruelty, neglect, and other stresses, has a direct correlation with violent behavior by those same children when they grow up.

Rape is any kind of sexual act committed against a woman's will.[9] Whether the rapist uses force or threats of force is irrelevant; rape is always traumatic. Surgically removing the "products" of sexual union and/or surgically incising women's genitals most certainly constitute a form of rape.
According to one account,

> It may be impossible for women to ever understand why men rape. When one looks at such a phenomena [sic] as rape, it is hard not to see the two sexes as very separate species. One wonders, too, whether some men are angry in the depths of their souls over women's access to the creative process of life and birth. . . . We do not know yet what desires or fantasies underlie the crime of rape, but it probably has to do with a masculine rage and alienation that goes very far beyond [the immediate past] . . . The rapist may be suffering from great metaphysical loneliness. . . . From the woman's point of view . . . it is a terrible desecration and denial. . . . of her holy potential to give birth . . . [which is] a spiritual and mystical peak.[10]

Phyllis Chesler remarks that women are blamed for anything that "goes wrong" in the universe. For example, she says, "A male rapist's mother is blamed by driving her son to rape by having been too cold. His wife is blamed for being . . . frigid. The victim is blamed for provoking . . . [the man's act of violence] seems a self-defense maneuver against the [guilty] female." Chesler maintains that we are in a woman-hating culture. Women are feared, hated, enslaved, overprotected, and impoverished instead of genuinely respected and supported.[11]

Savages? (Who are Those Masked Men, Anyway?)

Evolution argues that the male's body as well as his mind developed in response to the demands of the hunt. For the kill, he needed to tame his own fear of killing. Male aggression, we are told, became a matter of survival, and most scientists think that some form of aggression is built into the male system. "Put a group of males together, and once some dominant order is established, the group will either split into competing coalition units or seek some exterior object for collective 'masterful' action."[12] Dorothy Dinnerstein says that without a solid grounding in compassion (the light!) men will always find it easier to ignore or abuse the feelings of others and to dehumanize their victims. "And all too often their victims are women."[13] I would have said it myself. One medical student, writing a thesis on violence, states that "it is believed that a woman's moral superiority [is] needed to curb men's most brutal instincts."[14]

Chesler remarks that men are not socialized from birth to serve in psychologically nurturant ways, (although, of course, most men find ways to channel their "brutal instincts" into socially "acceptable" modes of behavior). They find ways to keep women "at bay": they adopt brusque, authoritarian styles.[15] Others agree. Kate Millet says that men's hostility is expressed in a number of ways. One is laughter, "which declines into ridicule and satire." Aggression is reinforced in his behavior, she says, and "[they] even vulgarly celebrate it: 'That guy has balls!'—as if being gutsy was related to the male gender."[16] Indeed, one woman who wrote to me said that her OB had told her that in order to get through labor "you had to have balls."

Back to the earth, for a minute. According to Mark Gerzon, Western settlers considered the red man's reverence for the land impractical and heretical. The Indians were shocked at the white man's lack of respect for the earth. They watched in horror as the land was exploited, destroyed, and mutilated. "We still do not treat her reverently, but contemptuously. We rape her." Gerzon says that we must replace man's desire to dominate with a willingness to learn humility, respect, and nurturance. Unfortunately, however, those qualities are not considered "politically sexy." They sound timid, ineffectual, and "cannot be described in terms of conquest."[17] As hunters (and then warriors defending the land in which they hunted—and then as soldiers), men had to embody strength and repress feelings of vulnerability. To embody courage, they had to repress fear. To show toughness, they had to repress sensitivity.[18]

In order to be prepared for war, other traits are sacrificed.[19] Tenderness, gentleness, openness, and softness become liabilities, not assets. What the soldier fears above all is cowardice: losing his reputation "as a man among men." Many of the supportive doctors who initially backed homebirth and who later reneged perhaps felt the strong clasp of their "comrades" and the admonition that accompanies it: to be supportive, sensitive, and understanding of women was a no-no. A doctor friend of mine said that the first time he had to cut someone open, his biggest concern was not letting his peers see how unnerved he was. After a while, picking up a knife became routine. Years later, when he decided that he was doing too many cesarean sections, he said that his concern was the same—alienation from his peers for being "too sensitive" to women. "Once, when I 'put the knife down' so to speak, and decided to hold-off rather than to do a section at that moment, I was told [by other staff members] that I was insane. In fact, it was the most sane moment of my life."

Tenderness, camaraderie, and affection—all emotions that are normally taboo between men are permitted and even respected on the battlefield. "Facing the foe, men could hug, exchange keepsakes, even cry. If one's comrade perishes, one could cradle him in one's arms, kiss his face, and admit to deeper feelings (love?) that in peacetime were forbidden. In uniform, men felt secure in their masculinity. They would permit themselves to become conscious of feelings that were otherwise too threatening.[20] Obstetricians and anesthesiologists are all in uniform; hospital maternity units often resemble M*A*S*H units, don't they?

Men raised by authoritative fathers look for the opportunity both to submit to the powerful and to retaliate against the powerless. (Birthing women are *not* powerless, but they often act that way, and are certainly viewed that way for the most part.) "These men are likely to describe all relationships as hierarchical; it is difficult for them to imagine an egalitarian relationship."[21] (Imagine going for your first prenatal and asking your doctor to tell you about his dad.) Some Germans claimed that they joined the Nazi movement innocently: "We were looking for a place where we could get together with other boys in exciting activities . . . We weren't fully conscious of what we were doing. . . . We felt important." Gerzon remarks that they weren't fully conscious, and "we cannot afford to pay the price of unconsciousness again."[22] Gerzon also remarks that the door-closing that goes on (for a cesarean section or an emergency birth, for example) is part of the hierarchy that arises among men ("I'm the one who is in charge here!") as well as a "convenient coverup" that protects men from exposing uncomfortable (i.e., feminine) feelings in each other's presence.[23]

Some psychologists state that, in order to cut a human body open, the surgeon must distance him or herself emotionally from the experience. To do so is to go unconscious. Surgeons are generally "not in their bodies," for to be there would cause great pain. But it's hard to talk to someone who isn't "there." "It would make doctors sick to see their cutting, so they devise an efficient and orderly bureaucratic system"[24] that supports the act. Since only one cesarean can be done at a time, no one has to take responsibility for the thousands done each week. Gerzon remarks that if the doctor is to cut, "I want him to perceive the [situation] accurately—to recognize it for what it is," not through a half-dazed brain, or "as a test of his manhood."[25]

Are Ewe in Wolf's Clothing?

The "good" obstetrician should have the so-called "feminine qualities: patience, restraint, gentleness."[26] Doctors today are in a quandary: they are supposed to be respected by women, but the women they see are becoming increasingly hostile. The manliness that women once revered because it protected them is now increasingly condemned because it endangers them. [27] Purebirthing women are indeed an endangered species. The "sharp-tongues" that women are so often accused of possessing are no match for the utensils men utilize.

The book *Growing Up Free* presents a chart of adjectives to describe behavior. [28] If a person is forceful, for example, a male is called charismatic, whereas a woman with this quality is considered domineering. If a man is efficient, he's competent, but the efficient woman is compulsive. Men are inquisitive; women are "nosy." Assertive becomes "pushy." Many men are unfamiliar with contempt or scorn; they are rewarded for ambition and drive. They are never referred to as "scatterbrained" (they are "absent-minded") or "gabby" (talkative or articulate). But note that studies show that female physicians spend more time with their patients and interrupt them less. Patients of female doctors seem to receive clearer explanations than patients of male doctors. [29]

The attempt to brand women as intellectually inferior is also not new. An "expert" can use his mind to pursue power. Whoever "knows" has more knowl-edge—power: data become a weapon, a political tool. "Unable to bear a child himself, the Expert achieved the next best thing: power over those who could. Master of the Womb." [30] Gerzon states that what is also striking is how the Expert appoints himself the supreme authority on raising children. He doesn't do the child care; he studies child development.

> Unlike the true seeker of knowledge, the Expert is often more concerned with protecting his power than with establishing the truth. When others disagree, he tends to dismiss them as emotional or irrational. He will say that they do not have the facts or that they are biased. His attitude is condescending. He considers himself indispensable. [31]

"Men are always supposed to have an answer—never supposed to say in wide-eyed amazement, 'Wow, I never thought of that!' or 'I'm really confused about this,' " says Gerzon. To do so was to admit ignorance and uncertainty: to appear vulnerable. A man was to appear well-informed, "even when he was not." If something touched him, his eyes might moisten, but he was not allowed to weep. He was never to admit to being depressed. [32]

No one speaks with more authority about the ramifications of women's "weak and delicate" bodies than American doctors. Gerzon says that the more they learn about the unique anatomical features and its hidden hollows, the more power they attribute to themselves. According to a learned professor addressing an American medical society in the late 1800s, it seemed that "the Almighty," in creating the female, had taken a uterus and built up women around it. [33] To cure women of their ailments—from backaches to nervous exhaustion—physi-cians would "probe the sexual interior." Dr. J. Marion Sims, whose disciples called him the father of gynecology, admitted he "hated . . . investigating the organs of the female pelvis." However, by knowing the intricate workings of the female body, perhaps one could control those workings as well. [34]

The field of obstetrics is no place for what psychologists call "exaggerated masculinity." If a woman looks pretty, she is taken seriously—that is, she's regarded as a sex object. If not, she is dismissed as unfeminine and therefore not of great value. There is a great deal of literature on woman as maternal being or sexual being—not both. These writings can be traced in part to religious teachings such as the Immaculate Conception. If men cling to their adolescent fantasies of women as sex objects, they will not want to see "with our own eyes that the vagina is not only our erotic playground but also a child's birth canal." By "witnessing the woman who inspired our passion become a mother, we may integrate more harmoniously our maternal and sexual images of women."[35]

Typically in our culture doctors have been viewed as gods. This attitude is changing, but His (the doctor's) word is still the word of . . . (as the saying goes). We worship "God," and since doctors are often regarded as all-powerful and all-knowing, our worship often extends to them as well.

Anne

Author Anne Wilson Schaef tells us that our white male society (WMS) controls every aspect of our culture. According to Schaef, few white men do not fit into the WMS. One myth propagated by the WMS is that it is the only thing that exists in the world; other systems, especially the female system (FS) are "sick, bad, crazy, stupid, ugly, and incompetent. Any difference of opinion is to be discounted or destroyed."[36]

Other myths about the WMS include the belief that it is innately superior; it knows and understands everything; and it is possible to be totally logical, rational, and objective. Members of the WMS spend a lot of time and energy telling women that females are by nature not logical, rational or objective: "Often they do so in highly emotional ways." In the WMS, there is always an underdog. One has to be either this way or that—superior or inferior. The WMS uses power to control, condemn, and stereotype.[37]

In the WMS, religion is the scientific method. The WMS concludes that it is possible to control the universe. Most other systems attempt to comprehend the universe so that people can live in it; the WMS wants to run it, not just live in it. The WMS believes that mastery over the universe is possible through better technology and better measurement techniques: if we can measure, we can predict; if we can predict, we can control; if we can control, we can be God. Many women instinctively distrust the "findings" of the WMS researcher— "and for good cause. They are simply data which have been interpreted to suit the bias of the WMS . . . and then used to reinforce WMS stereotypist myths." Feelings are immeasurable, so they have no validity in this system. There is no place for "soft research"—data gathering by observation, experience, and listening.[38] In the Female System (FS), Schaef says, it is possible to be different and still be all right. There can be two or more answers to the same question and all can be right, no one has to be wrong.[39] Part of the misuse of the scientific method is that it involves unquestioning faith in the validity of numbers. We become convinced that numbers are essential and are real. We can certainly begin to see how important understanding of Ms. Schaef's proposals are to birthing women.

To atone for the "original sin of being born female," that is, *inferior* by WMS standards, women become good and fair and follow the rules. We learn that our intelligence must never threaten men and that our competence must never overshadow that of men. Schaef says that we do not like or trust each other. In fact, as women living in a foreign reality, we frequently distrust our own perceptions. This makes us hesitant to express them, and when we do, and they are different from the way men see things, we are dismissed and ridiculed.[40]

Women know very little about female sexuality "because men have always been the ones to define it. . . . We let men tell us how we are supposed to feel, behave and respond. We let them dictate how we should experience our innermost selves." Never is this so apparent as in the obstetrician's or gynecologist's office and in the hospital at the time of birth. If men were left on their own, the planet would probably be blown apart. "If men cannot even take care of themselves—how can we trust them to take care of us?"

Men who stand up for themselves are considered competent and assertive. Women who stand up for themselves are considered obnoxious and aggressive. Schaef discusses the "fragile male ego" and control. "Who touches who first is the one in control." Think about it—who touches who first in the OB's office? At the hospital for birth? ("Let's just do a 'check,' Mrs. Morrison. Let's see how dilated you are.") She says that women are suppressed and angry and that we live in a culture that suppresses female anger.[41]

Seeing Red

In *The Dance of Anger,* Harriet Goldhor Lerner notes that anger is a signal that our needs aren't being adequately met, that our rights are being violated, or that something inside of us is being compromised. "Unlike male heroes who fight and even die for their beliefs, women are often condemned for waging a bloodless and humane revolution for their own rights." The direct expression of anger, especially at men, makes us "unladylike, unfeminine, unmaternal, and irrational. We become witches, bitches, hags, castrators." It is interesting, Lerner notes, that our language has not one unflattering term to describe men who vent anger at women. "Even 'bastard' and 'son of a bitch' do not condemn the man but place the blame on a woman—his mother!"[42] Phyllis Chesler says that we are accused of "uppity" behavior when we exercise our freedom of thought or speech.[43]

According to Lerner, when we are depressed, guilty, and self-doubting, we stay in place. We do not take action except against ourselves, and we are unlikely to be agents of personal and social change. In contrast, angry women may change and challenge the lives of us all. "And change is an anxiety-arousing and difficult business for everyone." We silence ourselves, she says, by questioning the anger: Do I have a right to be angry? What good will it do. The valuable questions instead are: What am I really angry about? How can I learn to express it clearly? (". . . for if not clearly voiced we may elicit disapproval instead of sympathy which increases our sense of bitterness and injustice—all the while the actual issues go unidentified . . . Nothing blocks the awareness of anger so effectively as guilt and self doubt.") What do I want to accomplish, change? What is the real issue here? It is amazing, Lerner says, how often we march into battle without knowing what the war is about.

Lerner says that when we fly off the handle, we are "written off." The other person becomes calmer and cooler and more intellectual as we become more infuriated and hysterical. "Whether we are nice or bitchy—the outcome is the same—we are left feeling helpless and powerless. Our dignity and self-esteem suffer. And nothing changes. We betray the self." Fear surfaces: we are afraid of transforming the anger into concise, direct statements lest we evoke that disturbing sense of separateness and aloneness that we experience when we take a stand. We are afraid if we take a bottom line stand ["I'm sorry, but I will not go to the hospital"; "No, absolutely no fetal monitor!"] we risk losing a relationship: "More often, and more crucially, separation anxiety has its roots in early family experience." We turn our anger into tears, Lerner says, which shifts defensiveness to concern and restores a sense of connectedness. We are told that women feel accumulated rage in direct proportion to the degree of submission. [44] The rules and roles of society make it especially difficult for women to handle negative reactions from others. We must have a clear sense of "I" in order to do this.

> We must separate ourselves from others' wishes and expectations in order to clarify our own values, evaluate our own choices and priorities, and make decisions regarding what we will and will not do. . . . Anger signals a problem but provides us with no answer. It tells us we need to slow down and think—yet anger can make clear thinking difficult. Our task is to achieve a lower degree of emotional reactivity and greater degree of self clarity. Using our anger effectively requires a clear "I"—and women have been blocked from selfhood at every turn. We must also observe and change . . . the patterns that keep us stuck. [45]

Back to the . . . WMS

In the WMS, time is perceived as numbers on the clock. Men believe that the numbers on the clock are real and that time itself is nothing more than what those numbers measure: 5 minutes = 5 minutes; 1 hour = 1 hour; 1 week = 1 week. One who accepts this, Schaef says, believes that it is possible to be early, late, or on time and that these concepts have real meaning. In the FS, however, time is perceived as a process, a series of passages, or a series of interlocking cycles that may or may not have anything to do with the numbers on the clock. The clock is frequently irrelevant and may even be seen as interfering with the process of time. Early, late, and on time are concepts that have no real meaning.[46] By the WMS, I am late with this book. By the FS, this book is being created *in its own time*. Obstetricians are scientists and it is difficult to claim our right to feeling in numerical terms. "Numbers can't really tell us about the depth and passion of an experience."[47]

In the WMS, the center of the universe is the self and work; in the FS, the center of the world is relationships. In the WMS, there is only so much power available. In the FS, power is viewed as love: it is limitless and when shared it regenerates and expands. There is no need to hoard it because it only increases when it is given away. In the WMS, power means to exert dominance and control others; in the FS, power is *personal* power, which has nothing to do with control over another. In the WMS, rules exist to control others and limit freedom; they eventually become sacred, taking precedence over the individual. In the FS, rules are developed to increase individual freedom. If a rule doesn't make sense, then it is changed. Rules never take precedence over people.[48]

Men think linearly. They go from point A to point B. Female thinking is "multivariant—it makes use of more data, such as feelings, intuitive, and process awareness." Men think with their heads—rational; and women through their solar plexus—intuitive. "When questioned about their processing, women can often do no more than throw up their hands and say, 'I just feel it,' or 'It feels right.' And men will respond, 'What do *feelings* have to do with *thinking?*' " [emphasis in the original].[49] In the WMS, logic is a tool one uses to win; in the FS, logic is a clearly balanced progression in which both grace and power are possible. In the WMS, negotiation is seen as manipulation and winning; in the FS, negotiation stimulates creativity and imagination and is used to facilitate solutions for everyone concerned. Women, Schaef says, are seen as poor negotiators. In the WMS, responsibility involves accountability and blame; in the FS, it means the ability to respond. A responsible person is one who does something when it needs to be done, and blame never enters in.[50]

As we have noted earlier, in the WMS, concern with the environment means controlling it; in the FS, it means conserving it and saving the planet—living in harmony with the cycles, processes, and seasons of the earth.

Schaef remarks that one of the major strongholds of the WMS is the AMA, which should come as no surprise to us. "Its myths and assumptions are almost identical to those of the WMS, and the difficulty many doctors have in differentiating between themselves and God is apparent."[51]

Chinese Feet

Chinese footbinding. Now what in the world could Chinese footbinding have to do with birth? Footbinding is a vivid symbol of the subjection of women.[52]

The practice began as a restraining measure. Men feared that women might easily "leave their quarters and therefore binding the feet made it painful and inconvenient for women to get about."[53] However, footbinding was, in fact, a sexual act: When the footbound woman walked, the lower body was in a state of tension, causing the skin and flesh of her legs as well as her vagina to be tighter. Rich men preferred bound-foot concubines because "they gave the same sensation of tightness in intercourse as a virgin."[54] Eventually, the custom spread. The injuring of a woman's physical being was regarded as beautiful.[55]

In order to get up to walk, the bound woman had to hold onto the bed and cling to a wall for support (sound familiar, anyone?). The woman was described as being forced to sleep only on her back (we can identify, can we not?), with her feet dangling over the side of the bed. The sensation was said to be like . . . [being] . . . punctured with needles. Footbinding caused gangrene; many women died of blood poisoning. Women described the pain as incomparable and unendurable. It was not denounced as evil until it crippled half the population, added to the misery of the poverty stricken, increased infanticide, preventing women from supporting themselves and from caring adequately for their children, "and confined women and her thoughts to the narrowest of spheres." Many Chinese women echoed the sentiments in *From Tiny Foot Lady*: "The agony of my feet penetrated the marrow of my bones and I am plunged into despair. The toes in my feet are broken and my heart breaks with them."[56]

Footbinding lasted for over a thousand years. Then it disappeared in a period of about twenty years or less, less than one generation, Levy states. How many years will it take for BIRTH to be normal again? I cried through much of Levy's book. There were letters and poems written by foot-bound women that touched me deeply. And someone out there will surely tell us that there is no correlation here with cesarean section and that it isn't the same thing at all, that our bodies heal, after all, and that we can get on with our lives just the same.

Sonia

In Sonia Johnson's book, she says that she suddenly realized that women were "deeply into male worship, a condition that tends to afflict even the strongest woman . . . [If this continues] and if there ceases to be a woman's movement, there will cease to be life on the planet."[57] Before you decide how you feel (not think) about that, please let me tell you more about Sonia's book and about her definition of the "woman's movement."

Nonhierarchy, she says, is the very nature of feminism. We exclude ourselves when we act like men in the woman's movement. "Our old methods of working for social change were never more than illusory accesses to power encouraged by the men in power to take up our time, and to confuse and distract us. To go out of our minds is to be truly sane: 'I trust in my own heart and in my growing ability to hear my own voice and to obey it.' "[58]

Feminism, she says, is about the rising spirit of half the human race. "Sprung, from the dark, airless little box called patriarchy . . . my possibilities were suddenly as the sunshine and the wind."[59] One of the most powerful taboos in our world for women has been the one against disobeying men. We have believed the message, "If you go against the men, you will surely die. . . . We *blossom* [emphasis mine] as we break the taboo . . . We must be free not just from the terror of breaking taboos, but from the garden-variety fear of social disapproval as well."[60] She says that she longed for a mass sloughing-off of old, dry nervous, cautious skin—in a mountaintop ritual, maybe, somewhere among the sunbaked rocks.[61]

More than anything else, Sonia says, women's organizations crave respect from the men in power. They want to appear objective and rational, and they long to be seated among them, making public policy. If apartheid applied only to black women, she says, no one would be paying the slightest public attention to it. It would be seen as a cultural matter only. However, there is a violation of men's human rights as well. She says that we get busy doing things and think we are actively achieving something, getting somewhere: "There's a grim complacency in that."

Sonia says that most woman's groups don't demonstrate sufficient seriousness; they don't demand courage, and they don't inspire courage: "We must step over the line and discover undreamed reservoirs of love and daring. . . . [or will there be] another season of silence?" We simply have to stop being afraid, she says, afraid of losing respect, afraid of losing credibility, and afraid of losing our lives. "I love life. I don't want to die and I don't want other women to die either. But if we want to move on to another place we must stop worrying about the possibility of death. . . . Fundraising, letter writing, lobbying, and demonstrating just isn't enough. Justice is never bestowed, it is demanded—now, if necessary at the peril of our lives."[62]

We are socialized to obey the law—to obey men—Sonia says. When we do, we live. But only when we stop obeying men do we truly begin to live. . . .

> We have such immense sources of untapped strength, bravery and daring—we are capable of anything!—and that's the truth as well as the necessity. Help us begin not to be so afraid—of our own burgeoning powers, of not being polite and nice—of not following the eminently "reasonable" leaders of organizations, of hurting the men in our lives, of speaking the truth more boldly. As we become less afraid we become more dangerous. Patriarchy can only exist so long as women are afraid.[63]

When we identify with ourselves in opposition to something, we become its unwitting accomplices. Sonia says that what we resist persists—we bestow our energy on it: we reinforce it as reality. In the very act of trying to wrest power from patriarchy, we strengthen it instead. By focusing our attention on obstetricians' attacks on us, for example, we collude in our own defeat. "But, if instead of focusing on the attacks, we redirect our intent and energy toward our own goals—think of where we are going instead of how to get free—there is a far

abstracted by Belita H. Cowan

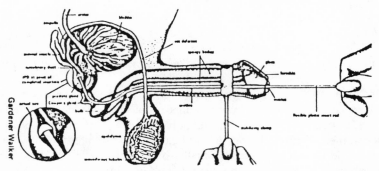

Gardener Walker

New Device Tested

The newest development in male contraception was unveiled recently at the American Women's Surgical Symposium held at the Ann Arbor Medical Center. Dr. Sophia Merkin, of the Merkin Clinic, announced the preliminary findings of a study conducted on 763 unsuspecting male grad students at a large midwest university. In her report, Dr. Merkin stated that the new contraceptive— the IPD—was a breakthrough in male contraception. It will be marketed under the trade name "umbrelly."

The IPD (intrapenal device) resembles a tiny folded umbrella which is inserted through the head of the penis and pushed into the scrotum with a plunger-like instrument. Occasionally there is perforation of the scrotum, but this is disregarded since it is known that the male has few nerve endings in this area of his body. The underside of the umbrella contains a spermacidal jelly, hence the name "umbrelly."

Experiments on a thousand white whales from the Continental Shelf (whose sexual apparatus is said to be closest to man's) proved the umbrelly to be 100% effective in preventing production of sperm, and eminently satisfactory to the female whale since it doesn't interfere with her rutting pleasure.

Dr. Merkin declared the umbrelly to be statistically safe for the human male. She reported that of the 763 grad students tested with the device, only 2 died of scrotal infection, only 20 experienced swelling of the tissues, 3 developed cancer of the testicles, and 13 were too depressed to have an erection. She stated that common complaints ranged from cramping and bleeding to acute abdominal pain. She emphasized that these symptoms were merely indications that the man's body had not yet adjusted to the device. Hopefully the symptoms would disappear within a year.

One complication caused by the IPD and briefly mentioned by Dr. Merkin was the incidence of massive scrotal infection necessitating the surgical removal of the testicles. "But this is a rare case," said Merkin, "too rare to be statistically important." She and the other distinguished members of the Women's College of Surgeons agreed that the benefits far outweighed the risk to any individual man.

better chance of breaking free. Concentrating on goal rather than on attack. When I don't struggle, he thinks he's won. Momentarily, automatically, almost imperceptibly, he loosens his grip. In that moment, I . . . extend toward my goal and escape.

> My partner grabbed my wrist. Using strength, I wasn't able to get away. . . . But when she grabbed my wrist and instead of concentrating upon her grip I thought instead of how I had to scratch my head, my hand flew out of her grasp to my head without any effort on my part.[64]

Imagine, she says, if we were united! If we refused to follow the pattern that men have cut out for women's groups—patterns of mistrust and hurting one another so much that some have to leave the group or the group has to disband altogether. Imagine if we could avoid the traps of jealousy, competition among ourselves, the backbiting, the suspicion.

In a chapter entitled "Women Against Women," Sonia says that peer pressure to follow the leaders blindly and to condemn any one deviate—and to regard any diversity of opinion as insubordination, even treachery—these were blatant hallmarks of cult membership (and of the WMS). One of women's serious acculturated disabilities is fear of acting; we are so afraid of public opinion and censure that we hardly dare to move. "We are afraid of freedom! We don't trust ourselves."

> We oppress each other since we know more about being oppressed than being free. As slaves, we have so completely identified with those in power, so sided with them against ourselves, so thoroughly internalized their values, that we have come to fear our freedom as our masters fear it. This dynamic functions unconsciously long after we have consciously understood and rejected our oppressed status. It is therefore not surprising that women have so bitterly betrayed each other for so long.
>
> Patriarchy is totally dependent upon our mistrusting, thwarting, and hurting one another—and so for this reason we have been deliberately, thoroughly, and fiercely indoctrinated from birth to hate and to hurt women. We must forgive one another and learn to resist this most central and deadly of all patriarchal mandates. . . .
>
> . . . [We must] cease to try to be like men, cease to pretend that their structures are our structures, their values our values, begin to love and be ourselves. . . . The woman's movement is the greatest cause for hope on Earth.[65]

Women, Coming Together

Freed from patriarchy, women do things differently. They throw away the podium, microphones, and rows of chairs. They sit close together in circles, light candles, sing, and share their wisdom. There are no evaluation forms or great debates. Johnson says that a woman could go into a room, lock the door, and not be seen or heard by anybody. But if she did it with purity of heart and lack of hatred, "light would shine out of that room that would be like a laser beam to the hearts of people. Women's ways of making change are different, but no less effective than men's—and often far more humane."[66]

And ALL the Colors of the Rainbow . . .

An authoritarian father can affect his daughter in many ways. As a daughter grows up, her emotional and spiritual growth is affected by her relationship with her father. He is the first masculine figure in her life, and he is the prime shaper of the way she related to the masculine side of herself—and ultimately to all men. The father-daughter wound, Linda Schierse Leonard says, is a condition of our culture, as well as an individual event. "Whenever there is a patriarchal authoritarian attitude which devalues [women]— . . . there one finds the collective father overpowering the daughter.[67]

We are told that when a woman really values herself, "creates in a way that is hers, experiences her own authority, she is then really able to dialogue with the masculine. Neither is she subservient to the masculine, nor does she imitate it."[68] Dialogue with the masculine. Dialogue with the feminine. Not kill them or beat them with a hairbrush or pummel them into the earth or cut them open/apart/out. The important thing to remember is that we are all made up of both masculine and feminine and that both are potentially positive or negative. (Someone who is sensitive, for example, can be seen as caring and empathetic (+) or high-strung and irritable (-); on a continuum, assertiveness can range from strength to aggression.) We must accept and balance these qualities within us, or, like Mother Earth, we will fall off kilter.

When men and women are in harmony on the planet, there is a balance of positive male and female energies (yin and yang). We have each integrated the best of those qualities which were once attributed to only one-half of us. There has been an exchange of our attributes for the betterment of humankind. Scientist George Land remarks that all living things have a common drive to grow and that all things grow in almost the same growth pattern—a three-stage progression: "The first stage is self-oriented and accretive—it defensively gathers everything to itself, like a baby does; the second stage is replicative and tries to endlessly duplicate those things that seem to work for it; the third stage is the most mature and the most *mutual* [emphasis in original]—problems and rewards are shared."[69] When we understand that the union of our energies strengthens us all, we are no longer afraid of accepting from "the other" and forming a whole. Our combined energies create life.

Through fate, choice, luck, or divine intervention, we find ourselves on the planet with men. Men must learn that other ways of knowing may bring wisdom and meaning that the rational will never know.[70] Betty Friedan says: "There needs to be a new kind of dialogue that breaks through—or gets behind—both our masks: women cannot [restructure society] by just talking to themselves."[71]

Men and women need to teach each other the very best of their individual qualities that will keep us all alive.

Reclaim the Earth: Women Speak Out for Life on Earth says, "We do not want the sickness transferred by the violent society through the fathers to the sons. . . . If we cannot affirm women and women's bodies and women's birthing and women's choice, we will go on bringing death to the planet and to ourselves. We cannot affirm life without affirming women."[72] At the same time, "We must believe that men have some virtue in them. Something honorable that can be appealed to. Every person has light within that responds to the light in others. We must blur the distinction between them and us. The person who sets out with some idealism once is still inside somewhere and can be reached.[73] Another source confers: "No boy is born with an evil thought in his head or a hacksaw in his hand. Even if aggression is in the genes, violence is not."[74]

"No religious doctrine is violated, nor is any scientific principle contradicted by the observation that we have been endowed by creation to do better than we're doing. Wrong choices can have catastrophic consequences. Now more than ever, we need to be informed and to participate in making decisions that will shape the world our children will inherit, for we can no longer afford the terrible consequences of behaving badly." Phil Donohue said that.[75] I liked it.

Mark Gerzon, talking to men: "As John Irving put it, 'We are obliged to remember everything.' Until we hear in our own voices the screaming of a hungry child; until we recognize in our own eyes the frightened look of an infant seeking its mother; until we can look at our hands and remember when our fingers clasped an open nightgown as we nursed; until we recognize in ourselves a baby totally dependent on his mother's care—until then, we do not know ourselves. We can no longer forget . . . we can't afford masculine myopia . . . patriarchal anesthesia."[76] You understand that when my doctor friend put down his knife, he was remembering. He was acknowledging and accessing the woman place inside of himself.

Gerzon says that in any encounter in which one dominates or is dominated, the gain is inevitably at someone else's loss; the failure is someone else's victory. No purpose is served by blaming one sex for the other's pain.[77] We are at a crossroad in time. It is our shared responsibility to break destructive patterns and to heal us all. Norma Benney, author of "All of One Flesh," tells us that liberty is a holistic concept: it is neither fair nor just to claim the freedom for one segment of the population without claiming it for others.[78] Another article echoes this message: "The genuine fulfillment of individual or group needs can never be purchased at the expense of other individuals or groups, for then the inhuman means negate the human ends of our seeking."[79] In *Reclaim the Earth*, we are told that women conceive of their struggle in the larger context of human liberation and, furthermore, "in the context of liberating the earth and all life upon it" as well.[80]

Although women have a history of little involvement with technology, we were, in fact, responsible for developing many of the early survival technologies for food gathering and preservation, shelter building, clothing production and healing, as well as many of the implements to carry out these tasks.[81] When technology is neutral—when it is a result of the balance of the masculine and the feminine, it will reflect the values of all. "Being able to bring a feminine critique could help lay the foundations [that would] make technology completely human. When masculinity is seen as an incomplete—and thus distorted form of humanity, the issue of making science and technology less masculine is also the issue of making it more completely human."[82]

"The crowning achievement of femininity is to be able to bring joy into life. Man values woman because she has just this capacity or power. Men cannot find this ecstasy alone without the aid of the feminine element; they must find it in an outer woman or in their own woman within. Joy is a gift from the heart of woman."[83]

We light our lamps. We offer others our joy. We can see from here to China.

8 *Bless the Beasts*

Each according to the dictates of his own conscience.

—Unknown

Instead of being angry with him, take pity on him. His habits are his disease.

—Gandhi

Physician, heal thyself.

—Hippocrates

A man does not begin to attain wisdom until he recognizes that he is no longer indispensable.

—Richard Byrd

Obstetricians cannot afford to allow women to see childbirth as the typically uncomplicated process that it is. If they did, most women would neither want nor need them. So they persuade mothers to think that a normal physiological experience is a life-threatening disease. They seek to control what they themselves do not fully understand, what perhaps is beyond our full understanding. In so doing they often acquire an attitude of arrogance, indifference, and superiority. "Obviously, the better the patient can be controlled, the more predictable will be the outcome. . . . And the more predictable the outcome on a population basis, the more effective the organization will appear to be."[1]

Basic Training

Medical training itself is largely responsible for many of the problems that ultimately affect the care given to the patients once the degree has been earned.

There are "grueling and sleepless years of specialty training that constitute a rite of passage into American doctorhood."[2] Many doctors believe this is a "toughening-up process" that is necessary for professionals who must deal with emergencies and late-night awakenings. Students, however, not yet indoctrinated, plead that the extreme pressures and the chronic exhaustion coupled with the enormous responsibilities exact terrible tolls. One third-year resident admitted to "nodding off" at the surgery table after 36 hours without a wink of sleep.[3] A study published in the *New England Journal of Medicine* by Columbia University researchers showed that interns make nearly twice as many mistakes reading tests when deprived of sleep as when they were well rested.[4] It is impossible to calculate the judgment errors made daily.

Some of the resistance of older doctors to easing medical training comes from a "macho boot-camp" mentality. Their mentality is, if I went through it, so can you. Belatedly, the AMA has begun to study the problems associated with stress, exhaustion, and undersupervision in residency, hopefully starting a new generation of training in which the humane treatment of students will result in more humane treatment of future patients. The medical profession, in its reluctance to heal itself, "may be forced to swallow the bitter pill of imposed reform."[5] "If they are neither kindly, nor pure, the power they have will destroy them and their system."[6]

Other articles echo concerns about physician training. Stephen Hall writes, "Even the AMA agrees that fatigue erodes physician competence. . . . Yet their position [on it] remains sacrosanct."[7] The "novitiate" must prove his worthiness to his superiors by holding up (i.e., staying up) until the bitter end—he's got to "toughen-up." Another theory, he says, is that the sleep-deprived intern acts out an unconscious wish widely held by physicians to attain abilities that transcend what is ordinarily thought of as human. Another source remarks that by instituting stringent requirements and extending training to maximal lengths possible, it is impressed on the public that "the mastery of the mysteries of the profession is difficult—and that professional knowledge can only be professed, understood, and applied by the initiated."[8] Medical schools are reluctant to flunk students— they lose money—and the Board of Censors hesitates to turn down applicants and lose their licensing fees.[9]

Ivan Illich gives us more insight into the matter. He discusses what medicine really does, "as opposed to the myth about it." Medicine, he says, has not justified the faith with which people have turned to doctors and to the medical system; the medical establishment, in fact, has become a "major threat to health."[10]

Illich discusses professional callousness, negligence, and incompetence, which become "scientific detachment," "random human error" or a "system breakdown," and "a lack of specialized equipment" in turn.[11] A military officer with a similar record of performance would be relieved of his command, he says, and a restaurant would be closed by the police.[12] He discusses the damage that doctors inflict with the intent of curing. "Under the stress of crisis, the professional who is believed to be in command can easily presume immunity from the ordinary rules of justice and decency."[13]

Until recently, Illich says, medicine attempted to enhance what occurs in nature. It "fostered the tendency of wounds to heal, of blood to clot, and of bacteria to be overcome by natural immunity." Now, he says, medicine tries to engineer.[14] He goes on to tell us that more health damage is caused by "people's belief that they cannot cope without a doctor" than doctors could ever cause by fostering their ministrations on people.[15] More often than not, we are reminded, the best a conscientious physician can do is what grandmother would have done, and otherwise defer to nature.[16] Our life span, he says, is brought into existence with the prenatal checkup and ends with a mark on a chart ordering resuscitation suspended. Between delivery and termination, this "bundle of biomedical care" fits best into a "city that is built like a mechanical womb."[17] Illich tells us that doctors' "power" and authority have encroached on and medicalized infancy and childhood through to old age. The time has come for the public assessment of medicine and also the disenchantment of it.

Anger and suspicion toward the medical profession are reportedly increasing.[18] Years ago, the doctor's "cheery manner and solicitous style" (not to mention his willingness to come to your home via his horse and buggy) compensated for his inability to cure or his uncertainty about a diagnosis. Increased depersonalization in a growing system of group practices, clinics, and HMOs promotes increased dissatisfaction and criticism. (Doctors themselves, we are told, have to create intimacy and at the same time protect themselves from it.)

"The hours are endless. The pay is paltry. The tasks are often menial and frequently terrifying. And for this, one must spend years slaving in medical school and acquiring a debt that [approximates the national debt]."[19] Young doctors often feel that their training has been "cruel and unusual punishment" that destroys any semblance of a normal, private life. By the time they are ready to hang up their shingle, they have already lost many of their "good" years. To help pay back the astronomical costs they have incurred for their education, and to help compensate for that loss of time, many find themselves interested in money—in having enough, or more than enough, to do all the things they were unable to do for so long. One woman wrote that her doctor's office was undergoing an "efficiency study." "I was told that I would have to make my appointments during the so-called "Afternoon OB Express." If she had questions that couldn't be answered in the time allotted, she would have to make another appointment, for which she would be charged extra. "In the hospital they poke their heads in the door and say cheerfully, 'Good morning, how are you?' That exchange is considered a consultation for which you will receive a bill for $75."[20] A doctor in the South remarks, "You can be a mediocre doctor and discount your fees enough to have all the business you want," rather than to be a very fine doctor and build an impeccable reputation.[21]

To eliminate the incentives for expensive and unnecessary practice, the nation's doctors could be placed on the public payroll and given a salary, adjusted for training, experience, and performance. "This would liberate them from such worries as malpractice and bill-collecting, and would let them devote their full energies to medicine's real purpose: healing the sick and promoting good health for everyone." We are reminded of all the other occupations that directly protect our lives and safety—policemen, firemen, soldiers, air traffic controllers—and reminded that all of them work directly for the government. "When your home catches fire, does it matter to you which fireman pulls your child from his burning bedroom? When a robbery is in progress do you specifically ask of Officer Jones to help you? Of course not. Our lives and safety are so important that such services have traditionally been kept separate from the marketplace and those motivated by private gain. That's because our need for these services is so great that their providers possess the power to blackmail us, to force us to accept terms they dictate to us because they know we have no other choice."[22] This is true to a point, but since childbirth is not a medical circumstance, we do have choices.

One More Strike and You're Out!

In Israel in 1973 the doctors went on strike. During the month it lasted, the Israeli death rate dropped 50 percent. There had not been such a profound decrease in mortality since the last doctor's strike, twenty years before. In Bogota, Colombia, the death rate dropped 35 percent during a two-month doctor's strike in 1976. That same year, in Los Angeles County the doctors went on a work slowdown to protest soaring malpractice insurance premiums; this coincided with an 18 percent drop in the death rate. Dr. Robert Mendelsohn writes, "When the strike ended and the medical machines started grinding again, the death rate went back to where it had been before the strike."[23] Emergencies decreased considerably; people became healthier. Oliver Wendell Holmes once wrote, "I firmly believe that if the whole [medical system], as used now, could be sunk to the bottom of the sea, it would be all the better for mankind—and all the worse for the fishes."[24]

Most pregnant women do not have to see a doctor at all during the course of their pregnancy, labor, and delivery. Illich reminds us that healthy people need minimal bureaucratic interference to mate, give birth, and die.[25] However, we live in a culture where, as children, we integrate a belief that we must be seen by a doctor in order to make sure we get a healthy baby. We learn early on "to be exposed to technicians who, in our presence, use a foreign language in which judgements are made about our bodies; we learn that our bodies may be invaded by strangers for reasons they alone know; and we are made to feel proud" that we live in a country that indoctrinates us into this theology.[26] The same concern was voiced as early as the 1830s: "Physicians have learned just enough to know how to deceive people, keep them in ignorance, by covering their doings under a language unknown to the general public."[27]

Martha Weinman Lear, author of one of my favorite books, *Heartsounds,* learned a lot about how to react to medical indifference:

> It was a moment of triumph born out of pain . . . I limped into a doctor's office and settled myself among other painracked patients to wait—and wait and wait. That is, after all, why it's called a waiting room.
>
> An hour later I dragged myself over to the receptionist and said, "I was here on time. Where's the doctor?"
>
> She glared. "You're not his only patient, you know," she said. "You have to wait your turn."
>
> "No, I don't," I said and limped out. And what made me almost forget my aching back was the soft, sweet call of another patient, saying, 'Attagirl, lady!' as I exited.[28]

"I don't take that kind of treatment anymore," Lear says. "I used to. Most of us do. We are so intimidated by authority and uniforms—especially starched white uniforms— . . . that we back down, accept whatever treatment we get and say, 'Thank you; sorry to be such a bother.' " Consciously or not, we are afraid that if we are aggressive we will be punished. Childbirth educator Luanne Lee remarks, "I can't figure it out. People refuse to take responsibility for their health care and doctors get angry when they do!"

We have a right to know, Martha Lear reminds us, and the doctor has an obligation to explain. In addition, we can expect caring medical care. "Most doctors are professionally competent," Lear says, "but many of them can't make a human connection. By my code, no matter how good the doctor's skills, if he or she is emotionally unavailable, that's not good enough."[29] Doris Haire writes that obstetric residents and practicing physicians are so pressed to keep up with technology that they do not develop—or they lose—their ability to perceive and interpret human factors and their contribution to pregnancy and labor. They increasingly turn to electronic and ultrasonic devices, she says, instead of to the mother, for information and confirmation.[30]

Author Jay Katz tells us that patients have always been asked to trust their physicians without question. "But only in recent years have doctors been asked to trust patients by conversing with them about medical options and soliciting their views on how to proceed."[31] He distinguishes between blind faith—passive surrender—and trust that is earned. Patients' participation in decision making is an idea alien to the ethos of medicine, he says, and "we need to inquire why physicians have been so insistent in their demand that all authority be vested in one party—the doctor."[32] He reminds us that practitioners, however competent or dedicated, are fallible human beings in an imprecise and uncertain world.

So Who's the Boss?

Katz remarks that physicians are reluctant to acknowledge to their patients and to themselves which of their recommendations and interventions are based on science and which on intuition.[33] According to Katz, there is wide diversity and much tension among practitioners, based on scientific principles, clinical experience, and judgment. He calls "the forcible and uninvited entry into bodily space" a "trespass."[34] Patients must be viewed as participants in decisions affecting their lives, but most doctors believe that a patient is too ignorant to make these decisions. Informed consent, he says, is a charade: he believes that many doctors inform their patients only to the extent that they deserve to be informed. Informing them about the uncertainties of medical intervention in many instances "seriously undermines faith."[35] And, of course, one cannot impart to another what one does not know himself.

The idea that doctors know what is best and can therefore act on the behalf of their patients "is so patently untrue that I can only marvel at the fervor with which this notion has been defended."[36] I am reminded of a woman who called me whose baby had died in utero. The doctor had scheduled a cesarean for her for the following day, without her consent. "He didn't think I'd want to carry a dead baby," she said. "I didn't. But I also did not want to have to recover from major surgery and grieve for my child at the same time. He was so upset with me that I had to change doctors." Katz continues by saying that the physician's personal and professional ethics and experience may dictate one course: the patient's needs, wishes, priorities, motivations, and expectations may dictate another. "Thus, health turns out to be an ambiguous state in which two parties conflict."[37] In most exchanges, the physician's and the patient's separate identities collapse into one identity and one, single, authoritative voice emerges—the physician's.[38] He says that any evaluation of perceived "irrational" conduct must take into account that such a judgment may be based on differences in values, life-style, and other personal matters.

Subtle psychological interplays may become subconscious motivating factors. Unconscious motivations and past history influence the decisions we make, and patients may abdicate their decision-making responsibility. "The doctor's promises can stimulate the magical hopes of finally having met the perfect caretaker [benevolent parent]."[39] Richard Selzer comments that often when he calls a patient in on a consultation, the patient will say, 'I want you to tell me what to do. You're the doctor.' The only unspoken word is 'daddy'; tell me what to do, Daddy."[40] Patients who think their caretakers will protect them as once-upon-a-time their all-powerful parents did are doomed to inevitable disappointment, Katz says: "there is a needle-fine line that good doctors must walk, a desperately sensitive balance to preserve, which consists of understanding for each individual patient: Does this person need to hear me discuss the possibility or need not to hear it? The patient's needs have to be reflected back off of the doctor's perceptions, and the skill of those perceptions will determine whether the doctor's word brings catharsis, comfort, or catastrophe."[41]

What do physicians mean when they ask a patient to trust them? To trust that the treatment they think best is indeed best? To trust that the physician has adequately considered all the different senses of "best," especially the non-technical ones, before arriving at a judgement of "best"? To trust that if he discusses all reasonable alternative treatments, that he will do so without exerting undue pressure to choose one treatment over the other? To trust that he will sort out any professional or personal motivations that might influence his selection? To trust that he will not withhold information? To trust that he sees the patient as competent? I could go on, but I hope these questions sufficiently demonstrate our collective ignorance about the nature and scope of the trust that should govern interactions between physician and patient.[42]

A new model of trust must be applied. No single right decision exists, Katz says. Physicians and patients bring their own interest and vulnerability to the decision-making process. Both parties need to relate to one another as equals. Physicians may know more about pathology but patients know more about their own needs.[43] The new model requires that doctors acknowledge the tragic limitations of their own professional knowledge; they must learn not to be unduly embarrassed by their personal and professional ignorance. As we all know, it is sometimes difficult to determine until much later whether the decision made was the "right" one. "If mutual trust were ever to govern physician-patient relations," Katz says, "the silent guerrilla warfare that exists will significantly decrease."[44]

Doctor Jerkall and Ms. Hide

The "warfare" that exists in the field of obstetrics erupts partly from an awareness, however unconscious, that doctors do not belong at normal births. You do not invite your plumber, for example, to wallpaper your living room; rather, you get the right man for the job. The trouble is that the right "man" for any job in obstetrics is not a man, as we will see later in this chapter, but a woman. Few men who had questions about their genital area would seek the opinion or expertise of a woman: chances are, they'd want to find someone with "similar equipment." It never ceases to amaze me how someone without a vagina can be such an authority on them. That we listen to men, who have never been pregnant, never felt a contraction, never felt a baby move inside—and that we follow their instructions and take their word as the gospel truth—is pure folly! It no longer makes any sense to me whatsoever. Janet Leigh says, "What we have now are many men who study birth from a variety of perspectives, who lack the principal vantage point—the ability to give birth themselves. . . . These men dictate the terms of birth and control the passage of women through territory that is uniquely feminine. How did we ever let this happen?"[45]

Since pregnant women are not "patients"—a patient is a person undergoing treatment for disease—an interesting conflict can develop. Disputes and skirmishes often occur when two diametrically opposed ideologies are in close proximity. When one "ideology" insists upon infringing on the other "ideology's" innermost boundaries, armed conflict is almost inevitable. Warfare also exists because the "fighting" goes on in artillery-laden fortresses (better known as hospitals); those occupying the fortresses are the ones in command.

Countless women are frustrated each year in their search for compassionate, quality medical care. We also learn that doctors treat women differently than they treat men, that they take women's complaints less seriously than men's. They often dismiss our symptoms as emotional or psychosomatic, even when the symptoms are identical to a man's. Sue Fisher tells us that women are viewed as sickly, hysterical, and ruled by their reproductive systems.[46] She believes that medical education helps perpetuate these stereotypes, a notion confirmed by a study conducted at the School of Nursing at the State University of New York. The study found that a number of gynecology texts written for medical students were extremely paternalistic and condescending toward women.[47]

Arthur Barsky reports that women consult doctors more often than men do and that they are labeled hypochondriacs as a result. In fact, Barsky explains, women are more sensitive to bodily changes and are simply less reluctant to seek help; in contrast, men are less willing to acknowledge suffering or weakness, but "true hypochondria is actually more prevalent among men."[48]

If we are seen as sick and whiny when we are not pregnant, we can only begin to understand the biases that await us when we walk into a doctor's office three months pregnant, tired, nauseous perhaps, and apprehensive because we do not wish to be cut open six months hence. I would like to share with you a number of examples of women who were met at the doctor's office or at the hospital with patronization, condescension, ignorance, anger, rage, sarcasm, and disdain and some of my responses to them. Keep in mind that these women were paying customers: abuse doesn't come cheap these days, it appears.

Helen's doctor said to her, "I will not allow you to enter into the decision-making. I insist upon a cesarean section. You are a reasonable person, I am sure, and I expect you will accept this recommendation." Helen wrote: "What country is this? I thought this was America where people have a right to make their own decisions, especially when it comes to their own bodies! I felt as if the very core of my privacy was being invaded! Damn right, doc. I am reasonable. To me, being sectioned when the risk of rupture is so small and the danger of major abdominal surgery is so high, is ridiculous and UNreasonable." Helen changed doctors and had a VBAC in spite of her "Y" uterine incision.

Mary said, "Dr. Williams came over to me and practically rubbed his hands in glee as he told me I had torn and did I want stitches? I told him that I didn't want them, but if he felt they were necessary, I'd agree. He told me it was going to hurt, and so I asked him to please use a local anesthetic for the repair. He refused, saying, 'I thought you didn't want any anesthetic.' I couldn't believe what a sarcastic, sadistic jerk he was."

Elaine said, "My doctor kept telling me that I was much too small to have a baby. Well, I went into the hospital so far along in labor that her head was crowning just as he walked in. She was over eight pounds. He threw his gloves

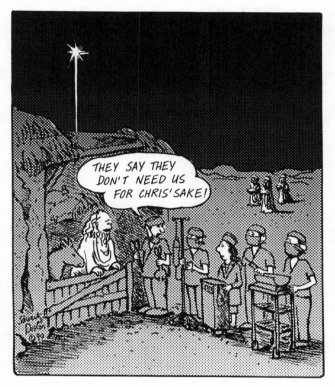

on the bed and said, 'If I hadn't seen it, I wouldn't have believed it.' He told the nurse to weigh the baby again. He said the scale was probably off by a few pounds."

Nora called me. "My doctor said, and I quote, 'I absolutely do not believe in VBAC.' " He probably doesn't believe in the Easter Bunny either! Any doctor who does not believe in VBAC is cutting women open unnecessarily. People who cut other people open unnecessarily are butchers. He doesn't have to believe in VBAC—it's not *his* body that is getting cut time and time again.

Deborah called her previous doctor to tell him that she had just had a VBAC— for a 10 pound 4 ounce baby. He had insisted that she had cpd and that any attempt at a natural birth would fail. "I told him that I wanted him to know this so that perhaps in the future he would consider a VBAC with another patient, instead of automatically sectioning her. Instead of congratulating me, or thanking me for the call, he said, 'You can thank me for a satisfactory surgical repair of your uterus. I hope you had a glucose tolerance test to make sure you do not have gestational-induced diabetes,' and he hung up. I was naive to think that he would reconsider his position. He just got egotistical and defensive."

Lori called her doctor to tell him she was in active labor and that she would soon be on the way to the hospital. He called her back five minutes later and told her that he had just checked her records. "I'm not delivering you," he said. "You haven't paid me in full." He explained that the $1,500 she had paid him was $300 short of his full delivery fee, and unless the bill was paid before the birth, he was unwilling to make an appearance.

Lisa said that she protested when the doctor insisted on general anesthesia for her section. "I want to see the baby!" she told him. "You told me I wouldn't have to have a general!" He told me that he had *changed his mind*, and that I wouldn't be allowed to bond with the baby even if I was awake—and then he instructed the anesthesiologist to put me under."

Joanne told me that she was "computerized." Her new doctor told her, even before she met him in person, that she was on his computer and was listed as "antagonistic," a description faxed over from a doctor she'd had a falling-out with.

Mimi said: "I'm beginning to feel insecure about the depth of my doctor's support for a pure birth. He seems to have a case of the "in-cases": we have to do this *in case* that happens; we should do this *in case* you go into shock, etc."

Bonnie told me her doctor ordered complete bedrest for her for a month. When she went back to see him, he said she could go onto "restricted activity"— vacuuming and intercourse. "I thought he was joking when he said that. He was dead serious!" Perhaps she could save energy, I told her, by doing both at the same time.

Susan wrote: "At my first office visit my doctor commented how hairy I was. It's a sensitive subject—he didn't help me feel too fond of my body, I can tell you that."

Ruby said, "My doctor's motto is 'As long as you sound like you know what you're talking about, it doesn't matter if what you say isn't true.' He told me that 95% of all women who don't have episiotomies have to come back for major repairs. He said there were no home births in our community (I knew of seven, right in my neighborhood). He said that amniocentesis had no risk, and he told me that you can't have a VBAC if your babies are less than two years apart. all this sh— he spouted as if he was Mr. Medicine-Man-Almighty. I call him Chief Lying Bull."

Michele knew that her doctor didn't even know who she was when she went back to him a year after her section. "He kept looking at his records, and it was clear that he had no recollection of our contact. I couldn't believe that someone who had had such a major impact in my life—and such a negative one at that, could look at me as if we had never met. He even looked at my scar, a thick, ugly, red, squiggly line, and said, 'I couldn't have done that.' "

Delia reached down to stroke her baby's head just before the actual birth. She said to her physician, "This is wonderful. I'm sorry that you won't have an experience like this in your lifetime." He barked, "Thank God I don't have to. I recommend vasectomies to men so their wives don't have to go through this." Delia's doctor is among a number of obstetricians who see birth as a predicament from which a woman must be saved. Other physicians are also frightened of birth, but equally jealous of the power and strength that reside within the woman at that time in her life; they oftentimes find this strength intolerable and seek to weaken the mother during labor in a number of ways.

The callous, unthinking remarks that so many doctors make to women never cease to amaze. Bernie Siegel says, "People do not go to medical school to become villains, yet most doctors kill people with their words."[49] (He also says that if you don't feel better after going to see your doctor, you have the wrong doctor.) Gerald Bullock writes that any doctor can sabotage the plans of any mother, "no matter what her preparation, no matter what her degree of determination, no matter how miniscule her level of actual risk. All it requires is a few well chosen negative phrases designed to undermine her self-confidence and to exaggerate the risks of her condition."[50]

Bitter Pills to Swallow

Tact 101 should be a required course in medical school. Unkind, unsubstantiated, unnecessary remarks hurled at vulnerable ears or at an already wounded heart can last a lifetime. The following are some of the comments made to women in my classes or workshops by their doctors.

Sure, go ahead and eat or drink in labor if you want to. I don't care if you throw up, breathe it in, and die.

It's your fault the baby had Down's Syndrome. You released a bad egg.

We have to do an ultrasound every six weeks. See, in a twin pregnancy, one twin sucks the nutrition out of the other.

Your complete lack of labor experience will get in the way of your being able to deliver the baby.

It is a myth that most women can and should breastfeed.

I'll give you a nice episiotomy: I might even carve my initials for you.

Shellshock

No, I do not expect doctors to be perfect, but when *so* many show so little respect for women, and little or no understanding of the birth process, then it's time to bid adieu.

Not all doctors are beyond redemption. Read this impressive account by a doctor who learned to face his mistakes with grace and candor.

In between seeing other patients in the office that morning, I make several rushed calls, trying to figure out what has happened. Despite reassurances from the pathologist that it is statistically "impossible" for four consecutive pregnancy tests to be negative for a viable pregnancy, the horrifying awareness is growing that I have probably aborted Barb's living child. I won't know for sure for several days, until the pathology report is available. In a daze, I walk to the hospital and try to tell Russ and Barb as much as I know, without telling them all that I suspect. I can't really face my own suspicions yet.

. . . The pathology report confirms my worst fears: I have aborted a living fetus at about 13 weeks of age. No explanation can be found for the negative pregnancy tests. My consultation with Russ and Barb [who have been my friends for years], is one of the hardest things I have ever done. Fortunately, their scientific sophistication allows me to describe in some detail what I have done and what the rationale was. But nothing can obscure the fact that I have killed their baby. . . . To make matters worse, complications after the D & C make it [impossible] for Barb to become pregnant again for two years.[51]

Dr. David Hilfiker, the courageous doctor who lived the tragedy and wrote the article, tells us that his guilt and anger grew. He spent weeks analyzing his mistakes (relying too heavily on one particular test, not being skillful in determining the size of the uterus by pelvic examination, etc.). He remarks that as physicians, the automatic response is to try to discover what went wrong and to institute corrective measures so that such things do not happen again. "This response is important, indeed necessary, and I spent hours in such review. But it is inadequate if it does not address our own emotional and spiritual experience of the events." Everyone makes mistakes, he says, and no one enjoys the consequences,

but the potential consequences of our medical mistakes are so overwhelming that it is almost impossible for practicing physicians to deal with them in a psychologically healthy fashion. . . . Painfully, almost unbelievably, we physicians are even less prepared to deal with our mistakes than the average lay person.

. . . Indeed, errors are rarely admitted or discussed once a physician is in private practice. . . . I am of at least average competence as a physician. . . . I assume that my colleagues are responsible for [a number of major and minor] errors. Yet I cannot remember a single instance in which another physician initiated a discussion of a mistake for the purpose of clarifying his or her own emotional response or deciding how to follow up. I do not wish to imply that we don't discuss the difficult cases or unfortunate results; yet these discussions are always handled so delicately in the presence of the "offending" physician that there is simply no space for confession or absolution. The medical profession simply seems to have no place for its mistakes.

. . . The only real answer for guilt is spiritual confession, restitution, and absolution. Yet within the structure of modern medicine there is simply no place for this spiritual healing. . . . Even if one were bold enough to consider such a confession, strong voices would be raised. . . . Malpractice lawyers urge us not to have any contact with the families. Even if a suit is unlikely, the nature of the physician-patient relationship makes role reversal "unseemly." Can I further burden an already grieving family with the complexities of my feelings, my burden?

And if confession is difficult, what are we to say about restitution. The very nature of our work means that we are dealing with elements that cannot be restored in any meaningful way. What can I offer [Barb and Russ] in restitution?

I have not been successful in dealing with the paradox.[52]

Heartburn

I remember a session in one of my classes when I asked the couples to fill in the sentences. I picked a card from the pile and read it aloud: "My obstetrician —————. From one side of the room, a woman yelled out, "is a sweet man!"; from the other side, we heard "sucks." You guessed it: they were both talking about the same person. The class nicknamed him Dr. Chameleon.

How subjective the choice of doctors is, and how loyal women are to their obstetricians, became more clear to me in two situations: one in which a doctor was accused of "gross misconduct and negligence"—endangering pregnant women and newborn babies—and another in which the doctor was accused of sexual misconduct. In both situations, the doctors were found guilty, and the women who had supported them found it almost impossible to believe that their OB could have been responsible for such crimes. Their vehement defense of their "knights" was unflappable. When they could no longer continue to believe in their innocence (either by his own admission, or by the testimonies presented by a number of other women), they felt betrayed, angry, and depressed.

Obstetricians touch, view, and examine our genitals. In order to make this behavior "acceptable," women often "fall in love" with their OBs. Their feelings of endearment excuse the fact that a man is touching them in places that are supposedly off-limits except in a love relationship. By "loving" the man, they can be touched without paying the internal (no pun intended) price of being labeled sleazy or promiscuous.[53] Many women report that they take extra time and care dressing and primping for their gynecological and obstetrical visits.

How deeply women are enmeshed in feelings of "love" (either the parent-child type, or the lover-paramour type) with their obstetrician is illustrated by the following remarks: "I felt like an adultress when I left him"; "The hardest part of moving to another town was leaving my OB"; "I thought I'd rather die than tell him I was leaving his practice"; "I felt as if I couldn't talk to him. I'd go into his office with a list of questions, but I was too afraid to ask. I'd get weak in the knees." [child: fear; adult: infatuation]. It was also interesting for me to learn that in some lawsuits a number of women did not come forward to testify against their doctors for quite some time. Although they knew their testimony might be useful, they had to work through feelings of embarrassment and dis- loyalty (infidelity), as well as to recover from the trauma and emotional pain they had endured as a result of their sorely or tragically invested trust. Some were too stunned and despairing to speak up. I recently heard that an obstetrician in Wyoming raped more than one hundred patients; however, only twelve were willing to testify. It took all twelve, and days of testimony to convict him. It is no secret that in a male-dominated society, woman are often seen as instigators or liars.

Many feminist books today help us to understand the male doctor/female patient relationship, with whatever romantic overtones, implicit or explicit sexual innuendoes, dominant-aggressive/passive-submissive qualities that characterize it. It is not within the scope of this book to continue a discussion on this subject. I find myself wondering, however, what kind of a man chooses to spend all the days of his life with his face—and hands—in women's vaginas. I wonder what percentage of the men who choose obstetrics do so because of a deep and abiding reverence for life, a respect and appreciation of women, a love of little babies, and a sense of humility for their own role in the process of birth.

Pink in White

Women doctors, is that the answer? They have vaginas. Unfortunately, many of them have never used them for childbirth; the fact is that female OBs have a statistically high incidence of cesarean section. Many of the women OBs who have children did not have a purebirth. "The pressure to perform, to know it all," said one woman obstetrician, "was unbelievable. At that point, I was just a woman, about to become a new mother. I had seen a number of labors, sure, although in retrospect, you're right—none of them was really natural. But I had never experienced a labor on my own, and let me tell you, I was nervous and feeling as if I had to keep it all together the whole time." Many women physicians meet with sexism and prejudice and, in an effort to be respected and included, begin to practice much like the men with whom they have studied and worked.

It isn't easy for these women, not by a long shot. Some of the comments: "There are astonishing events in medical school, like dissecting a cadaver. I mean, how do you deal with that? At most medical schools, there is very little encouragement for students to talk about their feelings. . . . [All these] very overwhelming experiences, and no space for talking about them"; "You have to work incredible hours, and you're deprived of sleep. I found myself being mean and hateful with patients . . . I would have to stop myself and say 'It's not their fault' "; "Surgery is the scariest. . . . You've got just one chance to do it right. If you screw up, you screw up big. The insecurity is the highest, so it brings out the worst in people."[55]

Maureen Katz remarks that women have many qualities that are essential to the healing process. (She cautions us, lest we are burdened by stereotypes: "I made it through my third year in medical school because my male lab partner was incredibly compassionate, and he cried, just like many women do."[56]) Those same qualities—warmth, sensitivity, the ability to connect with others—can be a liability as well as a joy. Alice Rothchild, an OB near Boston, talks about the many directions in which she's pulled. "I'm trying to figure out how to have a life, be a doctor, work a hundred hours a week, have a kid, have a relationship and have friends. It's hard to work 80 hours a week when you are pregnant. It's hard to have a kid and be pumping your breasts all the time and have to be with someone while she's in labor at three in the morning. . . . I mean there are easier ways to live."[57]

Perri Klass, a doctor, describes how she felt when she was eight months pregnant and sitting in one of her classes in medical school.[58]

> I sat there, rubbing my belly, telling my baby: "Don't worry, you're O.K., you're healthy." I sat there wishing this course would tell us more about normal pregnancy, that after memorizing all the possible disasters, we would be allowed to conclude that pregnancy itself is not a state of disease. But . . . most of us, including me, came away with a sense that pregnancy is a deeply dangerous medical condition, that one walks a fine line, avoiding one serious problem after another, to reach the statistically unlikely outcome of a healthy baby and a healthy mother.
>
> . . . As a medical student, I was spending my time studying everything that can go wrong with the human body. As a pregnant woman, I became suddenly passionately interested in healthy physiological processes—and I found myself rebelling as a mother and "patient."

Perri, bless her soul, read *Immaculate Deception*. She attended a childbirth class that was designed to teach couples how to be "bad patients." She enjoyed them, and learned a lot. Yet,

> they also left me feeling pulled between two poles, especially if I went to medical school during the day to discuss deliveries going wrong in one catastrophic way after another ('C-section! C-section!' my discussion section once chanted when the teacher asked what we would do next), then later to childbirth classes in the evening to discuss ways to circumvent medical procedures. As a student of the medical profession, I know I am being trained to rely heavily on technology, to assume that the risk of acting is almost always preferable to the risk of not acting. I consciously had to right these attitudes when I thought about giving birth.

Perri also found that some aspects of having a baby while in medical school were positive. Taking courses in anatomy, physiology, and embryology deepened her awe of the "miracle going on" inside of her. She says, "I want to believe that I will be a better doctor because I have combined medical school with the experience of having to choose and control medical care for myself. I also want to believe that obstetrical medicine will change, but I do not really believe that it will change from within."

Perri had her son in a birthing room. She had a long pushing phase. "Suddenly, I heard one of the doctors say something about forceps. At that moment, I found an extra ounce of strength and pushed my baby out. As I lay back with my son wriggling on my stomach, the birthing room was suddenly transformed into the most beautiful place on earth."

Yes, Ma'am, He's My Tootsie

Even *I* will admit that there are a few good obstetricians around. Not many, but a few. The ones whom I recommend have somehow managed to get through medical training without becoming dehumanized. Oftentimes, if they are female, they have had a natural birth themselves; if they are male, their children were born naturally. Perhaps they are "reformed," like Gerald Bullock, or "fed up," like one doctor who said, after performing seven cesareans over a three-day weekend, "I felt as if I was in a Stephen King movie. Blood, everywhere. I became determined to help babies arrive without using a knife." The better the obstetrician, the more like a midwife he or she becomes. As you will see later in this chapter, I have no greater regard for anyone on the planet than midwives.

An article in the *Boston Globe* a few years back presented us with "The Tootsie Awards," given to any man who, "in his efforts to understand and empathize with women, goes one step beyond and, in one or two cases, right over the edge."[59]

In my lengthy "career" in childbirth, spanning most of the states in this country, I have met only a handful of Tootsie OBs. I know that they are out there, quietly supporting home birth, helping to make changes in hospitals. Thanks, guys. Here are a few testimonies from women who have had positive, uplifting, warm, feelings about one of the "good guys."

> My doctor is wonderful. He really sticks his neck out for you. I had a homebirth after two cesareans. He agreed to back me up and said "Go for it, Debby!"

> My OB is a rare bird indeed. She is friendly, competent, confident, calm, a complete joy to work with. She gets a ton of "flack" from the largely male ob/gyn practices around here, but she holds her own.

> My doctor believes that the Golden Rule applies to pregnant women and newborn babies. When there is a situation that is of concern, he generally sits down and prays. He rarely intervenes, he just prays alot!

> My OB is a real human being. He was as sad for us as we were. That really helped. He cried right along with us. He was euphoric when our next baby was born healthy, and has remained in touch with us for a number of years.

> I like the way my doctor communicates. He takes his time, and listens carefully. His vocabulary includes please, thank you, I was wrong, I'm sorry, and I will support you. He has a wonderful sense of humor. We all laughed through the whole nine months, right into—and yes through (most of) labor!

> I went to see my doctor on my friend's recommendation. I couldn't believe he'd support me for a VBAC—I've had two c-sections. I found out he had been attending VBACs for years and not telling anyone—he didn't want to get fired. When I asked him if he would treat me any different than his normal mothers, he said, "You are normal!" His wife had trouble with her episiotomy for two years so he doesn't do them. He wears a shirt with rolled up sleeves to delivery, and "jams" in the summertime. When I asked him about a routine prep, you know, the shave

and enema, he said, "never done it in my life." Before I even asked him about position for delivery, he said, "I don't care how you do it—sideways, squatting, upside down, or on your head if it works. Just don't take me into the OR, ok?!" Then he said, "If I've done my job right, you won't even have noticed I was there." I pinched myself on the spot: I thought I had died and gone to Heaven. My birth was everything I had hoped it would be, and more.

Thinking you may have to switch at this point? Having trouble getting your current OB to talk to you, make eye contact with you, smile at you? Tired of the impersonal, assembly-line practice? It's never too late. Alice changed doctors when she was four days past her "due date," and Anne changed in labor! All the excuses why you can't change—not enough time for medical records to be sent (who needs them? They're a pack of lies or bits of inaccurate, rote, erroneous, subjective information for the most part anyway); you are considered 'high-risk'; you live too far; etc., etc., have all been faced by others before you. One woman lamented, "I want to change, but I haven't got the money! I asked her what she would do if her washing machine or refrigerator broke that day. "They're necessities!" she said. "I'd have to find a way to afford them. Okay. I got it. Say, are there any good OBs who take Master Card?" She switched doctors in her thirty-eighth week.

Prognosis: Hopeful?

We all recognize that there are many times when a doctor's training, skill, and intercession are not only invaluable, but essential. We cannot allow our anger to build such a gulf between us that there is no connection possible, for there may be times when we need a bridge. We must allow the best in ourselves to call out the best in those who offer medical care.

Ken Keyes provides me with a fit ending to this chapter. He says that we must replace the illusions of separateness with the emotional experiences of acceptance, cooperation, and togetherness. Instead of you *versus* me, it must become "you *and* me" on this planet together.

> However much our ideologies may clash, we must remember that nothing is more important for survival and for happiness in life than feelings of understanding and commonness of human purpose.
> . . . Whatever we expect to get creating hatred and separateness, even if it is 'justified' is purchased at too great a price. We can still want what we want. We can think it's only fair or right to get it. We can still put energy into trying to change things. But we must learn not to throw people out of their hearts.[60]

We must invite doctors to heal along with us. A Buddhist meditation of goodwill says, "Let us cultivate boundless goodwill. Let none deceive another, or despise any being in any state. Let none in anger or ill-will wish another harm. Even as a mother watches over her child, so with boundless mind should one cherish all living beings, [everywhere] over the world, above, below, and all around, without limit."[61]

9 *Divine Nonintervention*

And you can count on me . . .
and I will always help you . . .
And I will be the one
to help you ease your pain.
I will hold you in my arms
like a white-winged dove,
shine in your soul:
your spirit is crying.
Lean on me: I am your sister;
believe on me: I am your friend.

—From "Sister" by Cris Williamson[1]

In most countries, babies are brought into the world with a midwife in attendance. Midwives are known and respected as the most qualified people to assist
pregnant and birthing women. Although it is beyond the scope of this book to
give you a history of the almost virtual disappearance of midwifery in this country,
suffice to say that the obstetrical patriarchy spent decades bad-mouthing, black-
listing, and squelching any enthusiasm or trust for the profession. Midwives
became an endangered species. Thankfully, there has been a marvelous resur-
gence of midwifery over the past twenty years; however, there does seem to be
some confusion as to what a midwife really is and what she does.

Real Midwives

I'm going to let real (i.e., traditional) midwives speak in their own words, and
I think after a time, you'll begin to understand why they are so-named. Later,
we'll describe other women who pose as midwives.

Meg: I have an unfaltering confidence in birth, in a woman's ability to give birth, and in myself as a practitioner. No woman has ever looked in my eyes and seen doubt, and that unfailing encouragement is what helps to get stuck babies out. . . . This is what I love: I will always be reborn in midwifery, each day with each birth.

Mary: You know, there is always so much more to learn. When I observed [other real midwives], I saw them sitting on their hands and being supportive. I learn to sit on my hands, to trust, more and more each day. . . . A woman with four previous classical cesareans wanted a homebirth. Everyone thought she was crazy and that I would be even crazier for attending her. My heart said, "Do it. It will be fine." I always listen to my heart. It never lies to me.

Carolyn: Every time I saw an OB cut a woman's perineum, I felt my own was being cut. Finally, I said NO MORE. I put my hand in front of the OB's knife and said, cut off my fingers first.

Jillean: I learned early that patience is a virtue. Perhaps it comes from growing up in a large family, I don't know. Some women are just in that small classification of "long laborers." It took nine months to grow that baby and if it takes a while to birth it, so be it. The women thank me when their babies are born. I thank them. I relearn patience from them, time and time again.

Marie: I have been attending births for twelve years. The most important thing I have learned is—each pregnancy, labor, and birth is different. Each woman is different. Each child has its own "journey" to make, and the mother has hers as well. I used to feel as if I was a guide. I don't think that way anymore. I am really along on the journey, too. It is a privilege to be asked along on another's sacred journey, you know that?

Karen: My message is this: Be in love with the whole process and all the people involved. Keep the wonder of it alive inside of you.

Pat: To be the best midwife I can be requires that I must be clear in mind and spirit. I must take care of my physical body—respect it. Anger and hostility interfere with the work I must do. I learn, day by day, to relax and flow with birth.

Carol: I became a midwife because I had two cesareans myself. The small town where I live has a 47% section rate! With little education, few choices, and no support, the women give in to the doctors. I have become an outspoken anti-interventionist. No matter that 98% of my mothers—and I take a lot of the so-called high-riskers—have natural deliveries—I am considered a menace here.

Dee: The sight of a woman birthing a baby in a hospital is as foreign/unnatural/repulsive to me as anything I can think of. It really makes no difference if it is a "good" hospital. In fact, a "good" hospital says to birthing women, "You don't belong here!"

Lianne: Midwifery is definitely a calling. It's in my cells. It isn't my "profession"— it is a part of me. No, it IS me. There are no words to tell you the joy, the awesomeness of it all. It is a bit of heaven on this earth.

Here are some of the things that women who use real midwives say about them: They are gentle; they don't injure their clients; they don't use medical interventions; they are so kind to your bottom!; they aren't on a power-trip and they don't make you feel guilty or inferior or inadequate; they are patient; they know the meaning of the word "support"; they don't think the doctor's word is God; they understand your fears; they are willing to talk about death—not skirt the issue; they are strong in a very loving way; they love babies!; they love women; they know how to listen; they are intuitive; they explain things; they are emotionally accessible; their hands are soft, firm, and welcoming; they let me cry and complain; they are warm and compassionate; they are knowledgeable and wise; they know how to build confidence; they're very special, every one of them.

Real midwives don't "do" births; they attend them. They don't deliver babies; they assist them into the world. Real midwives are not medically trained; they are skilled in midwifery. Real midwives are not nurses. They do not work in medical institutions, since they know that birth is not a medical event. They do not put a time limit on labor. They are not dependent on doctors or hospitals for their instructions or their pay check. They don't wear uniforms or lab coats to look "professional." They live in the community where they work. Real midwives are among the people I most honor and cherish in the whole wide world.

In *The Midwife Advocate*, midwife Fran Ventre says, "Midwifery is a vocation, a romance, an addiction, a religion. It isn't something you dabble in; there's a part of yourself, of your life, that you give away." Many responsibilities come with the "territory" and the job brings many joys. A woman makes a commitment (and sacrifices) when she chooses to be a midwife: "You are always on call. And to your family, the promises are contingent upon whether or not you have a woman in labor . . . No wonder my husband keeps saying to me, 'Why don't you try something sane and reasonable, like becoming a fighter pilot?'[2]

In the mothering magazine *The Doula* (1986, no. 4), editor Liz Koch interviews Raven Lang, author of the *Birth Book* and a midwife for seventeen years:

> I think I was born a feminist. I was born wanting to be heard . . . wanting females to be as respected as males . . . I think midwives are natural teachers. They are women who can communicate, express themselves, carry ideas, extrapolate those from people who may not be as articulate, and work them out so that the women whom they help will have a more conscious idea of what their needs are, of what they are doing. . . . I've always been intrigued with birth and death, I think because I came in dying and birthing—I was born in trouble physically, or so the doctors perceived me to be—it was very much part of the same coin for me. I think midwives tend to play with that elemental energy of life-death and feel quite comfortable with it. You know, most people don't. Most people can't walk into a birth and see a woman deliver without falling apart. They can't see the blood, they can't hear the tears . . . they can't do that. They don't read it, they get it wrong. I've always felt really at peace, at one, with those energies. Most midwives do.

They know how to handle those energies and not be repelled or pushed away by them. They almost embrace them. They'll walk into a situation and put their hands right on it, whether it is blood or fear or sweat or death or life or tears—whatever. They're not afraid.[3]

Midwifery is also loving women; it is loving your sexuality at the apex. "Gestation, giving birth, lactation, that's really the essence of the manifestation of women's physical sexuality . . . this is different than emotional sex . . . this is more than biological sexuality I speak of." Raven shares a story about a birth she witnessed in which the doctor would not give the mother the baby. When she requested that the mother be given the infant, the doctor said, "Let me tell you, that motherly love kills more babies than bullets." Raven grabbed the doctor's shirt around his neck: "I violated his space—I told him I would smear his name like mud." He called for her arrest soon after that, but that was "the birth of my midwifery," she says.

Midwives are generally skilled observers. They are dedicated and self-directed. They usually have a political viewpoint, Raven says, and "they tend to be involved in life around them and they are smart." A person is "awakened" about childbirth for whatever reason: they had a baby, they saw a baby come. "Whatever it is that awakens that calling, that desire in them to find out about birth—is kindled."[4]

A number of the women whose letters are reprinted in Chapter 15 became midwives, are presently apprenticing or are attending births as LSPs (labor support people) or PBAs (professional birth assistants). They all speak of a passion inside that just won't go away—a deep, abiding, ongoing passion to be involved with birth, to assist other women at this time in their lives. I understand this passion; I began to train as a midwife myself and I loved every minute of it. (I got sidetracked writing books, but I've begun my training again!) There was a reverence, an excitement, a wonder about each birth that is indescribable. To be invited to someone's birth was *a privilege*.

There is an air of humility about real midwives. Ruth Watson Lubic writes that when she was in midwifery training she examined a woman in labor. "While I was rearranging the sheets, I smiled at her and said, 'Well, you are two fingers now and you aren't having your baby, are you?' With that she gave a great groan and there was the baby." Ruth remarks that her being on call that morning was "no coincidence" but "part of a grand design for dispelling . . . arrogance."[5]

Real midwives do not slap a "high-risk" label on a woman as a sentence from which there is no escape. They know steps that can be taken to reduce or eliminate risks. They do not use (as childbirth educator Jodie McLaughlin calls it) "gynegadgetry." Real midwives often consider a woman a homebirth "candidate" even when many others would not: her criteria include not only the physical and the physiological—but the nutritional, emotional, psychological, sexual, and spiritual, as well.

Real midwives attend the woman at home. They do not expect her, in labor, to take herself to a place full of strangers (and germs) and bright lights and equipment hiding behind paneled walls. Nan, for example, assisted a forty-eight-year-old woman as she VBACed at home. Mary attended a woman with four cesareans: another midwife attended a homebirth after six cesareans. Most of the midwifes I know have attended twin births, breech deliveries, VBACs, still-births, "overdue" babies, preemie babies—all at home. They believe it is the woman's choice where she gives birth, and although they will refuse to attend certain women at home, and do transfer others to the hospital at varying points during labor, they are also committed to homebirth whenever possible.

There are a few exceptions to the principle that real midwives come to you. For example, hundreds of women have gone to The Farm in Tennessee and been attended by midwives (such as Ina May Gaskin) there. Many of the women stay at the farm for a long time before their births, and so it becomes their "home." Other midwives invite women to come and birth in their homes or their centers—if the woman's own home is not conducive to birthing, or for a number of other reasons. Janet Jennings writes: "The definition of a midwife by the World Health Organisation is that she is the expert in normal midwifery. A favourite statement by many obstetricians and doctors is that no birth can be considered as normal except in retrospect, which conveniently disposes of the need for midwives at all."[6] Indeed, the list of women who are not candidates for home birth, by medical standards, is as long as a giraffe's neck.

Midwife Pat says that too many of the "midwives" she knows set up and follow masculine standards for midwifery. "The women compete in a male system and sacrifice some of their own female issues and instincts in order to 'pass the test' on male ground." Traditional Birth Assistant midwives, she says, are educated and skilled in depth in certain areas of obstetrics and neonatology, yet they acquire this information and expertise in a manner that meets female needs and have no masculine confines. They "exist in an ever increasing number and create a dilemma for the establishment and the midwives who are a part of that system."

Midwives help to prevent problems; wherever they are, the rate of normal deliveries increases. The countries with the lowest incidence of maternal and fetal morbidity and mortality have one thing in common: the use of midwives. Moreover, we all know by now that midwifery care is consistently associated with a dramatic decrease in low birthweight and prematurity and with increased maternal satisfaction and wellbeing. They have an important task in counseling and education—not only for women, but also within the family and community—this includes antenatal education and preparation for parenthood and extends to certain areas of gynecology, family planning, and baby care.[7]

In many traditional cultures, midwives are called in to handle emergency situations. They are considered the best qualified persons to handle certain situations because of their wide variety of skills.[8] A midwife has frequently been instrumental in demonstrating the art of breech delivery to obstetricians or in assisting "stuck" labors or babies. Elizabeth wrote that while the doctor was ordering a cesarean section, the midwife quickly instructed her to change position, and then firmly, but gently, reached inside and assisted the baby who was "caught behind the bones." The doctor said, "I have never seen anyone do that before." In countless incidences the presence of a midwife has saved the woman from unnecessary surgery, unnecessary interventions, episiotomies, and any physical trauma. One of Alabama's "granny" midwives says, "All my life I always did believe in helping people, and if I couldn't help 'em, I wasn't gonna harm 'em."[9]

Black and Blue?

Midwives—women assisting women at birth—were around from the beginning of time. It seems that this may very well be an instinctual part of our "animal" nature. I read that when an elephant went into labor in a zoo in the United States, the zoo officials isolated her from the other elephants. They believed that this was the safest thing to do. As the elephant's labor progressed, the animal became distressed and thrashed about so violently that she posed a threat to herself and to the baby. Zoo officials quickly telephoned a zoo in Europe where an elephant had successfully delivered just a few weeks earlier. When the Americans described the situation, the Europeans were shocked. "Where are the midwives?" they asked. "Where are the other female elephants to help with the delivery?"

The American officials immediately followed instructions from the Europeans. They allowed other female elephants into the same area with the birthing mother. They immediately began to assist the laboring mother, stroking her with their trunks, calming her with their presence, and helping her to complete her labor and give birth. While the new mother rested, the midwives cleaned the baby and stayed close by.[10]

It is no wonder to me that so many women in hospitals "thrash about" and are disoriented, upset, and traumatized at birth when we are deprived of women—midwives and friends—whom we know and trust. The results are often disastrous.

Bonnie had had a very long and difficult first labor that resulted in a c-section. For her second baby she selected a midwife and remained at home. She surrounded herself with soft music, crystals, and candles, and felt that she was laboring in a "sacred, magical space." Her labor continued for quite some time. Her midwife "hung out" with mellow energy for awhile and then, realizing that Bonnie was afraid to really "go at it" (because of her last labor), said, "You don't want to have a really long labor this time, do you, Bonnie?" No. The midwife replied by rubbing her hands together and saying, "OK, let's change the energy around here." They changed the music to reggae and started things on their way. As the contractions got stronger, Bonnie started saying, "No! No!" and the midwife, looking into her eyes, shook her head up and down and said, "Yes . . . yes . . . " Soon Bonnie was shaking her head up and down—yes, yes. The midwife kept reminding her not to fight it, to let it happen. Then she lovingly said, "Anytime that you are ready to give birth to this baby is fine with me." Within an hour, Bonnie's baby was born.

When a woman calls me and says that she can't find a midwife, we often talk about any fears or conflicts she may have about using one. When a woman is really set on having a homebirth, she locates an attendant. In some communities, it takes some asking around: as Jutta Mason writes, "Midwives play a quiet role in connecting families who form the new birth culture. . . . They become the witnesses of the community's experience, carrying painful stories as well as joyful ones and funny ones. . . . they help us rework a language that can express how women experience their bodies rather than what the experts tell them they experience."[11]

The NAPSAC books, as well as other books on midwifery, reveal that midwives are far more qualified to attend births than doctors. Why then do so many women flock to obstetricians for their prenatal checkups and deliveries?

Because we have been sold a bill of goods. We have been led to believe that birth is dangerous and that only medically trained interventionists can handle the delicate, serious problems that are bound to arise in the majority of situations. Those of you who are interested should read the sad history of midwifery in this culture in a number of excellent books. The slander of midwives is perhaps one of the best examples of male domination and female oppression in our culture. It exemplifies the patriarchal system under which we all live, day in and day out. Physicians, seeing midwives as strong competition, set out to destroy their reputations and "get the business" for themselves. As the organized medical profession and medical education system developed, "physicians increased their campaign against midwives. . . . Midwifery was maligned by physicians, and the public was led to believe that midwives were untrained and used unclean instruments. Although there may be a number of incompetent or uncaring midwives, there has never been any documentation that these practitioners outnumbered incompetent or unclean physicians. In most areas of birth, midwives have far better outcomes than physicians. Yet doctors have called midwives "baby-killers."

Doctors saw midwives as their servants. Doctors learn about illness: they are specialists in pathology and do not have the skills for facilitating normal birth.[12] Yet, they have managed to capture the vast majority of birthing women in our culture. They've worked hard to squelch the midwifery movement. Why? The answer boils down to this: egos, economics, and effacement.

According to Laurie Friedman: "Any physician whose philosophy is that he or she has the ultimate and absolute responsibility for all patients and outcomes, and therefore the right to make all decisions, will always conflict with a midwife who believes in shared responsibility. . . . Likewise, a physician who believes that birth is a dangerous event, usually accompanied by serious complications that require continuous monitoring and frequent intervention, will inevitably clash with a midwife who views birth as including many variations of normal, and

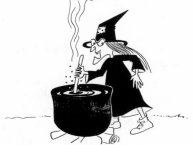

The material is copyrighted only to prevent its being misused.

who believes that even when complications arise, the fewer the interventions the better."[13]

Terry, a mother from Michigan, wrote that when she asked about VBAC, the doctor said he would have to consult with his three associates. He listed every intervention available as an absolute. "I mentioned that I had an appointment with midwives, and he changed his tune. He practically got on his knees and begged me to have the baby at the hospital with them. He said they'd use intermittent monitoring and a heparin lock, instead of an IV. This doctor, who had just insisted that he had three doctors that he HAD to confer with, all of a sudden could make this decision on his own."

Heat

In the Middle Ages, midwives were considered witches and were burned at the stake. Judith Hoch-Smith and Anita Spring write that despite their association with healing and nurturing, women were also seen as "the creators of illness." They are seen as "witches, [on which] the tensions of their society are scapegoated. The accusations that women witches harm babies, exacerbate illnesses of all types, cause crop failures and weather disasters—[are] all a perversion of the gynomorphized universe. Women still are very powerful through their mystical ties to nature, but men believe that on account of female envy, greed, or sheer evil, these powers are turned to world destruction and cataclysm."[14] Women, they say, are seen as potentially controlling the male-dominated society.

As a result, any effort to thwart this attempt is worthwhile. "Estimates vary as to how many midwives were executed [over four million at least], but it is certain that when the witch trials ended, medicine was completely in the hands of university-trained male physicians, and the "old religion" of the wisewoman [which is what midwife really means] had almost totally disappeared."[15]

In fact, the "witch hunts" and trials have not yet ended, but we'll get to that in a little while.

Raven Lang reports that one of the midwives whom she knew had no telephone: "Later that afternoon, she said, 'Feel the energy? Yep, my friend is going to have her baby. I gotta go and [assist]' . . . Sure enough, the lady was in strong labor." Years later, Raven was attending a birth and a doctor was present. He said that he didn't know how long it was going to take to have the baby. Raven said, "I do. The baby will arrive at three." The doctor looked at her with a big grin on his face and said, "Oh yeah?" Raven said, "Yeah." At three o'clock the baby came out, and he was amazed. The doctor said, "You know, it was hard for me not to interfere . . . but I was so intrigued by what you were doing that I wanted to see for myself." Then he said, "Listen lady, . . . who are you, where do you come from, and where are you going?" Raven echoes a number of other midwives who "sense" rather than feel how far dilated a woman is, "listens" to ascertain what phase of labor she's at, and uses the sense of smell as well. "Fingertips are only one of my five senses. My eyes are just as powerful as my fingers. My ears are just as powerful. So is my nose." And her heart.

The doctor who was with Raven at the birth was in his own feminine energy. He was not threatened by Raven; he learned from her. He was open to her suggestions and shared his expertise. This is not usually the case, however. Most doctors find it almost impossible to identify with, much less admit to, the "inner feminine." Robert Johnson writes that what a man sees as the evil element within is his feminine side—he is so "out of tune" that it frightens him. However, "when the man's feminine side is excluded, he often gets 'witchy.' Much of the . . . rejected element during the Middle Ages was feminine, hence all the witch hunting. . . . Instead of quelling his interior feminine aspect, he had to [exteriorize it—transfer it outward] and go out and burn [women]." He reminds us that we haven't gone far past the hunts yet: "Men are still projecting onto outer, flesh-and-blood women their relationship, or lack of it, to their inner femininity. In the ideal, the feminine and the masculine serve each other, are close to each other, and strengthen each other.[16]

For years the medical establishment made sure that predominantly male obstetricians controlled birthing, leaving midwives no role. Midwives are now seen as a threat to a doctor's practice. Doctors fear that women might seek the help of midwives "for help with all their 'female troubles,' and doctors would lose at least half their potential patients." Legislation allowing midwives into hospitals was not passed until 1977, after a decade of women's struggles to control much else in our lives.[17] Although midwives are tolerated in some areas and are "permitted" in many hospitals, they are still very much under the auspices of "the system." Antipathy toward them appears more the rule than the exception. The greatest fear surrounding them, and the hostility that follows, stems from the fear of competition. Upon hearing the prediction that midwives would gain popularity and continue to increase their number of deliveries, one well-known doctor replied, "Whether this prediction is fulfilled will depend in large part on whether [midwives] gain authority to practice independently. To avert this worrisome problem, family physicians and obstetricians must work co-operatively."[18]

Not Real Midwives . . .

Nurses, unlike midwives, are medically trained. They have come through the system, and they have learned to respect the doctor's authority. Unlike midwives, whose familiarity with the moon, or herbs, or tinctures or teas, make them appear "different," nurses know hospital jargon and are seen as benevolent healers. Nurses are a part of the "system"—their conversion to midwives was safe—the people trusted them, and the doctors knew that because of their enculturation (brainwashing?), they could be relied upon not to upstage them, control, them, or "take over." According to one source, "The traditional midwife is a competitor; her successor, the nurse-midwife, is not." Doctors want to prevent others from assuming a competitive entrepreneurial role.[19] Nurses and midwives are two completely distinct (and in many ways incompatible) professions. I have great respect for nurses in general, but if ever an oxymoron there was, nurse-midwife is it.

Molly, a nurse-turned-midwife, says "The consumer must remember that nurse-midwives are taught by the medical model. They rely heavily on diagnostics, lab work, monitoring, etc. for management of labor. They are also responsible for much documentation of labor progress and often have other clients in labor. These factors combined greatly decrease the quantity and often the quality of support given." Penny, a midwife who went to nursing school so that she could become "credible," was certain that she would not let the "system mentality" seep into her brain and damage it. She had trained in Kansas and had a strong sense of birth as a normal event. She found that it was impossible not to be affected. "I found myself thinking that something was bound to go wrong, whereas before, I just knew that things generally went right. I am on the road back to the belief in normalcy—I'm still shocked at the insidious way all that negative stuff creeped in."

Midwives who work in hospitals are not real midwives. They are nurses who have become midwives; they possess a medical training that has taught them that birth must take place in a hospital because "something might go wrong." If they haven't attended home births, they are not midwives and they don't know what real birth is. What they see as normal birth is the American (warped) view of birth. If they really believed that birth was safe, they would be convincing women to stay out of hospitals. They wouldn't be agreeing to ridiculous protocols and hospital/doctor ordained rules. They'd never be able to sit by and watch IVs routinely dripping into laboring women's arms. Until a nurse can say, "I am a midwife" and proudly feel that that is enough, it prevents me from giving her true respect. As long as she feels it is important to let the public know that she is also a nurse—that she is part of the system—she has identified herself first and foremost as part of the medical system that birth should not be a part of. When a nurse begins to be willing to identify herself with birth apart from obstetrical thinking, she will have taken a big step toward real midwifery.

Midwife Sloane Crawford writes that nurse-midwives are educated "in relative isolation within the classroom and hospital. . . . Learning is dependent on what a student can conceptualize and control. If transformation is seen as a radical change in consciousness, a restructuring of one's mutual and separated meaning integrated into and not apart from daily life,—then midwifery education can hardly be seen as transforming. It serves rather, to both limit and fragment the midwife and her relationship to the community of women she serves."[20] The education of the nurse-midwife "does not emphasize a new experience of reality in which the boundaries of the self become more permeable to an intensified contact with a transpersonal or spiritual realm. Rather, nurse-midwifery education merely adds further skills, technical and time management abilities to a nurse's repertoire." According to the American College of Nurse-Midwives, nurse-midwifery is the independent care of normal women and newborns, within a health care system that provides for medical consultation, collaborative management, or referral. However, it is not independent at all. "Many, many nurse-midwives spend their entire career working within the male-oriented medical model, dependent on the concepts and technology of twentieth century obstetrics to provide a woman with a 'safe' pregnancy and a healthy baby. Although midwifery education teaches that childbearing is a normal physiological event instead of the illness model that physicians work from, it is still too often isolated from family, community, and social contexts."

The midwife practicing in the medical model is a paradoxical outsider: she is an outsider because she is a woman practicing in a man's domain, but she is protected from her fear because her practice focuses primarily on the male reality of self-enhancement, responsible action, and an autonomous life of work. "She is a practitioner and not a healer."[21]

Certified Nurse Midwives (CNMs) do much good. Wherever they are, the rate of "abnormal" pregnancies drops dramatically, and the use of interventions decreases. No matter how valuable nurses may have found their nursing training to be, and although it served as their "ticket" into established midwifery in the United States, it was not a necessary prerequisite. Many midwives who are also nurses have said that in order to become real midwives, they had to unlearn much of what they first learned in school. They learned birth as pathology, right along with the doctors. One midwife said that when she told people she was a midwife, people would always ask, "Oh, are you a nurse?" She realized that it was the midwifery, in itself, that she wanted acknowledged and respected. She saw nursing care as helping sick people to get well (as well as prevention), and midwifery as assisting healthy women to have babies. Nurse-midwife has the same ring to me as ballerina-carpenter.

I call the women who do midwifery in the hospitals "FLAMES." Although they bear light, they are also *f*emale *l*abor *a*ssistants who are *m*edical-*e*stablishment *s*upportive. Their orientation/allegiance is within the obstetrical institution or close-by, within the framework of that system; and at the same time, they have a commitment to birthing women and a strong desire to assist them.

Hand-In-Hand

Sonia Johnson says, "We must conquer in ourselves the fierce pangs of competition and jealousy, and rejoice genuinely in one another's successes. We must know in our bones and blood that women are not the enemy. Whether we agree or disagree, we must give the highest priority to hanging in there with one another *no matter what*, with skins of unparallel thickness and the largest of hearts." [emphasis in the original].[22] Obstetricians in this country have nothing to worry about as long as midwives are divided. If midwives can't work together, teach each other, respect each other, and join together, then we all might as well throw out the baby with the bathwater.

A number of midwives groups have been founded, including certified nurse midwives, lay midwives or direct entry (or independent) midwives, and Christian midwives. There are also midwives trained by other midwives, midwives trained at midwifery schools or maternity centers, midwives trained through birth organizations, and midwives pretty much self-taught. MANA, the Midwives Alliance of North America, is working to bring all midwives together in greater strength and understanding, in support of midwifery at large.

Women, especially midwives, are not by nature competitive. They tend to be very sharing.

> I know that this is contrary to some of the thoughts about women in general. But if I know how to spin and you want to know, you come to my house and I teach you. If you weave, and I want to know how to weave, I come and look at your loom and you tell me how you set it up. Women give each other their knowledge. My baby has diarrhea, maybe your baby had it four weeks ago, and I call you up and you say this is what you did, a, b, c. That's what midwives do. They sit by the bedside of woman after woman and watch baby after baby. They join study groups among themselves and learn from each other.[23]

Our patriarchal system sometimes requires that a midwife attend a certain number of births with a physician in order for her to be certified. In turn, it seems to me that doctors should be required to attend many births at home with midwives before *they* are licensed. I know a number of naturopaths, homeopaths, and osteopaths, as well as a few regular obstetricians, who have attended homebirths. In all these situations, in order to provide the appropriate energy for birth, these people have put aside their titles, entered into the feminine, and become, pure and simple—midwives.

Any person who steps outside of the system may be lonely, isolated, and possibly hated. "A woman must want to be a healer in spite of the fear. She must activate her potential and break through her fear and cultural expectations to a new vision of herself, her strengths, her power, and her relationship with others. She must be transformed, both literally and figuratively."[24]

Midwives and VBAC

Some of the most transforming births among midwives have been homebirth VBACs. Jean, a midwife from Texas, writes,

I attended a young woman who had had two cesareans. She had been sectioned at age 16 by an impatient older doctor who admitted her in the latent "warm up" phase of labor, sent her for a pelvimetry, and cut her for a "slightly-flattened sacrum"—all other measurements normal. The second section was a repeat five years later by a different doctor who did a lower transverse incision. So she had an inverted T. In her eighth month, her husband suffered a head injury in a car accident. Afterward, he was not normal. The doctors said it might take a year or two for total recovery. This added much stress to her pregnancy, as you can imagine. . . . Okay, here's the birth story. She DID IT! Without any problem! there was a point at which no progress was being made. We talked for a long time about her last births, her husband, her fears. We squatted together and I started moaning. She moaned along with me. Ten minutes later, she said she had to push. I was never so delighted in my life. I just knew she could do this—needed to do this. She had spent enough time in a hospital, first with her sections, and then with her husband. The midwives in the community were worried about us all. Now they are all beginning to attend VBACs.

Midwife Peg said,

In my community, midwives are so far from public approval and respect that the added political risk of VBAC hardly matters. I attended a woman with three previous classical sections. I didn't come off a high from that birth for—actually, I haven't come off it yet! It has been four years. The mother is pregnant again and I am looking forward to attending her again so much!

A midwife from South Carolina wrote,

I have never been so excited! Everything pointed to a small pelvis—her first baby was only 6 pounds and it was a section. This time, she dilated in seven hours, pushed for three, and out came an 11 pound, 3 ounce baby!!! The joy we all feel is unbelievable. I am on a committee for a birth center here. I will fight to my death for the right to have VBACs there.

Cathy, a midwife from New York, says,

If I had to dedicate my practice to anyone, it would be to VBAC. I feel so drawn to these women! I feel such a pull to give them a fair shot. I suggest to any midwife who feels burned out or discouraged—attend VBAC women for a while—they are really something.

Valerie, a midwife from Michigan, received a dozen red roses from a VBAC husband with a note that read,

Thanks for giving me my sweetheart back.

Mary, a midwife from Ohio,

got a dining room set. The husband was a carpenter, and the wife had had two cesareans. The family was of limited means. As the head was born, he said, "Mary, I know you have wanted a dining room table. I'll build you one!" As the shoulders and arms were born, he said, "And two chairs!" And as the rest of the baby arrived, he said, "How about a whole set?!"

Gloria, a midwife from Canada, says,

I attend HBACs—homebirths after cesareans. The women are magnificent.

Midwife Ruby echoes:

My heart is so wide open to these women who have been so run over by the system. It brings me great joy to be at anyone's homebirth, but a homebirth VBAC has something about it that is just a little bit different because of the previous disappointment.

Midwife Mary writes

One of the most moving births I have ever attended was a VBAC. The woman was blind due to her own two months' premature birth. She was raised by everyone telling her how small she was, and told that her own children would most undoubtedly need to be born surgically. The die was cast. Her second child was born after only 20 minutes of pushing—a 7 lb. 5 oz. daughter. Her birth taught me a lot. I had to really think how it would 'feel' being unsighted in a sighted world . . . feeling insecure and defenseless on an operating table . . . not being able to see people's facial expressions, while they were examining you, not knowing what was to come next. . . . It would be unnerving and demoralizing, but this beautiful woman reached down into her depths and found the determination to carry her dreams out.

Midwife Lynn Richards, a VBAC and homebirth mother herself, writes

I have been privileged to witness the struggles, the pain, the frustration, the joy and the ecstasy of home VBAC mothers. I have seen women grow and change— give birth to themselves. These VBAC births aren't always easy. They are not always perfect, not always the birth of one's dreams. But the issue is not whether or not the baby comes out of the "right hole." The issue is whether or not a woman senses her own power and grows. Having a VBAC brings out the best in women. . . . I do not take credit for these outcomes. It is the woman who heals from her own cesarean, who works through her pregnancy and labor, who vaults the hurdles, who takes the leap of faith in her own body, who lets go and gives birth. I am only the midwife.

VBAC is a transforming event for the woman, too. Caroline, a VBAC mom after two cesareans, writes:

> You weren't listening to me, were you, midwife, when I told you cesareans didn't bother me, only the outcome counted? But you heard my heart screaming for my birthright. You didn't understand why I couldn't hear it. Those five years of screaming had deafened me to myself. It wasn't until after the birth, fulfillment of my birthright, that the screaming stopped. The silence frightened me terribly, and you remained by me, to comfort me, to help me understand.
>
> Both of you advised a hospital birth. Both knew your advice might be ignored. It was. Yet you didn't desert us. You stood by your convictions that the birthing couple has the right to choose the place of birth. It couldn't have happened in the hospital—all those strange ears listening to my screams. . . . We couldn't have stayed at home, unattended—those fierce contractions that reduced ME to scream-ing . . . I could have sworn my twice scarred uterus was rupturing, exploding.
>
> . . . Black stormy sea of miserable, screaming pain, lonely ship, pain-wracked ship. Two light-houses to guide me to safe harbour: Two midwives signalling from one: all is normal, you're okay, you can do it. You were there, telling us all was well . . . even the screaming, so, reassured, we went on. We went on to GIVE birth, to reclaim our bir-thright, to fall more deeply in love. You, midwives, made it possible for the doctor's daughter to be healed. I admire you. I respect you. I love you.
>
> Your courage allowed me to GIVE birth. Will you ever understand the full impact of what you have done for me? I can love life again. I can touch and be touched. My heart is silent, content again—full of love, life and laughter.
>
> The doctor's daughter thanks her midwives . . . she never thanked her doctors. Now she knows why.

With the joy that VBAC and HBAC births can bring, why do so many midwives still screen out these women? For the same reason that they screen out other virtually nonrisk situations: politics and fear. Some midwives have difficulty getting backup for "regular" births. Anything that is considered the least bit "fringe" is forbidden. As one midwife said, "We all want to be able to attend VBACs—and other births as we feel confident—without risking alienation from our peers, badgering from the state, or a jail sentence for practicing 'med-icine' without a license." Another said, "Personally, I have no problem with the thought of VBACs at home—that is where they belong if the woman desires to be there! My concern, my fear, is the same old question that crops up all over—politically, we are sticking our heads on the chopping block. My heart is torn." The difference between midwives who attend VBACs and those who do not seems to be location, backup, peer support, and their own birth experience. One midwife said that, although she didn't have a cesarean herself, her first child was pulled out with forceps. Her next baby wasn't born for twelve years—and she barely had to push and he was born. "But for all those intervening years, I carried the fear that I had an inadequate pelvis and that I might need a section, *all those years.*" This midwife gladly accepts the "cpd's" that arrive at her door.

One group of midwives wrote, "For a midwife to willingly attend a home VBAC would call into question her ability to 'risk-screen', to practice within her scope of [knowledge], and maintain midwifery standards. There is no international standard to use in her defense, and at least yet, no medical literature to support VBAC at home. This leaves her extremely vulnerable—even to criminal negligence! Politically, the whole movement would be at risk, at a time when midwives are misunderstood and struggling for recognition of their role and skills. The midwife would be painted as ignorant, careless; the parents as self-indulgent, misled fanatics, seeking 'experience' over safety. None of this is fair. However, after years in midwifery politics, we think it is real."[25] Midwives do not abandon clients, but once the situation is explained, most of the couples they counsel choose to go to a hospital. Michele Odent has said that the risk for the VBAC mother is emotional—to try and to "fail"; the risk for the doctor is economic—money out of his pocket; the risk for the midwife is the biggest of all—it is a political risk that can cost a great deal emotionally and economically.[26]

Midwife-author Peg Spindel writes that the first premise to which every point must refer is that midwives support cesarean prevention and VBACs "unquestioningly and wholeheartedly. . . . This assertion holds true whether or not a particular midwife is willing to attend home VBACs or not." One would be hard pressed, she says, to find a midwife who believed that because a woman has a scar on her uterus she is too high risk for midwifery care. However, "Midwives are in a bit of a moral quandary. . . . We are dedicated to both the individual and to the movement. Sometimes one is pitted directly against the other." The best hope for us all, we are told, is strong consumer support and lobbying.[27]

One such effort resulted in the formation in 1986 of an organization called Friends of Midwives; it began in Massachusetts and then networked across the country.

One woman found a midwife that was willing to attend her at home. "We couldn't tell anyone about it. Not our family or friends, and certainly not the doctor, in order to protect the midwife. I had nightmares that she was nabbed in the middle of the night because of us, even though things went beautifully. I hated the schizophrenia of the whole situation."

A number of nurses have remained in the hospital and become midwives. Some have left hospitals and become midwives. One midwife told me that she could no longer accept the protocols that had been forced on the midwifery staff where she worked. Another wrote, "I cannot work under conditions that make a normal birth almost impossible. It has become impossible for me to stay on . . . in the midst of a battle over basic maternity-care issues, when some physicians are choosing to exercise their power over midwives and other physicians in a manner I fundamentally disagree with." This woman was a midwife from the beginning. What frequently happens is that the really talented people, those who really need to be in the hospitals to save us all, often get burned out and discouraged—and leave, much to the satisfaction of most obstetricians.

Several articles I read stated that the doctors' view is that midwifery is invading territory that has for the past forty years belonged to them. But whom did the doctors rob it from in the first place? In some areas, the ashes still burn. If a baby dies at home, it is the midwife's fault. If a baby dies in the hospital, it

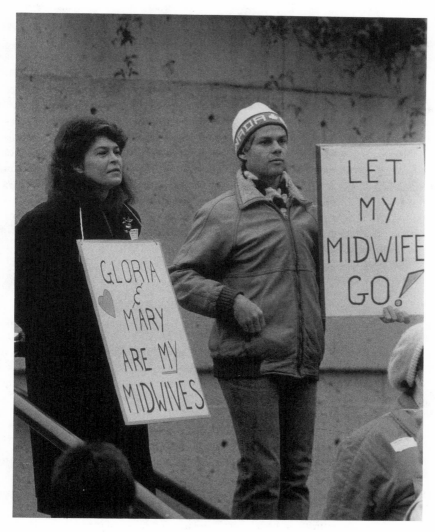

© DUNCAN BELL-IRVING PHOTOGRAPHY

couldn't possibly be the doctor's fault—he's absolved. If something happens at a hospital, it's "just one of those things." If something happens at home, however, doctors often accuse midwives of incompetence.

> Midwives are presumed guilty and must prove their innocence. In courtrooms, [we hear] bizarre and surreal tones that characterized a witchcraft trial. In court, expert witnesses are called to "enlighten" the jury. . . . If the midwife appears afraid this is sure proof—her conscience accuses her; if she does not show fear, this too is proof, for witches characteristically pretend innocence and wear a bold front . . .

she can never clear herself. The investigative committee would feel a disgrace if it acquitted [her] once arrested . . . she has to be guilty, by fair means or foul.[28]

Phyllis Chesler asks, "To what extent are witchcraft trials a means of keeping all women humble?" "When did the trials finally end? They never have." She reminds us that the men who sought to help the women were known as "witch lovers," or accomplices, and were executed alongside the women. "Eventually those who at first clamor most loudly to feed the [fires] are themselves involved, for they rashly fail to see that their turn too will come. Heaven justly punishes those who send so many innocent to the stake. . . . Judges must suspend the trials . . . or else burn their own fold, themselves, and everybody else for all are sooner or later falsely accused, and if tortured, are all proved guilty."[29] Mark Gerzon remarks that every witch hunt is sexual, and that sex and politics are always interwoven.[30]

One midwife, who was also a nursing supervisor, was suspended from her teaching job because the obstetrical group at the hospital "could not allow their patients to be exposed to one who advocates the home delivery concept."[31] (In a similar case, the judge admonished the medical profession to have enough "maturity" to accept different birthing practices.)[32] Plastered over newspapers in this country are accusations against midwives by local sheriffs' offices and state officials. These midwives are intelligent, skilled, qualified birth attendants. Some have been run out of town. They are scapegoats for the establishment's fears about birth and death. Yet, Margaret Atwood has said, "We all have this little fantasy of ourselves that we'd be brave and daring, but when the witch hunt is on the rampage, it takes extraordinary courage."[33]

Some midwives have tried to license midwifery, but there is no consensus among them as to whether or not this is the best "plan." Archie Brodsky, a staunch midwifery advocate, writes,

> . . . What good will it do if midwives continue to be regarded as having "less" rather than "different" expertise, homebirth as "just a little less safe" rather than arguably safer, and unmedicated birth as a perverse "extreme" rather than the norm?; if the medical monopoly can successfully portray those rejecting assembly-line childbirth as back-to-nature fanatics or self-indulgent yuppies?; if a new generation of consumers is conditioned to think that our battles have been won and everything is fine in the hospitals now?; if Third World countries and people of color in the U.S. give up traditional childbearing practices in favor of the status symbol of medicalized birth? In other words, what good will it do for midwives to be legal [or licensed] if they don't have enough clients to earn a living?[34]

"Women . . . are rapidly losing access to midwives through a complex set of factors such as increasingly conservative definitions of risk and intense conflicts between midwives and physicians over the management of birth."[35]

For those interested in the question of "To license or not to license," a recent book by Raymond De Vries may be of interest.[36] He tells us that state sanctions do not empower midwives: they merely formalize the dominance of the system

over them. I have read material on the myths, abuses, dangers, and miscon-
ceptions of licensure and on the benefits of it as well. I have spoken to midwives
who are very much in favor of it and to those who are vehemently opposed.
Either way, we are working within a system that is *totally* male, and we are "in
reaction" to that. We are trying to fit the proverbial square peg into the round
hole. Margot Edwards and Mary Waldorf ask, "How are we to resurrect a
profession that has been thoroughly vilified; and very nearly legislated out of
existence?"[37] Midwife Vickie Roy says, "There is so much controversy—and
now we seem to be fighting each other as well as the state departments!" Midwife
Lynn Richards says that, in truth, the whole medical-legal system must be
changed. She is right. It seems impossible to accomplish what we must within
its confines. Perhaps what we need to do is to disregard it completely and to
establish a system that reflects our own values and needs. (The best system of
all, of course, is one in balance—one that honors *humankind*.)

Jutta Mason has written two articles on licensure: "Reflections on the Alternative Birth Culture: Does Professional Midwifery Pose a Problem?" and "Licensed Midwifery: A Promise Betrayed." She says:

> We took on the gray, conservative heads of obstetrical departments and struggled
> with them in meetings, scandalizing them with our stubbornness. . . . Some women
> found that the project of restructuring obstetrics called for great ingenuity and
> strength of will, and provided a challenge they enjoyed; so they stayed with the
> task, practicing politics and changing policies, for years. Today some obstetrical
> units show astonishing evidence of the accomplishments of these patient, powerful
> women, working both from outside and inside the institutional hierarchy.
>
> But some of us found that the project of reforming medical obstetrics was too
> much of a vacuum, sucking up all time and energy, ultimately crushing imagi-
> nation—and de-railing us from our original intent, which was to put our women's
> neighbour-network back together without the mediation of meddling of medical
> men.

Jutta goes on. "We must be mindful of the dangers attached to the profession-
alization of the neighborly midwife and her admission into mainstream obstetrics.
I would like to talk about the dangers, not to the soul of the midwife, but to
the continued well-being of the alternative birth culture." She describes the "six
dangers of licensing" and what must be done to avoid them, (for a copy send
$2.00 and a SASE to her at 242 Havelock Street, Toronto, MGH 3B9 Canada).
She writes,

> Lots of people besides myself are uncomfortable with the direction midwives seem
> to be taking. In my opinion there is a lot of confusion in the thinking about this,
> compounded by a lightning-fast forgetting of even the recent history of the natural
> childbirth movement. There is a real danger that the alternative childbirth culture
> is going to be overwhelmed—swamped—by the newly renovated, revitalized twen-
> tieth century high-tech obstetrics. Midwives tell me that their clientele—part of
> it—is changing: more women are coming to them fully intending to have epidural
> anesthesia, with supportive midwives at their side ("They want to be pampered.")

Also, the midwives here are getting very complicated questions about the latest prenatal and labour technologies—the clients expect them to help them choose the best, the state-of-the-art options.

In most states, the Health Department or the Board of Medical Examiners oversees midwives and defines standards for them. Shari Daniels, who established the Birth Center for El Paso, Texas, says, "That means physical control. It's like Avis controlling Hertz."[38] Another quote: "Practice licensure perpetuates the existence of health care, which grants some providers more power and authority than they merit, while wasting the talents and skills of others, stifling upward mobility and making turf conflicts inevitable."[39]

Those who favor licensing midwives maintain that it will provide "consistent standards for gauging the standards of practitioners." In addition, it will allow insurers to reimburse midwives' clients for birth expenses. Even those who are in favor of licensure agree that it could severely restrict midwives from making autonomous decisions and could limit many women from homebirths.[40] No matter whether or not it is government regulated, state approved, or simply given some Good Housekeeping Seal of Approval, unless the issue of female oppression is addressed, it's not going to make a difference. After lobbying at the state house myself a few times, I knew that that wasn't where it was at for me. Yet I am grateful to others who have persevered and made some important legislative changes that have benefited many birthing women. Archie Brodsky, President of Massachusetts Friends of Midwives, says that one thing is for certain: It is time to stop the absurd usage of the legal system to intimidate and harass midwives.[41] If there is to be structure, it needs to be midwives—all kinds of midwives—together—assisting, teaching, sharing—not judging—others. Midwives must feel the trust and confidence in each other that they so easily inspire in birthing women.

Peace, I Ask of Thee Oh River

Doctors and midwives in England work successfully together. "They have an understanding and acceptance of one another's role. . . . It would be wrong not to acknowledge the role of the obstetrician, but not as being somehow superior or preferable to the midwife." This model of cooperative care with mutual respect is rarely found in the United States. Doctors here see women as "patients" with childbirth as their "illness." Most of these doctors have never seen a normal birth.[42] Dr. Edwin Hersh, an obstetrician who works with midwives at the Kaiser Permanente center in California says, "We work as a team. Some people have the mistaken idea that doctors and midwives must be in competition with each other, but that is not true." Gandhi once said that peace between countries must rest on a solid foundation of love between individuals. It seems to me that there is a lesson for us all, midwife-to-midwife, midwife-to-doctor, and doctor-to-midwife here.

Every unborn child and pregnant mother have a right, respectively, to be born and to give birth at home or in a woman-centered facility with any number of chosen "others" in attendance.[43] Friends of Midwives writes that those women who are truly high-risk, who choose hospital birth, or who have no out-of-hospital options available must have the right to "humane, empowering care."[44] As women bring forth life on this earth, they want the guidance and support of other women who themselves have labored to bring forth life. "So we invite our midwives to be with us . . . When we bear our children, we are not acting as patients ministered to by physicians. Neither are we consuming medical services. When we bear our children, we are living our lives."[45] I envision the women who choose hospital births going—not to an obstetrician's office—but to a "counsel of wise women."[46]

Clearly, cooperation among all midwives is needed. We all share the dream. We are, this time in a positive sense, "co-dependent." One midwife says, "We've gotta quit being so bitchy to our sister midwives, stop putting our noses down in condescension, start sharing more with each other, and break down the barriers to a place of love and honor. We are all in this together."

> It's the pain we dare to share,
> That's what knits us together.
> That's the bond that endures.
> We are guided to go deep,
> to caverns and dragons within,
> and to pain within,
> and to dare to let it out,
> to bring it out of dread and darkness
> into the healing light. . . .
> And during our days of daring
> we release some of that storming thunder,
> some of the kicking and the screaming and the sobbing,
> some of the feelings imprisoned for a lifetime. . . .
> Witnessing others confront their pain:
> ready to confront our own.
> Not one of us will forget the fire,
> Nor the light in each other's eyes.
> Amazing, is it not, that we know so little
> about the details of each other's lives
> and yet know each other so well?
> It's the pain we dare to share.[47]

And the joy.

Peggy Spindel, past president of the Massachusetts Midwives Association, says: "Midwifery really matters. . . . It is a natural and necessary expression of our deepest convictions about people, about nature, about women, about right and wrong, about what makes a good life and a good society. It is something essential, something worth fighting for, something not to be compromised away."

I've heard that in New Zealand, midwives are becoming an endangered species.[48]

It almost happened here. A world without midwives is a dark, cold, cutting, barren existence. Today New Zealand, tomorrow Australia? Then where? We cannot allow this to happen. Greenpeace will help to save the seals and the dolphins—we all must prevent the slander and the slaughter of these women.

10 *Hospitals: Cesarean Baby Factories*

"No, Mom, it's a *hostipal*, and you get there in an *ambleeance!*"
—my son, age 6

PART I HOSPITALS

Something vital is missing from American medicine, "and it isn't research or technology." Treatment in hospitals, we are told, is not only inadequate, "but humiliating and uncaring enough to break our spirits and even deprive people of the will to live. All our vaunted technology is brought to bear on us, but there is a lack of personal concern, humanity, and even simple courtesy."[1]

We know some things for sure about hospitals. They cost a lot of money. They're for sick people. For the most part, the food isn't so hot. They serve jello. They've got gift shops and hallways and special places for cigarette smoking. They've got a medical records department, operating rooms, and tons of equipment. They're dirty; a significant percentage of people get infections in hospitals that they didn't have when they arrived. Sometimes they're named after saints.

Recently, *The Boston Globe* reported that one of China's rare pandas had given birth.[2] "The watch on the panda mother ended when she could no longer stand the noise and human intrusions" from a logging area about fifty yards away, and so she disappeared into the forest preserve. This was a tremendous disappointment since the birth of a panda in captivity is a rare thing. "Gao Huakang went out to check on reported panda sightings and found the mother twisting around inside a hollow tree, groaning occasionally." The next day, a cooing sound from the tree confirmed the birth, the article said. Exactly one month after the birth, Momma Panda took the baby into the forests and "disappeared."

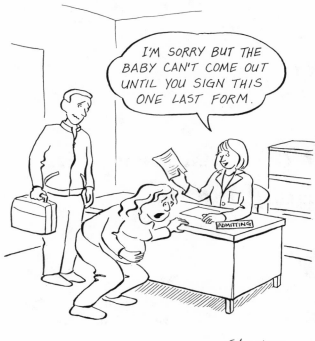

Schwartz ©89

In our culture, women flock to hospitals to have babies the way their mothers' generation flocked to Filene's Basement for a sale. They believe that the "noise and human intrusion" within spitting distance is just a part of the "inconvenience" they must ignore in order to "be safe" and get "quality" care. Some, in fact, do not regard the "necessary" paper work and check-in, the preliminary blood work, and the "getting settled into your room" a disturbance into their routine at all. They have been conditioned to believe that these are the normal things that go with having an easier birth and a healthy baby. Smart Panda, Stupid Women.

Ill at Ease

Rennie Stoltenberg, we are told, didn't choose her hospital because of the candlelight dinner it offered to new parents, "but she thought [it] would be a nice celebratory touch." Then she had a c-section and was in the hospital for six days because of an infection. "By the time we got the dinner, I didn't care. I just wanted to go home."[3]

Candlelight dinners are not the only "fringe benefits" that hospitals and birth centers are offering to "lure" prospective obstetrics patients these days; they often offer a wide array of prenatal and postnatal classes, pagers for expectant fathers who want to be alerted when labor begins, fashion shows of maternity wear, valet parking, designer labor-delivery-recovery rooms, and even, "for those who have prepaid their bill," a "Stork Club" in which new moms and dads can entertain their friends and enjoy fancy dinners with wine and flowers.[4]

These new developments are the result of two developments. First, the business climate for hospitals has become more competitive. Second, parents-to-be have become aware that they have options. In the past, a woman would automatically go to the hospital where her doctor sent her. These days, she can often select from two or three where her OB has privileges. Aware of this "shopper" phenomenon, hospitals are now marketing their services through advertising or other promotions.

Among some of the advertisements that have been sent to me from women across the country is one that says, in big bold letters: Hospital "X" introduces the kind of birth control an expectant mother wants. This, of course, gives a whole new meaning to the words "birth control," and is perhaps one of the key issues in birth today: Who is really in control of this birth, anyway? While everyone is mouthing the words, "Why, the mother, of course," opinions vary widely.

Martha Weinman Lear remarks that she has only begun to realize the enormity of the issues of authority and intimidation (present as subheadings under the bigger issue of "Control") in medicine. She talks about "hospital hierarchy." She says that a definite "totem pole of intimidation" exists and that we, the consumers, the patients, are at the bottom. "The weight is crushing."[5]

Another advertisement for a maternity unit at a local hospital warns: "The most hazardous journey your baby will ever take is only as long as this line. . . . one of the most traumatic times of your child's life occurs at childbirth. During this journey, through the birth canal, life-threatening distress can arise in an infant virtually without warning. Problems may also occur after delivery, endangering mother or child or both." The line is approximately three inches. There is the supine silhouette of a pregnant belly on the page, and the line is right above the middle of it. I think of those three, long, dangerous inches of the birth canal. It is hot and damp. The sun is beating down. The tropical birds are in the trees above, watchful, cautious. Yes, sir, there are alligators in this water. What they don't tell you, of course, is that the longest journey we women take, is the one from the delivery room into the OR. It lasts a lifetime. This particular advertisement represents the view of our culture at large: that birth is dangerous. In addition, the line above the abdomen is located in such a way that it looks like a classical cesarean scar. As to the dangers that await, lurking in the shadows, for the baby, we have only to open our ears and listen to the deafening sounds of newborn tears all across our land. Some people still think babies are supposed to cry like that.

More than one hospital now advertises epidural classes and epidural refresher courses. It's unthinkable that they are not only offered but are also popular enough that they keep being offered. A group of trusting, ignorant momdads who learn how to get numbed out by a dangerous, unnecessary procedure in order to have a baby.

Hospitals also make possible "every mother's nightmare": a maternity ward "mix-up" sending the parents home with the wrong baby. One of the articles states that when the baby was handed to the mother she said, "I didn't know if he was mine or not. But he was so tiny. He looked like he needed help." Another mother said she recognized her baby "by his fat cheeks and his hair."[6] Lots of babies have fat cheeks and hair. It is just so, so sad. . . .

A recent study done by researchers at Harvard University concludes that negligence "kills thousands of people in hospitals each year and injures many more." It is the most comprehensive study of medical malpractice ever conducted in the United States.[7] In an article entitled, "You can Say 'No' to a Hospital Stay," Inlander and Weiner tell us that most of us begin life in a hospital— naked, wet, and protesting. Most of us, they say, "unfortunately," will make at least one return trip as an adult, "in a similarly vulnerable position, vulnerable to poking, probing, and drugging for which we will be slapped with a mile-long computerized bill."[8] P.S. Check the bill. Up to 97% may contain overcharges.[9]

Sick and Tired

As many as one out of every three people who leave a hospital do so with a problem that was not there before they entered. Pregnant women did not have trouble urinating or gas pains, for starters. These are not generally the necessary sequellae of normal childbirth, although they have come to be expected in hospitals as the price one has to pay for having a baby. Before you become a statistic, "you need to consider whether hospitalization is really required *for your situation*. [emphasis mine]. Just because your doctor says you belong in the hospital doesn't mean you positively do."[10]

Laurence Cherry writes, "A hospital is no place for a sick person to be. Each year two million people contract infections that have nothing to do with the ailments they were admitted for. As a result, 300,000 die."[11] (Other "mishaps," he says—errors in medication, anesthesia mistakes, and accidents—may harm millions more annually). If a hospital is no place for a sick person, it is certainly no place for the well either. Pregnant women are healthy, normal individuals.

In an eight-year study at Cornell University Medical Center, 25 percent of patients who were told they needed surgery were subsequently told by a second doctor that they didn't need it. "Most chose to believe the second doctor and lived very nicely without it."[12] Four of the five women in the past years who have contacted me because their doctors recommended hysterectomies followed a number of suggestions I provided, including some excellent reading material on the subject, and found they did not need surgery. Remember, too, that second-opinion doctors recommended by first-opinion doctors do not represent a second opinion at all. Inlander and Weiner call them "professional ditto marks." Reluctant to disagree with a friend, or the colleague who recommended them, they are simply a "carboned school of thought." And, too, the more tests you have, the less chance you have of being judged normal by all the tests. "Some abnormality, however insignificant, is bound to surface [which] can lead to unnecessary treatment of a nonexistent condition.[13] Tests, however, cost money, and hospitals need more of it.

There is no such thing as minor surgery. "Sudden emergencies can and do happen during all types of operations" and procedures.[14] Anesthesia alone can produce grave consequences. Yup, hospitals can be dangerous zoos. A few big hairy gorillas and a whole lot of monkey business.

Commandments?

Most institutions have rules, and hospitals are no exception. They are called "policies," and it must be written somewhere that God Himself (in this case, definitely male) has established such commandments. Author Judith Herzfeld reminds us that decisions often have to be made under the pressure of time and physical stress, but "the protocols of one hospital are ridiculed by others" and "what was considered outrageous five years ago is now considered standard practice."[15] Years ago, I wanted to have my two children present for the birth of our third baby. When I spoke to the hospital, they said that they would be "instituting a policy of that nature sometime in the future." Since I was pregnant already, I couldn't wait for them to institute some conditional, provisional, or restrictive policy. At another hospital, the policy states that a child had to be at least six years old to attend the birth of a sibling. Judy wrote to her hospital, "This policy is ridiculous. I don't know any couples who voluntarily wait until their firstborn is six or more years old and few who would take their first to the hospital and leave their others behind. My daughter's age (below six) is optimal in that she is old enough to understand what she is told and to reason with, without being so old as to bring her own preconceptions into a situation."[16] Yet another hospital requires "psychiatric evaluation" of the attending siblings. The whole system is nuts.

A woman from Michigan wrote to the hospital closest to her regarding VBAC. She received the following reply from the vice president of professional services: "Your letter has been referred to me for a reply. Our hospital does have an established policy currently in effect which does not permit an attempted vaginal delivery following a cesarean section. This policy was enacted because it was felt to be in the best interest of our patients. I regret any inconvenience this causes you." Having an unnecessary cesarean is in the best interests of the *patients*? She changed hospitals, of course, and had a VBAC at *her* convenience.

Rules. You can't take the baby out of the hospital until the pediatrician has checked her, or you can't have visitors, or you can't do this—or you have to have an IV or you have to do it that way, all under the guise of hospital policy.

I have some rules too, some of my own "policies." You can't interrupt me when I am nursing. You do not have permission to take my baby away. I do not have to tell you how much I peed.

Harriet Tubman, I Need You!

Shifra writes,

> Everyone just accepts hospitals as part of the birth scene. I see them as a curse. Almost everything they do there seems criminal. I applaud your attempts to make radical changes. My experiences at two different hospitals were not too unpleasant; however, in retrospect, they are both crystallized in a single composite scene— that of my escape. I am running down a hospital corridor, clutching my newborn treasure. A doctor or nurse is in hot pursuit, shouting "You can't take that baby; he's not even two days old!" (I never even tried to escape on the first day.) Attempting to separate pursuer from pursued is my hero, my husband, getting away with all this only because he is a radiologist, a member of the hallowed brotherhood. He is saying: "Let me take them home; I'll be back here anyway and I'll sign the papers then." His facial expression, well-rehearsed, is eminently legible: You know how crazy postpartum women are.

At the hospitals I've visited, been in, and heard about, everybody thinks everybody else is in charge. "That's not my department"; "That's because of administration"; "We can't do it that way, the doctors won't allow it"; "Doctors run the show here? Nonsense! Those nurses walk all over us." Lear says the doctors are on top. "Then comes the house staff who are intimidated by the doctors; the nurses who are intimidated by the house staff; the aides by the nurses; the orderlies by the aides."[17] And the patients are intimidated by mostly everyone. The really good nurses, the "hot mammas" as one of the momdads called them, eventually get called on the carpet, and too often get the rug pulled out from underneath them.

Studies show that parents' first concern when searching for a hospital (or birth center) is the level of emergency care available. In many of the letters I have received, women were kept waiting for emergency cesareans (or what they were told were emergencies; in a few cases they were) for hours. Operating rooms were not "set up" or "available" or anesthesiologists could not be located. One father, writing about his wife's emergency, said, "There was panic. Not professional expediency and quick-action: panic. They had lost a baby a few weeks earlier and there was a big law suit going on. . . . It was a fiasco." Another letter says, "Our labor occurred on a particularly busy night in the hospital. At one point, the nurse hooked my wife up to a monitor and said as she walked out the door, "It's really busy here tonight. Watch that for me, will you? If it goes above that line, it's an emergency. Call me right away."

One woman wrote: "I am the wife of a physician. Nevertheless (and believe it or not, often along with my husband—he has a well-educated fear of surgery)

I have expended many millions of words trying to convince the faithful that hospitals are the greatest threat to the health of almost all who enter their portals. I have been to Israel: I believe I have a sacred obligation to refute [most people's] ideas about hospitals and to help them rebel against this powerful idol."

Hospital forms crack me up. One states, "We expect total cooperation from the husband and from the patient at all times." Another reminds us that those in charge have complete authority. Pregnant couples enter the hospital during labor (hopefully very active labor) and are expected to read forms, look at the fine print, and sign on the dotted line. Tomes of medical records are stored in "vaults" [read: medical libraries]; one doctor, the head of a department (one of the enlightened few, a VBAC father himself) told me that record-altering was common practice. "The truth," he said, "is worse than fiction." He said that he had asked for an investigation into the matter, "but it is the guilty people doing the investigating! It's like the pot calling the kettle black." I have been told that some doctors change the Apgar scores on medical records to "prove" that their interference begets healthy babies.

One woman wrote that she has been trying to get statistics from her hospital for months. She talked to everyone imaginable there, including the Chief of Staff, but to no avail. They all agree that the cesarean rate is "much too high," she says, but no one has been able to give her any further help. She said, "I talked to their Risk Manager (an apt title!) who advised me that 'this information could be damaging in the wrong hands.' . . . I get the distinct impression that they have something to hide." Another woman said that the hospital was unable to provide her with the data she requested about c-sections, because those operations were filtered into the information about surgery in general. I mean, can you believe it? She was told to ask her doctor about his own c-section rate. "Well, I asked until I was blue in the face and still haven't gotten a straight answer." This determined and resourceful woman has collected all the birth announcements from the local newspapers and is compiling a questionnaire to determine what's going on.

Yet another woman wrote that her hospital refused to give out statistics on cesareans, episiotomies, and so on, because "they have distorted statistics because they do all the high risk deliveries in this part of the state."

In hospital, the doctors are king, and all who come "beneath" him are his loyal servants. The birthing woman is by no means Queen; that position is reserved perhaps for the Nursing Supervisor. And all the little "royal subjects"— our babies—are being given the royal once-over under royal lights in the royal kingdom called a nursery. Funny, because they don't nurse babies there; they give them bottles of sugar water. Now's as good a time as any to remind you that the bright lights in hospital nurseries contribute to the development of a degenerative eye disease in babies. It just isn't normal for babies to be away from their mothers under fluorescent lights all those hours.

I used to recommend to women that they do whatever they felt necessary to get comfortable with their naked bodies. After all, a certain amount of nudity was probable at birth. Sit in front of a mirror! I'd say. Get a massage. Dance naked. Lately, I've changed my tune. It's not that I want women to be inhibited, quite the contrary. It's nice to have a back rub, or to feel the freedom to dance in the wind. But I now realize that I was asking women to feel freer not for their own internal growth and ease, but so that all the UFOs (Uniformed Figures who Observe) who appear in the delivery—or operating—room, nurses, technicians, residents, aides, and so on, wouldn't throw her off. There's nothing wrong with a naked body, but no one should have to display theirs to all those employed on the third floor of "County General." Robert Mendelsohn called obstetrical rotation in medical school a "peep show"—an invasion of privacy and a violation of constitutional rights.[18] Of course, if the birthing woman is going to be naked, in the OR for example, perhaps the only fair thing is for everyone else to be naked as well, except, of course, for hats, masks and shoe covers and gloves.

Baby Factories and AIDS

According to the one video on perinatal AIDS, "No hospital can be considered to be entirely risk-free."[19] Viruses have been isolated from tears, saliva, amniotic fluid, breast milk, vaginal secretions, urine and blood, all of which are a part of normal labor and delivery. (The tears, of course, are most often present at cesarean sections, and the semen most often at home births. Yes, Virginia, there can be sex at birth.) The video recommends that all health care providers who might get splashed in the eyes with blood should wear goggles. With all the cesareans and episiotomies done in this country, I urge you to buy stock in goggles immediately. On second thought, the economy's not great. Forget it. Besides, goggles aren't enough. Since the nose also has to be protected from the "blood splashing," you need a face mask.

Are there many among us who have not been touched in some way by AIDS? Unfortunately, it is something we all must consider when we make our choices about birth.

The Florences

You can't really talk about hospitals without talking about nurses. All the nurses whom I've ever met at any of my conferences or speaking engagements have been wonderful, great women—caring, concerned, and hard-working. But how can they be party to hooking laboring women up to unnecessary and dangerous gadgets, starving them, and giving them drugs? They must know at least how dangerous drugs are in labor. I know it's "doctor's orders," but some orders must be resisted. Moreover, most nurses rely almost totally on technology and don't know how to use a fetoscope. Many counter that they "can't find" the fetoscope, or that they "can't hear the baby," when in fact, either they are untrained to use one or are afraid that the doctor will be angry when he hears that the heartbeat has been recorded according to human ears rather than some machine. I know they're only human, but they're selling out, left and right.

Despite the nurse's natural diffidence in the presence of doctors, bitter confrontations do occur between doctors and nurses at hospitals across the country. "When a doctor who is used to being treated as if he were infallible runs up against a nurse who questions his decisions, the result is often a battle royal. In some situations, the hostility is so great, patient care deteriorates."[20] Those nurses who stay on the hospital floor, rather than advance professionally or become teachers or administrators, are often regarded by many—including doctors—as "handmaidens" whose main duties are somewhat menial. Doctors will often disregard their advice, even when they can be of great assistance to the patient. Doctors accuse nurses of wanting the doctor's power "but none of the life and death responsibility. . . . The situation resembles a family that is coming apart, and the patient—like the child in a divorce—is often caught in the middle."[21]

Nowhere does this seem more true than in obstetrics. I speak to nurses all over the country, and they are tired of being treated subordinately. Many of them truly fear the OBs they work for, for their paycheck is essentially in their hands. They work hard to please doctors, and they often feel unappreciated. "There are two doctors in the hospital I work at," says Christine, "who practice quite differently. One likes to be at the birth at least twenty minutes before the baby is born—he likes the fame and glory he receives for rescuing the woman at the end and delivering the baby. The other has 'had it' with obstetrics. He wants to breeze in as the baby is being born, just so he can get his fee. Then there are all the other OBs, each with their own little quirks about how things are supposed to be done. I get yelled at for not remembering which likes which, and how far dilated someone is supposed to be before the doctor gets his wake-up call."

One nurse said, "Where I work, a woman is not allowed to birth her baby unless a doctor is present." "What if the baby is just plain coming out?" I asked her. "We panic," she replied. "We yell down the hall, 'Get a doctor!' That usually—not always, but usually—slows the labor down."

Another nurse remarks, "I always thought that the doctor-nurse relationship meant two professionals working side-by-side. . . . I was stunned to be ordered about. . . . 'Do this; do that. Get out of here.' In front of the patients!"[22] This RN isn't the only one who feels doctors vent their anger freely. Several nurses told me that they had learned that the best way to 'keep peace' was to be "sweet, orderly, efficient, and compliant."

Lois Morris writes, "In nursing school, a nurse is instructed that her first duty is to the patient, not to the doctor. That means that she is supposed to question any order she feels is not in the best interest of her patient."[23] When nurses challenge doctors who have made a mistake, they often face an aggressive doctor as well as an administration that is more sympathetic to the physician (who brings in patients, i.e., money, to the hospital). The nurse is frequently right, but she gets little for her efforts except an embarrassed doctor on whose bad side she now stands.

Since nurses often feel powerless to confront doctors directly, they punish disrespectful, overly demanding, or unfair physicians by "subterfuge . . . passive aggressive behavior. They slow down, pretend not to hear orders, or insist on going strictly by the rules."[24] This, we are told, is an expression of the nurses' powerlessness because they are not being dealt with as professionals.

Making life difficult for each other is easy. Working out differences is harder, but Morris gives some hope. A national nursing commission for "peace talks" was formed a number of years ago, and in some hospitals group therapy sessions have been initiated in order to help communication between doctors and nurses. Arguments often erupt, "but this is good. Arguments erupt between equals."[25] Arguments that erupt at birth only help a birthing woman *on occasion*. More often, the tensions and upset that arise adversely affect labor.

Dis-Ease

According to Ellen Switzer, "Something vital is missing from American medicine, and it isn't research or technology. Whatever happened to *caring*?[26] Nurses sometimes take their frustrations out on patients, "particularly those who ask for what the nurses consider to be too much attention." In labor, women need love and attention far more than they need drugs or IVs or monitors or vaginal exams. We all know that. And babies need for their mothers to not have all that stuff. In this country we seemingly reward doctors for technology and procedures, not for wisdom and empathy. "More and more, doctors are paid by insurance companies and this alters the quality of care. After all, a physician can't submit a bill for an hour's conversation. But he can for a battery of tests. And the insurance company will pay, whether the doctor has been pleasant and concerned or clinical and indifferent."[27]

Many other non-professional staff (cleaning and kitchen) work part time and are not eligible for benefits. They are paid less than they would be in a profit-making business. "It is no wonder that many of these people feel no dedication to their jobs or . . . concern for the patients." If they drop a dinner tray in a patient's lap or forget to change the sheets, they are often more indifferent than apologetic: "After all, what's the worst that can happen to them? If they're fired, they can usually find a job for the same wages at the nearest fast-food restaurant or coffee shop." A hotel has to worry whether the service was satisfactory and wouldn't consider disregarding or insulting its guests; hospitals seem to operate differently.

The patient is usually at the bottom of the pecking order. This is an interesting finding considering that the health-care system is basically a service industry and the patients are the ones who pay the bills. She also says that some patients are more popular than others. Patients who are "cantankerous or emotional . . . get less attention than those who are attractive and polite."[28] Gail said: "When I was in labor, I looked like hell, I complained a lot, and I made sounds that must have approximated the mating call of some really weird goose. The nurses kept telling me to quiet down and stop all the noise. I felt as if they really hated me." But we should go easy on nurses; they have a great deal of responsibility but very little authority, "a situation that is guaranteed to sour anyone's disposition."[29]

Everyone, it seems, is a little on edge at the hospital:

> There is the admissions clerk, who is often curt, rude and concerned only with insurance, even when a patient comes in . . . in pain. There is the constant procession of interns and residents who poke the patient's body and conduct informal consultations as if the patient wasn't there. And there are the physicians who don't seem to have the time to explain procedures, nurses who don't answer bells, and aides who leave patients perched . . . for what seems like hours.[30]

Off to War?

It is into this environment that the unsuspecting pregnant American woman takes herself for one of the most important spiritual experiences of her life. Childbirth educator Sidney Mitchell writes:

> Yet our culture, in its overall lack of understanding, requires that we relinquish this vital process to medical jurisdiction by displacing our rite of passage to the hospital setting. There are many fine rationales for this . . . but there lies in this precedent an inherent congruency. As far as our psyches are concerned, having a baby in the hospital is as incongruent as birthing on the check-out counter at the supermarket where our contractions are "read" via plastic and metal electronic apparatus. . . . Automatically, our [output] is packaged and assigned to an individual steel cage on wheels, the bill is paid and we wheel our stuff back to the amorphous sphere of private living. . . . [31]

There are signs, of course, that things are improving. With a surplus of doctors and surgeons and too many hospital beds in some areas, "hospitals that alienate the community may face dire consequences."[32] There is also a growing number of hospitals for profit that compete for patients. The medical establishment itself has begun to realize the mistakes it has made, and is looking to combine technology with old-fashioned TLC. But most changes take a very long time, much longer than nine months.

We can get the kind of response we want from hospitals first by accepting responsibility in making the choice of hospital as birthplace. Often parents grumble and complain or display paranoia, or extreme docility and embarrassment in the hospital setting, simply because they gave little prior thought to their choice. "To later [place] blame wholly on the shoulders of a hospital staff is, in the majority of cases, a scapegoat maneuver of parents who are unwilling to admit their lack of preparedness."[33]

Next, we can gain an understanding of "the other side"—what the hospital represents in the minds of the health care providers on staff. Ellen Switzer reminds us once again that today hospitals are very much like any other large corporation—oriented, bureaucratic, preoccupied with labor-management co-existence, and permeated with group identity. Because of these dynamics, the hospital is the "homeplace" of the nurse, the doctor, the technician—the people involved have become a part of their setting. In this sense, even though the parents may not be enjoying a homebirth, the hospital staff is.[34]

We must cultivate the attitude of being "clientele" and approach health care providers as those whose sole function it is to accommodate you. "Whether or not they feel you are the guest in their home is beside the point, as long as your assertive approach to them elicits the properly hospitable response." We've invited strangers to participate in one of the most intimate processes available to human experience, and for this women had better be prepared.

Years ago, I couldn't imagine having a baby anywhere except a hospital. If I was pregnant now, I wouldn't be caught dead in one.

PART II   SMACK DAB IN THE MIDDLE: BIRTH CENTERS

I get letters from midwives who say, "We are so excited! After several years of planning, our center will finally open its doors next month." Then I get letters from other midwives who say, "Our center is shutting down. There just didn't seem to be any way to continue, given the politics around here. . . . "

Birthing centers are supposed to be that halfway land—that gray area between hospital birth and homebirth. Since you aren't really in the hospital, you don't have to worry about all the interventions that hospitals are known to push on you, but you aren't home either, so you don't have to worry about taking responsibility if something goes wrong.

A few large, well-known birthing centers seem to be doing very well. They have a fair degree of autonomy, and the midwives can make a number of "important decisions" regarding each of the pregnant women. In these centers, the cesarean rate is very low, and the rate of hospital transfer is also low. Some of these centers actually serve a "high-risk" population—low socioeconomic women who are considered poor candidates for normal birth because of poor nutrition, general health, and so on. Yet, these birthing centers get far better "results" than hospitals which serve matched clientele. Other birthing centers boast low rates of hospital transfer. These centers "risk out" those women who may potentially be "a problem." Their guidelines, which are generally mandated by the hospital with which they are affiliated, are restrictive. Once the "weeds" are pulled out, it is no surprise that the statistics of most birth centers are "good."

Birth centers serve a purpose for sure. They provide a "middle ground" for birthing women. They utilize midwives. They provide a sense of "security" for those who want an "insurance policy." There is always a medical facility nearby. ("Nearby" sometimes means across the street, or within a half-mile, or even in the same building, different floor.) They generally provide a more "personal touch." They generally counsel women in nutrition and natural childbirth in a far more extensive way than most hospitals. They are often the only place where residents can see "normal birth" in action.

But the majority of women I've talked to—both those who work in the centers, and those who birth in them—still have a number of concerns about them and wonder what will be their fate in the 1990s.

Byron wrote, "There was no real reason for my wife to have an ultrasound. She was healthy, and everything was fine. But you can't go to the birth center without one around here, so the midwife just penned 'Twins?' on our card and sent us over to the hospital to have one." If there are any circumstances that fall out of the head-down-medium-weight-within-a-week-of-the-EDC category, many centers are unable to continue providing care for the woman. Kay Matthews, midwife, says that there are many situations that are variations of normal births—not complications. Breech deliveries, multiple gestation, VBACs, and so on, are not supposed to be high-risk![35] But many centers will not attend women in these categories. It depends on "who" makes the rules, whether or not the center is "free-standing" (not associated with a particular hospital), and the politics of birth in that community at large.

"If you are only 'allowed' to take the absolute normal of normal women," one birth center midwife said, you don't have enough business to stay open. We'd say, 'This woman is a good candidate for the center': the doctors would find some reason that she was not. There are often differences in philosophy between centers and hospitals. Most of the centers that have folded cite rising costs, an inability to get adequate insurance coverage, and a lack of support from the medical community.

Is it any wonder? If birthing centers really caught on, if they became the rage, the 1990s answer to the cesarean epidemic—what would happen to all the doctors? What would happen to the fetal monitor salesmen and the pharmaceutical representatives? The anesthesiologists? They'd all be very lonely—and so broke. None of these people has an investment in seeing birth centers propagate and flourish.

VBAC women are still being screened out of some birth centers, which is outrageous considering that it is low-risk. If a birth center does not accept VBAC, you can be assured that the midwives there are not autonomous at all but are still puppets for the medical establishment. There is no reason why VBAC women should be risked out of birth centers—except economic factors and "power-plays" that force the centers to adhere to "doctor's orders." One birth center midwife said that her facility was not allowed to accept VBAC women until a number of smaller hospitals in the area closed down (due to regionalization of maternity care.) "Then the hospital here was overcrowded, so they said to us, 'Oh take your VBAC mothers if you want.' But now that they have added a new wing, they want the VBAC mothers back. It has been a battle."

I recently heard some statistics from a nearby hospital—their rate of cesareans was far lower than the national average. I knew there had to be something fishy going on. I learned from the midwives at the birth center, that the hospital had figured the center's low cesarean statistics into their own and was thus able to boast a lower section rate as their own.

The competition between birth centers and hospitals might at first appear to be a plus for pregnant women. If there are two facilities vying for the same client, those facilities will try harder to "woo" that prospective client. One hospital, upon learning that the midwives in the area wanted to open a birth center, appealed to the state. The state ruled that there was "unnecessary duplication of services" and no real "need" for the center.

Many women have experienced wonderful births in birthing centers. The issues are indeed numerous and complex. Many of them have to do with patriarchy, competition, malpractice, and fear. Some are women-to-women issues. The concept of a birth center is a good one, but if the centers are not free to make decisions on their own, then they are merely extensions of the medical model, beholden to the powers that be.

I have great respect for the women who want to move birth out of the hospital and to provide a safe and comfortable place for women to birth. There have to be a number of alternatives. I support their visions and hope that their centers will thrive. I want to see all midwives sharing their knowledge and expertise in birthing centers, not just those who are system-trained. I want to see birth taken as far from hospitals as is humanly possible.

Erica had her baby at a very nice birthing center. She said that she had no real complaints; everything went well, and the midwives were helpful and supportive. She said that a few months after the birth, she went to a zoo. "It was a very well-run place. In fact, zoos all over the United States are beginning to model theirs after this one. The animals are well cared-for, and as close to their own natural habitat as possible. Still, they all looked a little forlorn to me. The lions could stalk—except there wasn't much that was 'stalkable'. The buffalo could roam—but not too far. I felt sad—I just wanted them all to be back where they belonged!—in the jungle, on the plains—wherever. And then I realized that I, too, had been 'out of place' at my birth—I should have been at home in MY own environment."

One midwife who put years of her life's blood into planning, building, setting up, and running a birth center left a few years ago. "I stood back and looked at what was going on. Corruption! The hospital was running us, and nobody would admit to it or do anything about it. When I realized that this place was not good enough for my daughter to birth at—that I would not want her to come here to have a baby—I knew that I could not, in all good conscience, encourage other pregnant women to come here. They are all my daughters."

PART III   A PLACE IN THE SUN: HOMEBIRTH

Years ago, if you had ever told me that I would become a proponent of homebirth, I would have told you that you were off your rocker. I couldn't fathom how anyone in their right mind could stay at home and have a baby. I didn't change my mind overnight, of course.

My Own Story

After my cesarean, I figured that homebirth was pretty much out for me. Since I hadn't ever wanted one in the first place, it was no real disappointment. The fact that I couldn't (or didn't think that I could) have a natural birth bothered me immensely, but not being able to have a homebirth wasn't even an issue at that time.

Actually, my involvement with childbirth activism began the second the cut was made for my cesarean. It was as if my entire being burst open at that moment. At that moment, another Nancy was born. Unlike me, a veritable pussycat, she was a tiger—same species perhaps, but different genotype. Fortunately or unfortunately, I was never quite the same. I have read a number of spiritual books; I once read that there are "walk-ins" among us—beings who inhabit the healthy bodies of people who feel ready to exit the planet. I haven't the foggiest idea if this is true, but I do know that this new Nancy didn't walk in—she leaped out of me.

The more I learned, the more I observed, the more I read, the more I did, the more I thought—the more I realized how much I wanted a homebirth. This change of heart was born not only from the cesarean, but also from the vaginal delivery of my second child. Separated from my baby, unable to sit, bruised and battered from IV needles and an epidural anesthetic, I was told I should be "happy" about my birth. I was glad that it wasn't another c-section, but the womanplace inside of me was enraged. There had to be a different way. Calling me from very far away inside of my heart were tiny voices, almost inaudible, that reminded me of The Beginning (whatever that meant). The voices became stronger and stronger inside of me until they filled every available space. I came to know that I would never again step foot inside of a hospital to birth a baby.

I am friends with a doctor in my area (believe it or not) whom I respect and admire greatly. When I asked him if he would attend the birth at home, he deliberated for quite some time but finally said no. Later, he changed his mind, and said he might be willing to attend if I was sure to have blood in my refrigerator. But by the time he had begun to change his mind, I was already certain that I didn't want a doctor—any doctor—at my birth. I didn't want blood in my refrigerator: somebody was bound to use it as salad dressing.

I became pregnant and my search for a midwife (I was not into do-it-yourself births at that time) intensified. It was not easy. Having been involved in childbirth work, I had contacts all over the country by then, and not one person knew of a woman who had stayed at home after having a c-section. Of course, I had had a vaginal birth with my second child, so I was not technically a VBAC. But this was years ago, and no one would listen to me. I searched extensively, and I interviewed midwives everywhere. Because of their inexperience with VBAC (which was still so new) and political ramifications of homebirth even with "normal" women, no one wanted me. Indeed, I felt like a leper.

But I wouldn't give up. Finally, after months of searching, I found a midwife who said "yes." My husband thought she must be either insane, money hungry, or deaf: had she misunderstood when I told her my situation? He went with me to meet her and found her to be one of the most well informed and likable people he had ever met. We found out that she was incredibly experienced, well respected, and not even very expensive. The only stipulation was that I would have to find another midwife to attend as a secondary caretaker; all midwives with whom Janet worked thought she was crazy for taking me on as a client and told her that they had refused to work with her on my birth.

The months passed. My husband eventually agreed to a homebirth. You can read his story in *Silent Knife*. Once he "came around" his support and encouragement were unfaltering and now, eleven years later, that experience stands among his most treasured and proud moments.

I had my last visit with an OB (not my friend) when I was six months pregnant. By then, my husband had agreed to a homebirth. The doctor, whom I had chosen for his liberal attitude and sensitivity as well as his good judgment and excellent reputation, was concerned, and shared his views. He did not try to talk me out of my decision (and perhaps was even secretly relieved that I wasn't going to hound him anymore). He called the day after the birth with congratulations; he was not the least bit pompous, and he seemed sincerely happy for us.

Just fourteen days before my due date, Janet called, clearly shaken. The political climate for midwives in Boston, which had been "perking" was now boiling over. For months, her peers had asked her to reconsider her decision to attend me. It wasn't just Janet they were concerned about, but midwifery as a whole. If one of them did something "stupid", they would all suffer the consequences. If word got out that midwives attended VBACs they would all be thrown in the frying pan together. Under the circumstances, she felt she could not attend my birth. She was truly sorry—for everyone.

I hung up the phone, stunned. I wasn't angry with Janet per se. I knew her well by now and knew that the decision had been difficult for her; she was a woman of commitment and integrity. But I felt that the entire world had now forsaken me.

Fortunately no one was home. My children had gone for the afternoon with friends. I sat on the bed for an hour, shaking like a leaf. I decided I would have to make some phone calls. For the next three hours, I called every midwife within a hundred and fifty mile radius. Most of them knew me because I had called them months earlier. None of them was willing to attend my birth. I fell onto my bed, crying unmercifully. I had done everything right. I had eaten well, and I swam every day. I had attended homebirth classes and bought my "Chux" pads. I didn't know why this was happening, but still I knew I wasn't going to the hospital unless it was absolutely necessary. If I had to birth this baby on my own. . . .

No, that wasn't a possibility, I decided. I was too scared. Or was I? As I batted that idea back and forth in my head, the phone rang. Great, I thought. Another lady in need of VBAC help. I just don't have it to give right now. The voice on the other end said, "My name is Kay. I have been trying to get your number for a few weeks. I finally got it this morning, and your line has been busy all day. I am a midwife from Vermont, and I heard you speak at a conference that I also spoke at. I need some reference material from you." I sighed deeply and ran downstairs to get the information she wanted. When I returned, we talked for a moment. It didn't even occur to me to ask if she would attend my birth; she was much too far away.

Just as we were hanging up, Kay said, "You know, you sound a little funny to me. Are you all right?" Within a millisecond, I was crying. "No, I'm really not all right. I am nine months pregnant and I wanted a homebirth. But my midwife is unable to attend the birth because of the political garbage around here, and I can't find anyone who will attend me!" I barely got the words out, I was choking. There was a very slight pause, and I heard Kay say, "I'll come."

I couldn't believe my ears. "What?!" I shouted? "Do you know I'm a VBAC? How can you come to my birth, just like that? You don't even know me!" "Of course I know you're a VBAC," she said, "I heard you speak, remember? And I just called you for VBAC information, which you gave to me in a split second. I have a car that runs most of the time, I don't mind driving down to Boston [more than three and a half hours] at all, and I've been attending VBACs for years." I tried to thank her, and she said, "No need."

Janet called the next day to see how I was and to see if she could help me locate a midwife. When she heard about Kay's call, she rejoiced with me, and she offered to be the secondary midwife (which Kay had not required but was happy to accept). Having Kay there was a key for her to come through the door. After all, she wasn't the primary midwife, she would just be there to 'help out.'

Kay drove down to see me the very next day. We talked, she listened to the baby's heartbeat, and we had lunch. She told me to call her in early labor. Poor thing, "early labor" lasted four days (she drove down and back three times), only to have things slow down and all but stop. I invited her to stay overnight, but she wanted to be at home in the interim. She never once made me feel stupid or bothersome for not knowing when it was the "real" thing. She said that all labors were unpredictable, you just never knew. She assured me that the contractions I was having were doing something important and that I shouldn't be discouraged. "In time, at the right time, your baby will be born." If I had been in the hospital, I'd have been sectioned three days earlier for failure to progress.

The rest is history—or *my* story. As fate would have it, the labor "took off" so fast that Kay didn't arrive until thirty minutes after Andrea was born. I had been reluctant to call her a fourth time, and so I waited until things were moving along pretty nicely. She wasn't the least bit upset that she had driven three plus hours at one in the morning only to find everything all done; she was just delighted that everything had gone well. She stayed for a little while, gave me a hug, and drove back home. She said that she was just part of a bigger plan and was happy to do her part. Kay, you know I love you. You are never far from my heart and I am grateful to you beyond words.

Janet lives fairly close to me. She arrived about forty minutes before the birth. She said she had a feeling all along she'd be my midwife. What a time! A hurricane with gale winds and record tides. My labor was so intense that I felt that I would be 'whisked away' yet there was an undercurrent of peace and calm. I will never forget Janet's sweet voice, calming me, soothing me. She made a few suggestions: Try this, see if it works for you; I think you'd be more comfortable on your other side. "Seems as if you're going to have a baby soon, Sweetie," she'd say. "Just open. Let go." Her gentle hands guided our baby into the world— part way. When Andrea was almost born, Janet told me to put my hands down and lift my baby. What a baby. Talk about cute!

What a midwife. Talk about beautiful. My connection with this woman, who was destined to be at this VBAC home birth goes far beyond the physical into the spiritual where love doesn't need to be expressed, because Love is all there is. Janet has since gone on to be a Joan-of-Arc among midwives. She has challenged the state on a number of occasions and has offered a strong voice for homebirth and women's rights for many years.

The Joy and Comfort of . . .

In the appendices, you will find a page called "Values Clarification." Cut out each of the options and place them in order of importance. As you read books, as you talk to people, as you look inside yourself for the answers about your next birth, you can see whether the order has changed or remained the same. It is a good exercise to see where you are in terms of priorities for birth.

An "Informed Homebirth"[36] fill-out sheet that is passed out to couples has a number of questions that I found very interesting and useful. For example, one of the questions is: "On a real gut level, the birth attendant that I could trust the most would be   (fill in). At this point, the birth attendant I have chosen is   (fill in)." Then it says, "If the birth attendant you could trust the most is not the one you have chosen, list four reasons/advantages of choosing a birth attendant you could not fully trust." Likewise: "On a gut level, the birthing environment in which I would feel the most "in control" would be   (fill in). At this point, the birth environment I have chosen is   (fill in). If these are not the same, list four advantages of choosing an environment in which you feel less in control."

Mary, a woman from Wisconsin, wrote: "You told us that each of us would know where we wanted/ needed to birth—if we just listened to the womanplace inside. I did just that right there at the conference—and knew that I wanted to be at home. It was something I had totally rejected intellectually before, being a nurse, I 'knew better.' But there it was, clear as a bell, I felt it."

A planned homebirth is an idea that frightens some people, horrifies others, and draws criticism from the medical profession. Yet, "for the [many] women who elect a home delivery each year, it is a decision that brings great peace of mind."[37]

There are many excellent books on the subject of homebirth. Even if you don't think you are interested in pursuing the idea, I strongly urge you to read the NAPSAC books and to get their annotated bibliography on the safety of homebirth. Dr. Lewis Mehl's "Matched Population Study Comparing Hospital Birth with Home Birth" may also be of interest, as are the books by Peggy Spindel and Elizabeth Davis. If you finally decide to birth in the hospital, you are going to need all the information you can get about normal birth anyway, so all the reading won't be a waste of your time. There are many homebirth groups; surround yourself with people who have birthed at home, and see if you find yourself being excited and confident. I want to emphasize one point in particular: homebirth is safer than hospital birth. Doctors will try to tell you otherwise and will use all their scare tactics to convince you so. When you learn the facts, you'll know how to respond peacefully inside of yourself, and not necessarily debate the doctor or refute him. Homebirth is an informative, intuitive, heartfelt knowing. As more and more women consider this option, more and more "bad press" begins to appear. Cynthia Duffy says, "The obstetrician has seen his profession slowly lose its grip on women and [is making a] last stab at regaining control via surgical interference. After all, can you do a home cesarean?"[38] Sue wrote:

> My husband gets a quarterly dividend check in the mail that was given to him on his tenth birthday. The amount of the check is eight cents. It costs twenty-five cents to send the check, not to mention the cost of the envelope, the check itself, and the labor involved. Too much time, money and energy expended for so little return.
>
> It dawned on me that this is true in terms of obstetrics. Monthly schleps to the doctor's office, waiting in the reception room, hiring a babysitter for my four year old. . . . Gas money, paying for his office help, its upkeep, stirrups, paper robes. The exhaustion of it all just so that as the baby's head is crowning he can waltz into the room for a few minutes. I suppose I'm paying for his expertise and all that, but I think I'll switch to a homebirth and take my chances that there'd be someone "on call" at the hospital if I really needed them.

Doctor's Back (is) up?

Many women who plan homebirths do have doctor backup. A growing number of doctors are more than willing to be on call for midwives and homebirthers. Some of these physicians are "underground"—there is enormous pressure not to back up homebirth. This book is not the place to discuss the many political, economic, and psychosocial factors surrounding the doctor-midwife controversy. However, it seems to me that it is time on this planet for us all to allow for different schools of thought: If you want to birth in the hospital, I respect your innate intelligence and inner wisdom that tells you to do so; I also respect the source inside of me which bids me to birth at home.

The truth is, very few births of healthy women require a doctor's services. We have been frightened by statements such as, if medical care is needed, it is usually needed rapidly, lest the mother or child suffer serious harm. In fact, most home-to-hospital transfers are not "emergency" situations. I'll leave the experts to tell you all the details; suffice to say that we have been fed a lot of myths. One physician opponent of homebirth remarked, "There are things that can go wrong quickly and when a woman is in the hospital, we can intervene quickly." No mention that the interventions that have already been perpetrated on Mrs. X are most probably responsible for the mess she's in anyway. No mention that midwives are generally more qualified to handle most birth emergencies than doctors and that doctors' wives are notorious for having numerous medical interventions and a high rate of cesarean sections.

One doctor says that homebirth is "nice"—romantic and all that, but not "smart." Another doctor cites all the things that can go wrong at birth and then spends the time telling us that birth is so simple it can take place anywhere—in cars and taxicabs and even out there in the African bushlands. Diane Mason remarks that homebirth is not just a setting, but a philosophy.[39] When you have incorporated into your belief system a number of thoughts and attitudes that are conducive to normal birth, the decision to stay at home becomes an easy one.

Home (Un)Sweet Home

I received a call from a woman in the West. Sherry wanted a homebirth very much, but her husband was dead-set against it. It almost wrecked their marriage. In fact, they separated twice during the pregnancy. We talked a number of times by phone. We talked about decision-making and assertiveness and compromise and no compromise. We talked about resentment, power, control, decision-making, and responsibility. And we talked about love and fear.

Sherry said she was terrified that her marriage would end, but even more terrified of what would happen to her and to their relationship if she didn't "follow her heart" on this matter. I felt unqualified to help her, and I told her so. I told her that somewhere inside she would find the answers that were right for her, and that I would be thinking about her situation and praying that it all worked out well. I didn't hear from her for a long time. I wrote a letter to her but did not receive a response. Months later, Sherry called me. Her baby was already standing and starting to talk. She said that it had been a rough go for a while. She made the decision to have her baby at a friend's house—without her husband. This had been a deeply painful choice, but one that had ultimately felt like the best, all things considered. I have read a number of articles that say that pregnancy and birth bring out deeper issues in relationships—some that can be handled and healed and some that can not.

Keeping House . . .

Another woman, Wendy, also had a husband who was vehemently opposed to homebirth. Day after day, she was frustrated and discouraged, "trying to change his mind and make him more comfortable with the idea of homebirth. I didn't think that anything I was saying or doing was having an effect. But it was all worth it in the end. We had our baby at home and it was great." Wendy suggests the following: "Know yourself—know why you want a home-birth and research and educate yourself until you are certain that this is the best thing for you. You may have to work out your own uncertainties to become strong in your convictions. When you have no doubts yourself, you can better present your case to someone else. If you believe that what you are doing is right and not wrong or crazy, then you will also not try to deceive your partner or 'trick' him in any way. You will always be honest since you are being honest with yourself and having nothing to hide or feel guilty about."

When Wendy's husband saw how much a homebirth meant to her and how far she was willing to go to educate herself and learn what she was doing, and when he saw the statistics (left in the bathroom in place of the *Newsweek* magazine, of course), he began to believe that it wasn't as risky as he had originally believed. He told her that it was her body, and she had the right to make the decision. He said that it was the most fulfilling and exhilarating experience of his life. Incidentally, they had had two previous c-sections.

It has been my experience that when a woman really wants to have a homebirth she can usually convince her partner to go along with her. In the instances when a woman calls and says to me, "I want homebirth but my husband won't agree/ allow it," 99 percent of the time it is really the woman herself who is ambivalent or too frightened. Most of the time in the course of conversation, she is able to admit to her own fears and hesitations, and to begin to own them as her own

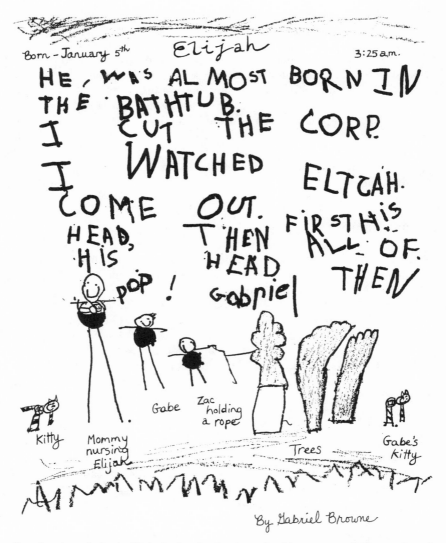

Born - January 5th   Elijah   3:25 a.m.

HE, WAS ALMOST BORN IN THE BATHTUB. I CUT THE CORP. I WATCHED ELTCAH. COME OUT. THEN FIRST HIS HEAD, THEN ALL OF. HIS HEAD. THEN pop! Gabriel

Kitty

Mommy nursing Elijah

Gabe   Zac holding a rope

Trees

Gabe's Kitty

By Gabriel Browne

(for the time being). This is the beginning of taking responsibility, a key for positive birthing.

A slightly different situation occurred when one of the dads in my class, Rob, wanted a homebirth and his wife, Holly, did not! Interestingly, they had also had two cesareans, and Rob had "had it" with hospitals. He tried to convince Holly to stay home, but she was most reluctant to do so. In the end, they stayed at home and had a nine pound daughter. It was an extremely long labor; we have no way of knowing if Holly's conflicts contributed to this, or if she would have birthed in less time in a hospital (or had another cesarean). No matter. It was what it was. Holly said that on some level at least, she must have wanted to stay home, much as she had protested.

Paula—et al.

Paula handled things differently. She'd had four sections (she had labored with babies #1 and #3) and was planning a VBAC in the hospital. But when labor started, she just couldn't seem to get motivated to get dressed and out the door. She kept stalling: first she told David she had to take a bath. Then she said she had to pack a few more things. Meanwhile, David was getting more than a little apprehensive: they had an hour's drive minimum to the hospital and his wife had had four previous c-sections! The midwife whose services they had engaged for the hospital was cool. She figured that what would be would be. Paula describes the scene: "David's out in the car. He's yelling, 'Paula! You get out here right now!' I look at the midwife; I know that I have to make a decision because the contractions are coming pretty fast by now. David yells once again. I turn on the water, take off my dress, and climb back in."

David came back into the house. He left the engine running. When he saw Paula in the tub, and the midwife sitting on top of the toilet seat next to her, he about died. They were singing at the top of their lungs; they were singing this baby out! Not until that moment did he know that this was going to be a homebirth. He quickly turned off the engine to the car and supported Paula the rest of the way. Paula and David not only had a VBAC after four cesareans, but a homebirth. Not only that but this child was a girl, after four boys. Paula said that the bliss she felt has never left her, even after all these years. Now THAT's a happy ending! [Note: Not exactly the end! Paula's fifth and sixth children were also born at home.]

Heather, a VBAC mother from Ontario, planned a hospital birth but also ended up staying at home.

> I was coming to know that it was me who had to birth the baby. No midwife or doctor could do it for me . . . The best exercise I took from the VBAC workshop was imagining that I was alone for the birth and I had to do it myself. Sometimes I even wished that could happen because I felt I would have to be strong enough if there was no one around to lean on. Sometimes you are braver when you are by yourself. When labor actually arrived, I was scared. But then I went beyond scared to just doing it. I was laboring, not thinking. There we were in our own bedroom with only a bedside lamp on: my memory is as of firelight in a cave. What a wonderful primal setting for such a primal experience. I could now see the birth canal as a pathway into the world, not as a closed lump of flesh and bone. I felt I had rejoined all the other women in the world.[40]

Caroline Sufrin, who is the head of the VBAC organization in Canada and a close personal friend, writes:

My cesareans were 'good' cesareans and I was 100% sure at the time that they were necessary. Then I read *Silent Knife* and I was 99% sure. Perfectionist that I am, the 1% really bothered me. A lot. I began devouring books, calling almost every doctor and midwife in the city. To be honest, your book perturbed me. It seemed so full of emotional "hype." And you even contradicted the exalted professors I had contacted at the University here. I set out to prove to myself for once and for all that my cesareans were necessary. The end result? A homebirth and one phenomenal transformation. What happened to this conservative logical beast? I love life and I really didn't before! I've become rather surprisingly social since my fall off the (high) horse. You earned my respect—a remarkable feat in those days. I've earned my respect, too. People look at me and say, "At home? All that pain! You poor, brave girl. You wouldn't do THAT again, would you?' "Yes, YES I would. I would do it again and again and again."

Clare was afraid that she wouldn't have the courage or assertiveness to buck the medical establishment in the hospital and avoid another cesarean. She was afraid that if she did and something went wrong, she would feel guilty the rest of her life. She thought that she had worked out enough of her fears to stay at home. The night that she went into hard labor, though, panic set in. "What if I couldn't do this? What if something was wrong with the baby? What if—? No, the decision was made, and although it wasn't carved in stone, it was at least etched—in my writing. It was time to get on with the task at hand. And I did, one contraction at a time."

Anne-Marie was a nurse. She didn't want to have her baby in the hospital, but she wasn't ready, she knew, for a home birth either. She left to go to the hospital very late in labor; Kyle was born in the car not a quarter of a mile before they arrived. Anne-Marie told her husband to turn the car around, and they went home.

A Refrigerator-Full

In class we talk about the experiences in our life that prepare us to birth—events or occasions that have provided us with feelings of openness, self-worth, courage. When we bring those experiences to the forefront of our minds, and then step into them, we actually create feelings of courage and self-esteem in the present moment.

Marilyn said she couldn't think of anything she had done in her life to make her think she could do a homebirth. We suggested that she do something between now and the time her baby was born to help herself feel strong. We also reminded her that it wasn't necessarily what she did, but what she thought that could assist her. We did some work about changing thoughts. In the interim, Marilyn signed up for—and walked in—The Walk For Hunger—a twenty mile walk benefitting the homeless.

Empty Hearths, Grateful Hearts

A woman from the Southeast had a homebirth VBAC. Her baby died. She and those around her were convinced that nothing more could have been done in a hospital to have made the difference. She believes that the baby's gift to her was the gift of a vaginal birth. Deborah Duda says that "No one dies before the purpose of his or her life is fulfilled, even if we cannot understand that purpose."[41]

Charlene wrote that she knew ahead of time that her baby would be born with serious problems. She and her husband made the decision to birth at home. "I wanted privacy and respect. I wanted intimacy and closeness. No strangers touching me, no one interfering. I held my daughter for 10 minutes while she lived."

One VBAC mother decided to have her baby at home after her sister was in a fatal car crash. "It was a beautiful, clear day, not slippery and wet, and someone had a stroke and crossed the median strip and hit her head on. It hit me: You can die. You can die at any time at any place. When your time is up, it is up, wherever you may be. If it is not, *it is not.*"

Robert Mendelsohn told us that when a doctor asks us, "Do you want your baby to die?" your immediate response should be, "No! That's why I'm having it at home!" Judith Goldstein tells us that there are many ways to aid the mother in delivery, to help the placenta be born, and to assist the newborn: "None of these need a hospital setting!"[42]

Send in the Clowns

Babies die in the hospital, and rarely do doctors get blamed. "They did all they could; it wasn't their fault." If a baby dies at home, the county sheriff's office, the department of homicide, or the local bureau of investigation is at the front door before the placenta has had a chance to see the light of day. Norma wrote that it didn't matter that two babies had died that same week at the local hospital (fetal distress and dystocia). When a baby died at home that week in her community, it was plastered all over the front page of the newspaper. Some couples who have lost babies at home have been charged with child abuse, homicide, you name it. Doctors are touted as heroes, but midwives are baby killers. Doctors are thanked; midwives are arrested, tarred and feathered or raked over the coals. Centuries ago, they were burned at the stake.

This one killed me: A letter from a midwife in the Northwest said, "I attended a home delivery that was a stillbirth. We knew something wasn't right. The mother chose to stay at home. She knew something wasn't right, too. She'd say, 'The baby doesn't 'check-in'.' Her son was born, beautiful, large—and dead.

The investigation was initiated because "there had been a little girl murdered in town and the medical profession have equated these two together." One mother told us they kept referring to "the remains," and another said they kept saying "the kid." Will we go to jail for choosing our place of birth? Will we find *The Handmaid's Tale* one of truth rather than fiction? As the article "Home-birth on Trial" reminds us: We are fighting for the right to choose.[43] Homebirth is not a criminal act; doctors are supposed to be healers, not jailers. And we as birthing parents are not incompetents or murderers.

The article "Childbirth 2000"[44] contains a horrific and stunning futuristic story. It seems that Susan and her husband have decided on a homebirth. They are relaxing in their home in the woods of Vermont when a helicopter swoops down and lands in their backyard. A doctor and a policeman emerge, producing a court order authorizing them to take the unborn baby into protective custody. They force Susan into the helicopter and take her to a hospital suite decorated with houseplants, flowered drapes, and a bedspread. Susan learns that during her one and only visit to an obstetrician, her pregnancy was registered with a perinatal center and a tiny receiver was implanted in her vagina—along with a device used to track down migratory animals.

In 1977, the American College of Obstetricians and Gynecologists declared that homebirth, "a growing trend, constitutes child abuse and maternal trauma." Their position has not changed very much in recent years. We know of one woman who was forcibly taken to the hospital during labor, and another whose baby was taken from her after birth. The helicopter nightmare, Corea tells us, is a real possibility.[45]

Home Equity

The Linders had a homebirth. Susan needed medical attention after the baby was born and was transferred to the hospital. If she had had a hospital delivery, the insurance company would have paid almost the entire amount. A typical hospital birth with all the trimmings (anesthesia, episiotomy, newborn nursery, silver nitrate, etc.) costs a mint. By delivering at home, the couple saved the insurance company quite a bundle. (Of course, this was not their motivation for staying at home, mind you.) They wrote to the insurance company, asking that their rejected claim be submitted to the Grievance Committee. Stephen wrote, "This admission was for an emergency health need that arose while my wife and I were pursuing our dreams, and living our life the way we believe best. This is why we have health insurance. We weren't asking the Plan to approve of our way of life; only to insure us against unforseeable outcomes. If a person were advised by his doctor to stop smoking, would the Plan not pay for his emergency heart attack because you disapproved of his life style?" Stephen then stated that he and his wife were people of very limited means but were nonetheless prepared to see the matter through to its absolute end. They informed the Plan that an attorney had been consulted and that this letter was being copied and sent to a number of other interested peoples (including Senators, the Governor's Council on Women, the State Insurance Commission, the secretary of Consumer Affairs, the attorney general, and the Massachusetts Midwives Council, to name a few). Two days later, Susan and Stephen received a terse letter from the Plan stating that benefits would be provided for all charges associated with their hospital admission.

Of Telephones and Soapsuds

Iris wrote:

> I never considered a homebirth until I heard you say that you opened your refrigerator during labor and said, 'Now, lemme see . . . what do I want to eat? . . . ' Then you said that you threw in the laundry at one point during your labor and the phone rang and you couldn't run up the stairs because your water was dripping, so you waddled up with a towel between your legs to get it. I laughed when you said that it was a computer on the line and you swore your head off to "him" that you were in labor and to leave you alone!" I pictured myself in the hospital or in a birthing center, with perhaps a heparin lock or just a few minutes on a monitor. It just didn't compute anymore. I wanted birth to happen amidst the natural flow of life in my own home. Dammit, if the hormones dictated, *I* wanted to be able to throw in a laundry, too!

One women talked to her sister long distance through the entire labor—ten hours!! Another took out her easel and painted (until the contractions got really intense, and then she flung paint on the canvas). Other homebirth moms have done everything from relaxing and rocking in a chair to finishing up a sweater for the new baby. Some couples cuddle up; a few make love. The sky is the limit when you are under that patch of blue that is uniquely your own.

Just the Two of Us

Marilyn Moran believes that "midwives and friends are not participants in the covenant of love. Only the husband and wife are. . . . For them to be there is to interfere with what is transpiring between husband and wife and to defile a sacred act. . . . What goes up comes down and, when it comes to marital relations, what goes in comes out," Marilyn says. She says that birth requires no more outside observation or management than conception.[46] A growing number of couples have opted to birth their babies in the privacy of their own homes on their own. Their shining accounts are recorded in a newsletter called *The New Nativity*.

Mirror, Mirror

I should probably have something extremely profound to say about homebirth at this point, but I don't. I remember the words of a woman, Rita, whose cesarean had left her with a well's worth of tears: after her homebirth she said—quite simply and not without a touch of surprise—"I didn't cry!" Then she added, "And neither did the baby." I remember the words of a song by Robbie Gass, "Your life has been a perfect teacher since you were but a child."[47] I don't know why those words come to me now, but they've been circling inside my head since I started writing this chapter, so I offer them to you, here and now. I realize that when I type "homebirth," it all has to be one word for me and that there is no pause between the syllables when I say it. I share with you a note from Rosalie's letter: "I went to church yesterday and saw all the people that had opposed our homebirth. Their mouths hung open with awe at how cute the baby was. I think they expected him to be ugly or something."

11 *"The Tears are the Healing"*

PART I DYING/BIRTHING

It has been said that the fear of death is the beginning of wisdom. How dark and puny a wisdom born of fear! The truly wise accept death as companion, so that they may know life.

—Dane Rudhyar[2]

What we hold in our hearts, we can never lose, and all that we love deeply becomes a part of us.

—Helen Keller

You walk into your first childbirth class at my house. Arranged in one corner of the room on the floor in precise rows are shoe boxes, painted grey. The rectangular boxes are closed, standing on one end. There are four rows and five boxes in each row. There are flowers next to some of the boxes.

Written on the front of each box are words. One of the boxes says simply "Jonathan." Another says, "Rest in Peace, Little One." The next: "Caroline. April 14, 1985." One reads, "We hardly knew you, Michael. But we LOVE you." A box in the back row says, "Jennifer Lynn. Nov. 3, 1989–Nov. 6, 1989."

A cemetery. A cemetery in a birth class. A cemetery at the first birth class. What is this? We came here to learn about birth, and you've got this cemetery staring us in the face. I don't talk about the cemetery at the very beginning of that class. It just sits there while we are talking about other things. I'm sure some of the people think I must be a little crazy or that I'm decorating early for Halloween. Often eyes dart in the direction of the boxes, curious to read what they are beginning to realize are epitaphs.

Note: "The Tears Are the Healing" is the title of a song by Karen Riem.[1]

At some moment, never planned, when the time feels right, I stop what we are doing and tell everyone that we absolutely cannot talk about birth without talking about death. I apologize profusely: I know that some of them are going to be uncomfortable.

I have experimented with a number of different ways to teach that first class. I have found none to work better for me than to begin discussing the subject of death early on. I understand that there is wide diversity on this subject; some childbirth educators believe that to teach about complications is to invite trouble. One said that she did not want to impress upon her daughters the feelings that might occur and the specific coping skills they might need in certain difficult situations. "There are some things that must be faced when they happen and resolved according to the life skills we have developed."[3] To skirt the issue of death, however, is to be an ostrich. When couples fear losing a baby or the pain of labor, or whatever, the fear creates a screen that blocks other information from penetrating. When we can remove the screen, or even poke holes in it in various places, information can get in. When we free up space inside of us that was once occupied by fear, we have room for excitement and calm to reside.

I ask the couples in my class to stay with me on this. I ask them to promise that they'll come back to another class before they make a decision whether or not to continue with the rest of the sessions. I ask them to trust me and to evaluate whether that trust is earned.

Most people really love that first class; I love it too. It's real. Chris said, "At first, I thought you were off the wall. I wanted to get out of the room, but somehow I was riveted to my seat." Another woman said, "I felt nauseous and started to break out in a cold sweat. It dawned on me in that same moment, that I had had the same symptoms during my previous labor. I knew right away that there was some important connection for me in all of this. I was eager and ready to hear what you were going to say."

In fact, I say very little. The couples do a good deal of the talking during that first class (and many of the others). I tell them that I believe that everything that we do around birth in our culture is because we are afraid of death. We allow ourselves to be hooked up to monitors and IVs and all of the latest fashionable apparatus because we are afraid that we or our babies are going to die. We ourselves are tested to death in order to ensure that nothing happens to our babies to cause them to die. We have it wired up that if we are in a hospital and something goes wrong, we'll be saved. "Anything! Anything!" a woman will say. "Do anything to me, but save my baby!" The desire to bring the life inside of us to Life is so all-encompassing that we seem unable to think apart from medical minds when technology is offered.

Author Deborah Duda reminds us that "fear keeps our hearts closed."[4] If we cannot begin to decrease our fears surrounding death, we will find it more difficult to birth. She says that the amount of emotional pain and suffering around dying is directly related to the fear around it. This, of course, may be true for birth as well.

My "teachers"—for now that is what my "students" become for me—talk. They talk about death, about God, about faith, about religious beliefs. There are no rights, no wrongs, no judgments. There is just a connection between people who want to be free of fear in order to make clear decisions surrounding this time in their lives. We talk about the kinds of things that we would do for someone else if their baby died or something went wrong, and what we would like people to do for us if we were in a tragic or unfortunate situation. We talk about people in our lives who have died who have influenced us in some way, and how we preserve the memories and keep that individual "alive" for us.

Teach Us, Little Ones

During the discussion, I direct the energy to the gravestones. I take one of the covers off the coffins. Inside is a little doll, with sweet little cheeks and closed eyes. I gently ask her permission to hold her. I lift her from her place of rest, and ask her if she would be willing to tell us some things that might be helpful for us to know. She'd be happy to. She might tell us that she needed better food in order to grow better, or that she passed out and passed away because of the alcohol that her mother consumed. She might say something altogether different than that.

One of the coffins contains a doll that is very small and sickly looking. Later, we are able to discuss prematurity, or intrauterine growth retardation and the things we can do to help ensure that our babies will grow well and give us the best possible chance for a successful outcome.

I opened one of the boxes during a class and took out a Raggedy Andy doll. One of the women in the class, Elaine, burst into tears. She had had a baby who had died just twenty-four hours after birth several years earlier, and when he was buried, she had buried a Raggedy Andy along side of him. I invited her to sit in the middle of the floor, and we all gathered around her in a circle. I asked her the name of her son and if she would like to tell us a little about him. She was reluctant because no one had asked her about him in years and because she thought that people just didn't want to hear about such things. She talked to us for a few minutes, and then I asked her if she thought her son had any "words of wisdom" that he would want to tell her about pregnancy and birth if he could speak to her. She lifted the Raggedy Andy. Tears were streaming down her face as she "listened" to her baby "speak to her." She told us that he said, "Mommy, sometimes people do everything right, and still things don't work out. You did everything right. You fed me good food, and you took care of yourself. I think it just wasn't time for me to be here, that's all. I'm sorry that you are sad. I love you."

If there was a dry eye in the room that night, I can't tell you. My own were too wet to see. Here were people who had never been together before, who hadn't even been introduced to one another, supporting each other and holding each other as if they had known each other for years. Elaine said she felt better, more peaceful, than she had since her son's death. I gave her the Raggedy Andy, which she presented to her new baby as a gift from her firstborn.

Women who have had miscarriages or abortions often have "stuff" to deal with during this class which are better addressed, or at least acknowledged, during this time than while in labor or on an operating table. I have come to know that people do not bring up things unless they are, on some level, "ready" to begin handling it. The good news is that it doesn't all have to be neatly handled, 'tied up in strings' as it were, in order for healing to occur. The fact that it is up, that it has been expressed rather than stuffed down, often "clears the pathway", allowing an open channel for the next birth experience.

Death: You Teach Me About Life

I have never lost a single momdad in all the time I have presented my cemetery. They not only return, but they often tell me that they couldn't wait to get back and see what the next class would be like. One woman said: "I was so excited after last week's class! When I attended hospital classes, I felt stupid and scared. I kept forgetting the word symphysis pubis. This time we all participated in a deep and meaningful discussion. Talking about death made my husband and me realize that one of us is going to die someday. After class, we held each other for hours, and it was really great."

Dad

My father died a little over four years ago. He died at home after a difficult and lengthy illness. My mother, my sister, and I were at his bedside for those long, painful days. Afterward, I realized that the hours spent with him, particularly the ones closest to the moment of death, had felt familiar in some ways. I was struck by the fact that the "energy" that was "in the air" as we awaited "the moment" felt akin in some ways to the energy present as one awaits the moment of birth, at homebirths, at least. There was a quiet anticipation, an intangible feeling of spirit, and a respect, acceptance, and wonder about the process itself. There was tremendous pain, but as the moment of death arrived, no fear. It was calm. We had let go, all of us. My dad was an incredible man, a teacher among teachers. He taught me as much in his dying as he had in his living (and that's a whole lot of sardines and chocolate milk, Dad. Thanks).

For Those of Us Who "Failed"

And what about us who "failed"?
The ones whose birthings were not the finest hour
of their womanhood?
The ones who did not defy all medical intervention?
Those who have no heroic defiant story to tell?
Where do we fit in?
We can't all be the ones that change the system,
but are we less a part of the sisterhood of those
who have given birth?
To those that have shone at the hours of birth,
remember those of us who have not.
Will we, like the Vietnam vets, be recognized
too little and too late?
We experienced giving birth too.
Less nobly than some maybe,
but a noble experience nonetheless.
You all say you honor choices.
Can you really honor mine?
I will always honor the process which
brought forth flesh of my flesh.
I honor your births too.
Can you ever honor my experience, or will I
forever be a part of your statistics on
the way things shouldn't be?
Remember me.

Anonymous

Last Breaths, First Breaths . . .

There are so many questions as death approaches, and they are often the same questions that are asked at a birth. How long is this going to take? When will it be over? How much pain will there be? Will it be difficult? How can I best help? And the answers are often the same: It will take as long as it takes. It will be over when it is over. It may be difficult, it may not be; much depends on attitude, support, different circumstances. You can help by respecting the person's wishes; offering suggestions of things that might ease any discomfort; and mostly by bringing your love and peace into this room.

If you can't talk about death, you will not be able to talk about birth in any meaningful context outside of the barriers of fear and intimidation. There are some babies who are just not going to "make it" no matter how many tubes, tools, drugs, machines, or devices we use, or even when everything is done "right" (whatever that means). Following doctors' orders and hospital policy does not ensure a live, viable, healthy infant. One woman's family was astounded when she decided to have her second baby at home. Her first baby had died shortly after delivery in a large hospital. "If this baby was going to die, too, I preferred that s/he die in the comfort of my arms. I had done it everyone else's way the first time, had a monitor and the other interventions, and my supposedly healthy baby died anyway. This time I was going to choose what felt best for me." She had her next baby at home. She said there was no fear. The worst thing that could have possibly happened to her, she said, had already happened. She could take responsibility and handle anything now.

Terri told me that in an effort to save her newborn, the doctors went "all out." "I think they wanted me to be grateful to them, for that, but frankly, I wasn't. I couldn't bear all the procedures that were done to her, and all the needles they stuck into her. She was so little, and every time they drew her blood I was sure they were going to suck her dry. We all knew that she was going to die, and I *wanted them to allow it!* I feel truly as if they prolonged her agony, first and foremost, and mine as well." Like any crisis manager of a bank or state, the doctor "commandeers resources, which, in their uselessness and futility, seem all the more grotesque."[5] Doctors often refuse to recognize the point at which they have ceased to be useful as healers.[6] Death is failure to them, and for the most part, they find failure unacceptable.

Living/Dying/Controlling/Flying

I recently read about a couple who were indicted on a charge of manslaughter. The "man" they had "slaughtered" was their two-year-old son, whose illness they had tried to cure through prayer and spiritual healing rather than medicine. Doctors in the area heard about the child and wanted to intervene; they believed they could save him. A battle ensued. The child died in the meantime, and the couple was charged.[7]

Medicine is not the only form of healing, nor is it foolproof. Whether or not the doctors could have saved the child is not even the issue. There are times when doing nothing-at-all is preferable. (A "hands off" approach might have saved the person.) We will never know for certain what would have happened. The issues involved are, among other things, control, decision-making, perceptual differences, fear, faith, and letting go. The largest issue, of course, is death itself. As a spokesperson from a Christian Science church said, "No one would think of prosecuting grief-stricken parents in the hundreds of sad instances where children have died under conventional medicine. What is on trial here is not the action of individual parents, but a public policy, a healing practice, and a way of life."[8] In addition, there is the not so subtle attempt to squander freedom of choice and establish a single line of acceptable thought.

Joseph's dad, Steven wrote,

I looked into his closed eyes as he lay . . . motionless. . . . A deep choice had to be made, a choice about life and death, a choice so deep and overpowering that it bent my shoulders and burned a hole in my soul. Then I took one step closer to the edge. A voice spoke and all it said was "Let go." I took one more step and leaning, nearly fell off the dizzying edge. I saw Truth. . . . In that instant I realized this choice was Joseph's and not mine. I let go and knew we would love him and respect him no matter what he chose. With that I took the final step. We flew.[9]

I know a doctor who was diagnosed with cancer. She endured chemotherapy and radiation treatments, to no avail. "On a whim" she left her hometown and moved to the southwest. There she lived with native American Indians. She had heard about some of the healing work that they had done and figured it was worth a chance. When she arrived, she asked how long their "treatments" would take. "As long as necessary," she was told. "And if they don't work?" she asked. "Then they don't." "How will I know if they've worked," she asked, since it was obvious there was no blood lab in sight. "You'll know."

One morning many months later, my doctor friend woke up and said she did know. She just felt different. A few days later, she left the reservation and returned to her home in Michigan. The doctors who had treated her were dumbfounded when tests confirmed what she already knew: there was no sign of cancer anywhere. I met this doctor several years later after she had been cured. She had opened a whole health clinic and was open to all kinds of healing—whichever suited the person and/or the disease. This woman had had a number (more than three) of cesareans and believed that working through some of her upset about them had been a key to her wellness.

We've all heard stories like these. Miracles, cures and poor diagnoses. My friend Fredelle lived eight months longer than doctors said was humanly possible. My dear friend Sylvia has twice looked death in the eye and said, "Not yet." And yet, I also know a number of people who have died without a moment's notice. Poof, they were gone. THE TRUTH IS WE JUST NEVER KNOW. Each, according to his/her own time.

Doctors' hopes to control the outcome of specific diseases gave rise to the myth that they had power over death.[10] Like all other rituals of industrial society, medicine takes the form of a game. The chief function of the doctor becomes that of umpire, with the duty to make sure that everyone plays according to the rules. "The rules, of course, forbid leaving the game and dying in any fashion that has not been specified by the umpire."[11]

Physician Perri Klass writes that doctors don't face death with serenity or acceptance; when you train people to think in terms of doing everything that can be done, it becomes difficult for them to turn off those attitudes, "even when all their aggression and energy are clearly doomed to failure." Doctors need to "resolve" mortality somehow or other, she says, since they have to face too much of it to leave it nagging at them. Deborah Duda remarks that often there is panic at death "And then everyone shuts down. Compassion is lost."[12] Duda's book *Coming Home* lists a number of advantages to dying at home;

interestingly, many are the same advantages as birthing at home. [Another recommendation: *Caring for Your Own Dead* by Lisa Carlson.]

A Loaf of Bread, a Cup of Tea, and Thou

Birth, like death, is not fully controllable. We weren't meant to understand birth or to control it. We are meant to take responsibility for the parts of it that we can, and then just experience it. Those who think it is possible to understand it try to make it fit into their own predefined slots. In so doing, they foolishly begin to believe that they can make it turn out exactly as they will it to be. Yet we all know inside that we cannot know and that we cannot guarantee, but we pretend we can and we hook ourselves up to fetal monitors and screw electrodes into our babies' scalps in order to avoid a possible death. In doing so, we display an innate mistrust of the Grand System. We confuse our bodies and make it difficult for them to do what they know how to do, left to their own design. In spite of all the technological paraphernalia to which we are attached and the numbers of medically trained people we surround ourselves with, we still quake in our little hospital gowns and shoe covers. At some point, we must let go and allow the process to be. Faith is not belief without proof but trust without reservation: I know this because my tea bag tag told me so.

PART II   GRIEVING

Alice in Wonderland went on shedding tears until there was a pool all around her. I have heard from so many thousands of "Alices" in the past eighteen years. Given the kind of birth that so many women in our culture are subjected to, it isn't any wonder that they feel anger, frustration, grief, and upset long after they have left the hospital. Women in our culture are, for the most part, discouraged, despondent, and downright depressed after their deliveries. Many of the women who write have had cesarean sections, but lately, more and more, I am hearing from women who have had vaginal deliveries. Almost apologetically, they say, "I didn't have a cesarean, but my birth experience has left me with feelings of upset and despair. I wonder if you would have the time to read my story." I would like to share with you excerpts from some of the letters I have received.

Alices

Now that the time has come to start thinking about another baby, all my old anxiety and feelings of helplessness are flooding back and threatening my serenity. What do I do with all this emotional baggage—all these tears?

I find it next to impossible to forgive the medical profession. I have suffered gross mistreatment at my doctor's hands. My feelings about doctors have turned to hate and mistrust which is poisoning me. I went and spoke to my priest and he said he would pray for me.

I'm going to have myself sterilized when I get the money. I couldn't go through another birth experience like that again. What little faith I had is totally gone.

They gave me pitocin, then morphine, then more pit, then demerol. My baby was 8 lbs. 9 oz. and had difficulty eating and breathing for "unknown" reasons. I was severely suicidal postpartum and everyone wondered why.

The expense of the c-section was tremendous because I had a wound infection. I was in the hospital for weeks. Now that all of this is over and it has been a year since I had our baby, I'm still surprised at how I feel emotionally. I want more children but I am afraid. I have a feeling of impending death. Physically I'm still not back to normal. I used to be active in Nautilus and now I'm lucky if I walk up a flight of stairs without the feeling of my legs going out. It's scary to think: What if I become pregnant again and I'm not physically able to survive the complications? What will happen to the child I have now? Who will be his mommy?

My cesarean experience was more than unpleasant. The surgery was done not only unnecessarily and not only without informed consent, but without my consent at all! I am sixteen years old. It's been 5 and 1/2 months and I have very strong suicidal thoughts. Every month it gets worse. I try to tell my mother but she doesn't understand. She doesn't care to either. While I was in the hospital I had to bend over the sink to wash my hair because that's the only way it would get done. Excuse me, I know I am talking in circles, my emotions get the best of me and I can't write fast enough so I come out sounding like an idiot. By the way, my doctor told me to stop breastfeeding because the baby had jaundice. I called a few weeks later—I still had a trace of milk—to see if I could nurse. She said, "Oh sure! There was really no reason for you to stop!" Thanks for telling me that now!

Babies may "arrive" as far as others are concerned. But, from a mother's point of view, birth is a little like having a child go off to camp or to school; although one welcomes the progress that allows greater independence and farther flung relationships, something is lost in the process and one at least wants to be able to see the child off. Looking back on it, the most difficult thing about my daughter's birth was not the pain of labor or of recovery, but the fact that she was born out of sight and touch, independent of my efforts.

They told me if I tried to give birth naturally, my baby would die. Even with a section, he wasn't given much of a chance. . . . When I came to, they told me that my son was born, and he was alive, on a ventilator, he weighed 1 lb. I can't begin to describe the horror and pain of the months that followed. He had to have surgery for a heart duct at three weeks. They said he would die, yet he lived. He gained weight, he opened his eyes, he smiled. He got better, he got worse, we rode this roller coaster for months. He had every invasive medical procedure done to him that is known to mankind! I held him in my arms every day and talked to him, and poured my love into him. I pumped my breasts so that he could have milk. I believed that my love would give him the will to live. I anguished and argued with the doctors and their diagnosis. It's such a long horrible story. Then they told me he was blind. He never smiled again. But he still had his own way of communicating with me. He developed [an infection]—the cure was more deadly than the disease. He died in my arms, he was 6 and 1/2 months old, and weighed 8 lbs. He was just beginning to look like a normal baby, instead of an elf. I know he knew how much he was loved, and I felt his love for me. He died many months ago and I am just beginning to feel alive again myself. I have begun to think about the future, but needless to say I am traumatized and terrified. I've been told I would have to have another cesarean. I could handle that if I had to, but what I'm terrified of is letting the ICU get a hold of another of my babies.

It was so hard. Everyone was so impersonal. I remember looking at the screen and seeing the baby. I asked if they didn't have the ultrasound that showed the baby moving and the technician told me that was what I was looking at. I saw no movement and my brain was starting to realize what my heart already knew. The radiologist entered and said, "There's no movement," and left. The doctor came in and uttered the same words. I asked him what that meant and he said, "The baby's dead." Period. Just like that. I asked if there could be a chance that it wasn't and his reply was "astronomical." He walked out then and refused any further comment. We had to make an appointment to come in the next day to talk. We were sent home and I cried like I've never cried before. It was Halloween night and what a horrible trick had been played on me. For nine months I had been consumed with thoughts of the baby. Everything I did was done for her and then suddenly, she was gone. My belly was so quiet. I kept wishing it was a dream and that I would feel a kick. It was the darkest part of my life. No grief I had ever experienced could approach what I felt.

Our five year old son recently went through a ten-day assessment program. He has a number of learning disabilities and although I doubt it could be proven legally, I'm sure as I'm sitting here that at least one enormous contributing reason is hypoxia in labor for the number of hours some #*#! doctor made me lie flat on my back. I could kill the whey-faced coward, the incompetent. The thought of my child suffocating by degrees inside me while those jerks kept me on my back in hard labor—and they are so damn respected! Medical professionals, small-town elite, turkey [poop]. I vascillate between wanting to dynamite this poor excuse of a maternity center and wanting to force them to learn about normal birth. Why couldn't I have known five years ago what I know now? It would have meant the difference between normal development and slow, painful changes and coping. I keep going back in my mind to where I was on my back wanting to turn over and get up on all fours. In my mind, I do it, never mind the wimpy docs. I doubt I'll ever be able to forgive them without contempt and spiritual nausea. I need God badly now. I don't think that most doctors are reachable. Maybe the sane thing to do is to leave them to their own devices and go about your own psycho-physical integration. Which is a journey, I suppose, if taken far enough, that entails forgiveness. Perhaps I'll never make it that far. I hurt too much.

Do you feel like crying? Now you know why there is a box of tissues in every room in my house.

"It Hurts"

Silent Knife had a chapter on grieving and healing. It would be helpful for you to read that chapter before continuing with this one. There is a description of grief, and suggestions for healing. We list many books on the subject of sadness and loss; one that I particularly recommend is *Ended Beginnings* by Claudia Panuthos and Cathy Romeo.

Many of the women with whom I work are deeply ensconced in grief. They feel as if their rights to a decent, let alone exhilarating and empowering, birth have been taken from them. If they believe the interventions or the cesarean was unnecessary, they have one set of issues to deal with. (Why didn't I know better? Why didn't the doctor know better? Where was my support?, etc.) Even if they believe they were/it was necessary, there are issues. (Why didn't my body work? What went wrong? Will it work the next time?) Always, they are concerned about the effects of the birth on their babies.

Some tiredness after birth is normal. The body has exerted great effort, and there is a baby to nurse and cuddle. But somehow in this country we seem to be far worse in the energy department than many of our foreign sisters, and it is no wonder considering the kind of births most of us have had. In addition to being physically tired, most women are grappling with birth-related issues that contribute to the exhaustion and make healing, in general, more difficult.

American women on the whole are a sad lot after birth. Our births have left us so depleted and regretful that we barely have the energy to shuffle from the hospital to the car. Whether because of a cesarean section or an episiotomy the size of a gerbil's tail, we are a group of bent-over and bummed-out beauties.

Physical healing is a primary goal. It isn't easy to care for a baby after major surgery or other body assaults. Good nutrition is important, and yet it becomes difficult for many women to eat well. "I felt so yukky," said Paula, "that some days I wouldn't eat at all. Other days, I'd 'pig-out' on junk food." She felt guilty, knowing that she wanted to have another baby in the future, but she was unable to find the reserve to go to the supermarket, shop for groceries, and prepare a meal.

Anger

The women who contact me are tired and sad. They are also angry at the physicians and the technicians, the anesthesiologists and the nurses, and the way in which they were manipulated. They are angry about childbirth classes that didn't prepare them to do battle. They are angry at themselves and their partners and at the injustices they endured. They want a reason for what has happened, something they can put their finger on. If they can understand what went wrong this time, perhaps they can make things different for the next birth. Sometimes there are no answers, and sometimes those that make sense don't suffice. When their feelings are misunderstood, ignored, or minimized, they get angrier still. Or they begin to feel there is something wrong with them, or that they must be crazy.

Some women use their anger to spur them onward. Susan painted furiously for months after her son's birth; Kathy sketched; Karen wrote music; and Pat ran a race. Many women have used the strong negative feelings they have to start childbirth groups and to right wrongs. In this way, anger can assist healing. However, anger is motivating, to a point. It may feel constructive and energizing at first, but after a while it is depleting. I have learned that releasing anger frees up energy that until then was unavailable.

Many years ago I attended a lecture given by a childbirth therapist. I asked her if she would help me to be as effective as I could be dealing with grief in my classes. She knew about my work with cesarean prevention and VBAC and was more than interested to oblige.

Mary told me that in order to help others heal, we must continually heal ourselves. I figured I was pretty well healed. It had been almost eight years since I had had my cesarean. I had managed to pick myself up and live my life. I didn't feel particularly angry or sad, although I did feel a drive to "save" every pregnant woman within shouting distance. Mary asked if I was interested in healing some of the birth upset that I was obviously (to her) still carrying around.

She asked me to make a list of all of the people whom I'd been angry with around the time of my c-section. I listed them: the doctor, the labor assistant, and surprisingly, the woman who had come into the room to prep me. Anyone else? Well, my husband. And myself.

Mary asked me which of those listed I was least angry with. I was surprised that I had even mentioned the prep lady; I hadn't thought about her in all those years! I was asked why I was angry and I blurted out, "Because she didn't even look at me, not once, and the water was cold! I felt so humiliated by what she was doing. She even turned me over and shaved my rear end! I don't have hair on my rear end!"

Mary had me role-play the part of this woman. In my mind, I was asked to imagine that I was this woman. I was to close my eyes and imagine the house she lived in. It wasn't a house, I said. It was a really dumpy apartment. It was cold, cluttered, and dirty. It was in a poor neighborhood. Yes, there were cockroaches. She asked me to imagine that I was getting up for work that day. I put on the white uniform (in my mind's eye) along with white stockings and white shoes, rubber soled. I imagined that I was coming in to work; I had no car so I had to wait out in the rain for a street car. On the street car, I felt okay; I was in a uniform, and I could have been mistaken for a waitress, hairstylist, or nurse. No one had to know what I really was. The other occupations had class. I was qualified for none of them.

All day long (in my mind's eye of course), I went from one room to the next (this was a big teaching hospital) shaving hairy bodies. Mary asked me if I was looking at the people I was shaving. Timidly, I answered her: No. Why not? she asked. "Because I can't," I said. Why not? Because I hate what I do and it is too humiliating! I want to be something else! I have no education and this is all I can do to earn a living—shave the hair off of women who are going to be cut opened! I practically tripped on the words as they came spilling out of my mouth. I could feel the despair and embarrassment that woman felt. I could understand perfectly well why she hadn't looked at me.

From that moment on, I had absolutely no anger toward this woman. I had only compassion and understanding.

I felt great. I'd released anger. All done, right? Wrong.

The next time I saw Mary she asked me who I was the most angry with. The doctor. She had me role-play him. Let's see. . . . He got up in the morning in his beautiful split level home. (I'd driven by it once, so I knew exactly what it looked like.) He drove his nice car to the hospital—there was a space reserved just for him. He did his rounds, flirted with the nurses, popped in on his c-section moms, most of whom adored him, and then went to his office in a new, modern office building. "Mary," I said, "this isn't working. I don't feel more compassionate. I feel even angrier!" Why are you angry with him? she asked.

"Well, for starters, he cut me open unnecessarily. Two, he brushed me off when I went back to him at six weeks, three months, and a year to tell him I was depressed. He said, 'Oh Nancy, you are such an emotional person—it stands to reason your postpartum depression would last a while!' I was brushed off, Mary!" I listed more and more reasons why I was angry at him. I felt betrayed. He hadn't intervened to get my baby for me after recovery. As the list grew, I realized that feelings I had stuffed down for a long time were beginning to surface. I wasn't sure I liked this healing business, after all.

My homework assignment for that session was to go home and write the doctor a letter. I could be as angry as I wanted to be, since I wasn't going to be sending it. Why not? I thought. If I was going to the trouble of writing it, why not let him see how that hour in my life eight years ago had affected me. I was beginning to feel really angry now.

I brought the letter back to Mary the next week. I was proud of what I had written—it was clear, businesslike, not too brusque, but just enough to know I meant business. Mary read it and then proceeded to rip it up. "Why did you do that?" I asked. It had been neatly typed and "ready to go." "It was a puny excuse for an angry letter," she said. "You were so polite, I could puke." Great language for a therapist, I thought. Polite? I thought I had really socked it to him.

"Nancy!" Mary screamed at me, and I jumped a foot off the floor. "The guy cut you open! It wasn't necessary! He told you you were too small to have a baby! That's bull#&#*! He induced your labor for his convenience—you know how dangerous induced labors are for the baby! And he miscalculated your due date, to add insult to injury!"

I started to cry. Mary threw up her hands in disgust and said, "Oh get out of here. You are a lost cause. You can't even get angry. You pull the Scarlett O'Hara number and start to wimper." "What do you want me to do?" I asked. "It's over. It's done with!"

And Mary said: "Yes, Nancy, for your doctor it is over and done with. He is out driving around in his fancy car and taking vacations. For him, it was ten minutes in his life and it is over. For you, unless you release it, it will never be over. This has nothing to do with him! It has to do with you! Do you love yourself, honor yourself enough to get rid of the anger that is inside of you? Or do you want to carry it around with you for the rest of your life? My sense is that you have to allow yourself to get angry about it before you move away from it. Now go home and write him a letter! Get those words that have been stuffed in your body for eight years out of your body and onto paper."

So I went home and wrote. Did I write! I told him I thought he should be hung on the Boston Common by his you-know-what. I told him I wanted to see him in a movie where his blood and guts got ripped out. I told him I thought he was ugly. I said I wished his doptone would infect him with lice. I said it all.

I went back to Mary again. She had me read the letter to her. Better, she said. Better? Only better? She asked me to read it again. This time she mimicked me. I would read, for example, "I think you're ugly," and in a sassy whiny voice she would say, "Oh I'll bet you're really upset, Doctor. Nancy thinks you're ugly. Sticks and stones and all that jazz." She did this several times. Do you know how infuriating it is to be mimicked? Try it out with one of your kids. My blood was beginning to boil. Then, as I was beginning to read it for a third time, she began to poke me on the side of the arm, as if she was trying to push in front of me in line. "Stop that, please, Mary," I told her. "Stop that please Mary," she mimicked back to me in that aggravating voice, as she continued to poke me.

Finally, she said to me, "That's it! You flunk healing!" she said. "You are a sorry case. People can poke you and scream at you and you just take it like a little mouse. You cannot set boundaries and you have no limits. It comes as no surprise that you had a c-section—and frankly, I am surprised that you managed to have a vaginal birth at all. You are a mouse and you will get mousier and mousier until all you can do is squeak and eat cheese."

I'd had it. She'd pushed me too far. I screamed out, "Well, this mouse roars!" She handed me pillows and I punched them and swore and beat them and yelled loud enough to wake the neighborhood. I don't know how long this lasted, but it was a fairly long time. I couldn't believe the amount of energy I had stashed into this fairly compact body. I was blown away by the noises I was making and the intensity of the pillow pounding. When it was all over, there was more. I just went at it again! And again! Finally, I fell over onto the couch. After a few minutes, I started to giggle and laugh and laugh and laugh. How did I feel! I felt wonderful. I hadn't felt wonderful in a long time.

Mary told me that all that energy that had been stored inside me to keep the anger down was now available for other things—for loving and for my family and for helping others. I'd had a lot of energy even with all that blockage; I could only begin to imagine what I'd do with all this newfound space. I could breathe—my lungs felt clear and my chest no longer felt constricted. I hadn't realized how much my body had been involved in holding anger until I was through this exercise and could feel the difference.

Mary said, "If you send an angry letter to someone, they may not be able to hear what you have to say. Their defenses go up, and they shut out anything that they don't want to, or can't hear. If you had sent that letter to your doctor, he'd have confirmed what he already believed—that you were an emotional nuthouse. He'd have written you off in a minute. When the anger has dissipated, you can then write a letter that has a better chance of being understood. When you are ready to write to him, if you feel a need to be in touch with him, write one that you would be willing to read if you were him. And write it for you, because you need to heal, not for him. You have no control over his response. Do it, when you are ready, for you."

I wasn't ready at that point. Months later, I was in the west doing a two-day seminar. I had met yet another group of incredible people—alive, excited, enthusiastic. We had had a wonderful time together, and I was feeling that old familiar   "I-love-these-new-friends-I-want-to-bring-them-all-back-home-with-me!" feeling. A tune started to float in my head: "A million tomorrows shall all pass away, 'ere I forget all the joy that is mine today." "God, have I been blessed," I thought. That night I wrote the following letter to the obstetrician, which I sealed and mailed the next morning:

Dear Dr. S., [I wasn't using first names at the time!]

I've been wanting to write to you for a long time and decided that the time to do so was now.

I have experienced many, many different emotions since the cesarean section delivery of my first child. I was at first grateful to you, as you know, for "having presented me" with a healthy child but then was filled with rage—as you also know—because the more I learned, the more I was convinced that the section was unnecessary. Later, I was again grateful that I had had a vaginal delivery—"your" scar had held up "nicely"—only to be enraged again for reasons too numerous and now unimportant to mention here.

The experience of cesarean section and my subsequent VBAC led me, as you know, not only to a homebirth with our third child—which was a pinnacle experience in my life—but also to the work that I do. I have learned, grown, and changed in ways I might never have if my first births had been different. I have met wonderful people, traveled to parts of the country I never expected to see, and found my "earthly path." I take responsibility for the part I played in the cesarean—you could not have sectioned me without my "permission." You know what they say about hindsight.

I want you to know that although you and I will probably never agree about the subject of birth, and may never understand each other on the subject—and although you may have wished never to hear from me—I am once again grateful to you in many ways. I hope that you will forgive me for any unkind thoughts I have had along the way. I truly wish you well and carry you with special thoughts—and love—in my heart.

If I were to write the letter today, it would be a little different. But I have never been sorry that I sent it. I feel no animosity toward this man whatsoever, and I feel peaceful inside. I believe that the more loving "vibes" we send to people, the sooner the planet as a whole will heal. Whole people do not cut up other whole people unnecessarily.

I received a copy of a letter that a woman had sent to her doctor. She had written: "I thought you might like to know what I think of you. Even if you don't, I'm going to tell you. I think you are a pig and a butcher. I would wish you a miserable, cruddy day, but I am afraid that if you have one, you'll take it out on other, unsuspecting, trusting women, just like I was. So have a nice day." I saw the woman about two years later and asked her if she had really sent that letter. She said, "You bet your bottom dollar, I did. I've felt great ever since!"

Susan wrote a letter to her doctor urging him to "remember the magic of birth. Charts and graphs are limited, but the human potential holds all possibilities. We cannot know the outcome of any birth—we can only assist in the process." Her doctor had predicted that she would have a repeat cesarean—in fact, she had a 5-hour home water birth. He wrote back, congratulating her and thanking her "for the enlightenment—I needed it." He promised never to tell a woman she was "too small."

Sadness

The next session with Mary and its aftermath was one of the most healing experiences of my life. She explained to me that underneath, or at least alongside of anger, there is always sadness. "You say that you are angry about your c-section, Nancy. I know that you are also sad. You haven't allowed those sad feelings to surface. Your anger felt strong and powerful. The sadness felt weak to you. If you are ready, you can bring the sadness up and get it out."

I told Mary that I had cried millions of tears after my cesarean. She explained the difference between the kind of crying where you just cry and cry, but don't feel better—unproductive crying, as it were—and the kind of crying when you really get into it and feel a whole lot better afterward—a releasing cry. I knew the difference.

Mary said, "We're going to do your cesarean again. This time, you will get a chance to do whatever releasing crying you did not do." I think my heart stopped in that moment. I had spent years putting the birth behind me, and now I was to do it again? Yet, I trusted Mary. I knew the work she did, and I knew that whatever work we did together would benefit me in some way.

Mary asked me to begin by telling her some of the details about my section. What time of year was it? What was the weather like? How did my body feel? "Pregnant," I said, "very pregnant." She instructed me to close my eyes. "Can you feel you're pregnant?" she asked. Yes, I could. That was easy. I loved being pregnant, and I could remember the feeling of Eric inside of me as if it were that morning. I began to feel sad, knowing what I was going to be visualizing in the next few moments.

Mary asked me to describe the operating room. I told her I had been on a narrow table. She guided me to her coffee table, and I lay down on it. Since I had told her that the room had been cold, she opened the window. When I told her there was a light above me in which I could see the reflection of the anesthesiologist, she arranged a light. It was getting kind of real. . . . I began to shake (I'm shaking as I type this!) just as I had before my section. I had been so scared! Mary asked me to begin describing what was happening. I said, "Well, they put a sheet up so I can't see my abdomen," I said. "Speak in the present tense," Mary said. "Okay, they put, I mean, they are putting. . . ."

That did it. Lying on that table, describing my cesarean as if it were happening at that moment I remembered how awful getting the epidural had been. Oh, this was hard! Mary asked me to keep the words coming, "They are swabbing my abdomen with something called betadine, and now they are poking me with something sharp to see if I am anesthetized. Now they have made the first slice. . . . ," and I began to sob. Mary was with me, talking softly, guiding me. "Good, Nancy, keep it up. You're doing really well." They were the same loving words that I have often said to a woman in labor. I later asked Mary why she didn't hold my hand. She replied that I had told her that my hands had been strapped down.

My heart started to race. "They are pulling back tissue or something, Mary, I can feel it! They're talking about—French restaurants! I can't believe it. My body is cut apart, and they are talking about croissants and mousse and duck l'orange! How can they do that, Mary, how can they?" I must have sounded like a five-year-old child, crying my eyes out in abandonment, fear, and grief. "They're unconscious, sweetie. People have to go unconscious to some degree when they cut another person open. It's okay. You're going to be fine. I'm here with you this time."

Finally, we got to the time when I asked the anesthesiologist when the baby would be born. "If you were paying attention," he said, "you'd know that your son was born a few minutes ago." I had a baby! I was a mother! For a fleeting second, I felt absolute joy, followed by complete, total, utter panic. Where was he? Going to the special care nursery? Why? Wasn't he okay? What was wrong with him? I kept asking questions, over and over again. The anesthesiologist said, "He's fine, but if you don't quiet down, we're going to have to put you out." I begged them to let me see Eric. They passed him in front of my face for not more than a few seconds. Then he was gone.

He had been wrapped up in a blanket already. Why was he in the special care nursery? What was wrong? In fact, nothing was wrong. He was okay. But at that time, all cesarean babies went immediately to the special nursery. It was just a routine hospital procedure. To this day, I still don't understand why someone in that operating room couldn't have told me that. One lousy sentence to explain the policy might have saved me hours and hours of sheer terror. I was certain they were lying to me. I was certain that he was in bad shape.

I was sobbing. I felt like a complete zero. I cried and cried and cried. At this point, Mary was holding me. I felt as if she was Mother Earth herself. I felt love and healing radiating out from her. Not only had my baby been taken away, but my husband had not been present for the birth. I had known Paul since I was thirteen years old; for years we had discussed how we would be together when our child was born. Because of hospital policy, my husband was two floors down and one building over. Yet, with Mary stroking my brow and whispering to me ("You did the best you could. You wouldn't have allowed your body to be cut open if you didn't believe it was in the best interests of your baby. The love that a mother and baby have is sacrosanct; Eric knows he has that love even when he is in the special nursery, Nancy."); the healing began. On and on, she soothed my bleeding heart. It might have been hours. I was cradled in her arms. I think she would have stayed with me for days if she had to. In time, the tears stopped. I realized that I am who I am partly as a result of my cesarean experience. It was what it was. It was Okay.

Play It Again, Mom, or, Legos, Legos, and More Legos

There's more. Mary had me relive the cesarean one more time. This time, we began at the point where Eric was born. At that moment, she instructed me to insist upon having the baby. "You don't have to be hostile, just clear and strong. This is a gentle birth, one in which your needs are respected and met." So in my mind's eye, I imagined that I was asking for my son. Into the "un-strapped-down" arm, she placed a doll. I didn't see the doll, remember, my eyes were closed. I just felt Mary put what I knew was a "baby," wrapped in a blanket, into my arms.

"Here is your child, Nancy."

I hugged him to me. Oh how I cried! Mary said, "now you have an opportunity to tell Eric all the things that you wish you had had a chance to tell him when he was first born, before he was taken from you. I began talking to him, and brought him close to my face. A while later, I opened my eyes and realized that she had left the room, left "Eric" and me to be together alone. I felt so peaceful, so happy, so filled-up. I laughed when I looked at the doll—it was an old "Curious George" monkey and it was wrapped in a tee-shirt. ("It was all I had. I had to improvise!" Mary said later.)

It was suggested to me that if I wanted to take this process one step further, I could go home and do this with the real Eric. A few days later, I went into his room. "Eric," I said. "Would you do me a favor? I didn't get to hold you when you were brand newborn, and I'd like an opportunity to hold you now and tell you all the things I didn't get a chance to tell you when you were a baby." He looked at me as if I had finally, once and for all, gone bonkers. "You've got to be kidding," he said. "No way. Nooooo way."

The kid is tough. I actually had to bribe him. He drives a hard bargain, but finally we reached an agreement. He was going to get a Lego set that he wanted—an Expert Builder's Set—for five minutes in my arms. As he was about to lay down, he renegotiated. "I want the power pack, too." He lay in my arms, stiff as a board. He clearly just wanted to get this over with. I started to talk to my son, and my eyes welled up with tears. "Oh how I love you, Eric." "I know that," Eric said. "Quiet," I told him. "You are a newborn baby. You can't talk yet!" After a minute or two, he relaxed in my arms. He would catch himself and stiffen up, only to get kind of newborn floppy again. I took off his socks and counted his toes. I turned him over and looked at the little place on a baby's head where all the hair spirals together—I love that spot! I've always loved my son with all my heart. But something subtle occurred when I held him that day. A wound that had been opened eight years earlier was closing.

It Doesn't Hurt Anymore

Women who have had vaginal deliveries often feel a need to "replay" their births, too. One woman's baby was delivered by forceps. She replayed the birth with her daughter, who was six at the time. Her child had had frequent headaches from the time she was very little; after they replayed the birth peacefully, her daughter's headaches completely disappeared. My own daughter Elissa and I had a delightful afternoon when she was five years old; we pretended she was born naturally. I made pushing sounds and after quite some time she popped out from under the blanket and said "It's hot in here. I'm ready to get born!" Having been pulled out by forceps, she seemed happy to be able to decide "birth time" for herself this time.

It Never Did

Having had so much fun and success with my first two birth replays, I decided I'd better do one with Andrea, who was just over a year old at the time. I picked her up and waited for some words to come—the words that hadn't had an opportunity to be expressed at birth. There were none. Everything that I had needed to say to her at her birth had been said. There had been no drugs to make us groggy, no separation, no hurts to heal. It came to me then: birth is not an experience that should even need a healing! If anything, it can and should be a healing in and of itself.

A number of couples in my classes have gone home and talked to their children about birth or done something new in an attempt to heal a hurt. Most of the time, they've felt good about it, although the mountains didn't rumble and the seas didn't part. Two letters that I received from people in my workshops, however, are noteworthy.

Patti writes:

First, a little background information. When Sean was born I was literally strapped down and unable to touch him. He went to the special care nursery and I didn't get to hold him until some 15 hours later. He was taken from me because I had developed an infection. I was allowed no contact with him for three days. Last month, I settled into bed with *Silent Knife* and read the visualization for a separation. I did the visualization. You suggested we imagine a gift that we could "give" to our babies as they were taken to the nursery, something that would symbolize our connection, and their safety. The gift I saw myself giving Sean was a blue ribbon. The gift I received from him was a heart. I felt so much more peaceful after this. But the really wonderful part is the speed with which changes took place in Sean's and my relationship. The next day I could see a difference! Since then, we have been all over each other, hugging and kissing. I can't tell you how good it feels. Thank you.

An interesting sidenote to this story is that a few days after I did the visualization, I received a heart necklace as a gift from my mother. Then, the next week, I bought six bunnies for Easter. They were packaged; when I took them out I just grabbed one to put in Sean's basket. I noticed for the first time that the bunny had a ribbon around its neck. I checked the other bunnies. They had yellow or pink ribbons. Only Sean's had the blue ribbon. You'd better believe that I saved the ribbon.

Michalene wrote:

I had an interesting experience tonight that showed me how well healed my emotional scars from the cesarean are. I was in the bathtub with my little boy. I was ready to get out and I held him tight and kissed him. It flashed into my mind that we were all wet and how much like his birth it had been. I wondered if in his subconscious he was remembering his birth too! It wasn't until after I was out of the tub that I remembered: Curtis' birth was nothing like that. For the first time, I had actually forgotten that I'd had a cesarean. My heart had integrated a different experience that I now live with on a day to day basis. It was a deeply moving moment. I think my son felt it too.

PART III   HEALING

Now when it rains, I let it.

—Judy Collins

For some reason, I picture the scene in "Gone With the Wind" where there are wounded for miles, as far away as the eye can see. A cast of thousands.

Instead of men with bandages around their arms, there are women, women everywhere, with bandages poorly wrapped around their torsos. The less wounded are caring for the more badly bruised; the few that survived intact are ministering to the most battered.

In order to begin to heal, we must believe that we deserve to do so. We must feel deeply committed to our own emotional well-being. We must open ourselves to healing on all levels—spiritual, emotional, and psychological as well as physical. One woman, eager to begin mending her wounds, said, "I want to pray, but I don't believe in God. I'm going to pray, 'To Whom It May Concern!' "[13] Another woman went to a cooking class to learn how to feed herself in a healthier way. Linda, never the outdoorsy type, began to take walks in the early evening. We owe it to ourselves to do everything we can to get to a place of wellness. This is not selfish: a culture without whole, energetic, healthy, alive women is a darkened culture, indeed.

I Like Me

In my classes, I begin early on to help women feel good about themselves. When we feel bad about ourselves, we contract. We roll up into a little ball inside of ourselves. It is difficult to birth a baby with an internal position of contraction. The worse we feel about ourselves, the larger and tighter the ball becomes. It eventually has the ability to clog the passageway for birth. Every time a woman in my class gets down on herself, I pick up a piece of black yarn and start to wind it into a ball. Interestingly, by the time the first classes are done, the ball is usually about the size of a grapefruit. I then take out the box of other yarn balls that I have assembled and add it to the lot. Weeks later, I demonstrate how this ball of negativity fits neatly into the opening of the cervix, making it all but impossible for a baby to "get out." We all know that birth is not simply a physical event. Our thoughts and feelings influence our bodies. Negativity tightens us, closes us off. We want to open to birth our babies; in order to do so, we must be open.

When I ask my momdads to make a list of the things they do not like about themselves, the pencils really start moving. Too fat. Too tall. Too nonassertive. Too much cellulite. Too nervous. Too self-centered. When I ask them to tell me some of the things they did "wrong" or "bad" at their last births, the negativity really flies. "I didn't push right!" (yarn); "I couldn't remember the breathing. I lost control" (yarn); "I didn't give her enough support" (yarn) "STOP!" I command. "No more of this!" It is hard to birth a baby when all these little black yarn balls are everywhere in your body. Even if they are small to begin with, they move around like the mercury from a broken thermometer and coagulate. Eventually, they form a ball the size of an orange or a grapefruit. The bigger the ball, the less of a psychological opening, so to speak, is available for birthing. "If I had asked you to tell me the things that were wonderful about you and the things that you had done well, then what?" "Oh, that would be much harder," they say. "Impossible. I didn't do anything right."

So we begin. I demonstrate to them the internal position from which I believe birth emanates. I stand up. I tell them that I am in a place of neutrality. I begin to think bad thoughts about myself; I'm too short; Sometimes I'm self-righteous; I'm getting a zit. With each of these putdowns, I feel less tall, not only physically, but inside of myself as well. I begin to contract slightly, to close up, to wilt. I continue: "I had no guts at my cesarean. I didn't even open my mouth to ask questions. I just listened to the doctor (contract, roll up a little more). I starved myself before doctor appointments so he wouldn't yell at me for putting on weight, and then pigged out afterwards (more contraction); I allowed my son to be circumcised even though I knew it was the wrong thing to do (a big, gigantic contraction that rolls me up right in front of their eyes). I am so tight, so constricted in this position, that I cannot visualize myself standing tall inside myself. The internal "me" is also rolled up into a ball. There is no room to stand in an open and tall position in my mind's eye. You just cannot birth from this position.

I then begin to think good thoughts about myself and the things I did: I'm creative. I'm funny. I care about people. I insisted that they bring Eric to me— I was unrelenting to the point where they wrote on my chart that I was making them crazy. I started a childbirth organization. With each affirmation of the good that is me, I begin to stand taller. As I continue to do this exercise in front of the class, I open, much like a flower blossoming in time-lapse photography. Within a very short time, I am standing as tall as I can be, with my arms extended and my head up high. My entire body feels expanded. I breathe more fully and I feel good. I believe that this is the internal position from which birth emanates. Then all passages are open and free and clear. I am a channel. The life force that brings a baby to this planet can pass through me in this position from head to toe, without being challenged or blocked.

Each of the people in my classes is required to stand up at some point during that class, or during the remainder of the classes to come, and to tell us the good things about themselves. By doing so, they become more open and breathe more clearly. Without exception, they report that their bodies feel different, better, freer. They are asked to say their name, and then they tell us good things. For example: "I, Pat, walked down the hallway two days after my cesarean to get my baby!" (At first, she had been down on herself. She thought she should have been able to get herself to the nursery sooner.) We all applaud and whistle and really get into it. With each opening in the room, each of us gets to experience it inside of ourselves too. At first, Pat was reluctant to get up. After a while, she said, "This feels great!" She didn't want to sit down.

Little kids often love to get up in front of other people and perform. When asked what they like about themselves, preschool little girls can usually rattle off a list of admirable qualities: "Well, I'm very pretty, you see. And I can draw— want to see my picture? And I can ride a bicycle. See how I do ballet? And I do fun things in school." But something seems to happen to us when we get into school, something that tells us it isn't okay, or it's conceited, to like yourself. We go from admiring ourselves to picking apart every little aspect of our physical and psychological makeup. It hurt me the day I watched one of my daughters, who had always enjoyed looking in the mirror, and who had a fairly good self-image, burst into tears as she looked at her reflection. "Oh I am so ugly!" she said. From that point on, she became far more critical of herself than complimentary. Although this has begun to change as she gets older, I often wonder what we do in our society to foster this disillusionment with one's self. Pablo Casals tells us we must teach our children well. "We must proclaim and demonstrate to each and every child his/her uniqueness and beauty. Do you know who you are? You are a marvel. In the whole world there is no other child like you in the millions of years that have passed . . . Yes, you are a marvel." ("Yes, you are a marvel. And when you grow up, can you then harm another who is, like you, a marvel?")[14]

On at least two occasions this class turned out to be very different than I had expected. The first was a class in which one of the women was quite a bit overweight. She was unable to find anything about herself that she liked. She went back in her mind to the time she was four or five, but evidently had even begun to feel poorly about herself by then. I explained that even if it was something little, it would be a beginning—the first brick next to which others could be placed. She was at a loss. She had had her feelings of self-doubt and inadequacy so long that she was unable to think of anything.

Her name was Diane. We put her in the middle of our circle. She faced one of the momdads. One by one, she rotated around the circle while we told her the things about her that we loved. "You are warm and compassionate," she was told. "You are intelligent." One of the men in the room said, "You are big and marshmallowy and like a pillow." (My immediate reaction was to shoot the guy. But he had said it with such honest caring that Diane took absolutely no offense.) By the time she had rotated around the circle, her cheeks were pink, and her eyes were beaming. She stood up and began to speak. "I am Diane and yes, well, I guess I am intelligent. Well, most of the time." By the time we were finished with her, she was standing on a desk, shouting out at the top of her lungs, "I am dynamite!"

I quoted a few passages that night from Geneen Roth's book, *Breaking Free from Compulsive Eating*: "At what point are you going to be willing to stop eating and say, 'I want to feel good. I want to feel good about myself. I want to take care of myself'; When you are not putting food down your throat, it gives words a chance to emerge. . . . When we find ourselves engaged in an activity designed to produce numbness, a voice is present and struggling to be heard; When you push away an emotion, it remains in the wings of your heart."[15] We talked about weight and nourishment and ended up talking about parents and memories. There was so much support in the classes; we were all together, healing each other. Diane's personal victory that evening was a victory for us all. She later said that that night was a turning point for her. She bought Geneen's book and began to take charge of her life in a new way.

The second occasion involved Laura, a very pretty woman about six months pregnant. She was unable to think of anything at all that she had done that was good concerning her cesarean. Nothing. "Something small, Laura?" I coaxed. No, there was nothing. She felt completely worthless. Her body was clearly in pain; she was taut, and her lips were sealed tight. She looked as if she was biting her tongue behind them.

"Stand up, sweetie," I said to her. She did. I went over to her. "You are so lovely inside of you, but it is hard for me to see that right now because your inside Laura is all rolled-up in a ball." I asked her if it was alright if I put my hand on her belly (by that class we had discussed limits and boundaries, and I know she would have felt perfectly comfortable saying no if it wasn't alright). "This baby," I said, "will want to come out in a few months. Help, if you can, Laura, by standing up inside of yourself—by beginning to create a pathway. I know you did something good, something you feel tall about, at your last birth. And if you can't think of anything, then so what?! We'll just make something up!"

The tears were flowing down Laura's cheeks. "You don't need to make anything up. I have something," she said. She was beginning to shake. In a meek voice, she said, "The anesthesia paralyzed even my hands. I was told that I had to keep my head perfectly straight, and so the only thing that I could move was my mouth. When my baby was born they did bring her over to me. I wanted to hold her so badly I was practically out of my mind! I tied to move my fingers, but they wouldn't budge. I couldn't see Marissa's face well enough. They said to me, 'Well, there will be plenty of time to get to know her later on!' and started to take her away. Without even thinking, I said 'No! I am not finished seeing her!' " Lucky for me, they responded. I think they were surprised I had spoken up, I'm not sure. They brought her closer but it wasn't good enough. I told them to put her next to my face. When they did, I don't know why I did this, but. . . . " she hesitated, "I started to lick her. I mean, not just a little lick, but great big tongue swirls. When they realized what I was doing they were freaked out. 'Stop that!' I was told. The next thing I knew, I was knocked out cold. They thought I had gone crazy."

We were stunned. The room was absolutely still. Then, almost without thought, the entire class got up and gave Laura a standing ovation. She was sobbing by now.

"That was incredible!" I said. "Goodness, how many of us wish we had had the presence of mind to make some kind of contact with our infants! Your 'womanplace' was alive and strong, Laura—she was certainly not anesthetized! But in Heaven's name, why did it take you so long to tell us this?"

Laura then told us that her baby had gotten an infection. She was hospitalized for several weeks and was quite ill. When she bumped into the anesthesiologist, he said, "Oh yeah, I remember you. You're the mother cat. Why do you think your baby got infected?" Laura was mortified. For three years, she had carried the weight of believing that she was responsible for her baby's illness.

We assured her that what she had done was an incredible, instinctive, loving, creative act. We were so proud of her! More important, she was proud of herself.

Adhersive Tape: Bonding, Binding, and Becoming

As you can tell, feeling good about oneself is a key issue in my classes. From a place of confidence and strength, new options can be explored and considered, and new decisions can be made.

One of the questions I ask in my classes is: What would you need to feel whole inside of you right now? What quality or qualities would you need to possess in order to feel ready to birth this baby?

"Courage!" someone inevitably calls out. "Trust," someone else might say. "Sexiness!" So, we exchange qualities.

Carol felt she needed bravery. Vickie said she felt brave. I asked Vickie if she was willing to share some of her bravery with Carol. "Sure," she said. So, we did a little ceremony in which the exchange was made. First, Vickie had to bring her bravery to the forefront. She had to "own" it. You cannot give something to someone else unless it is yours to give. She remembered occasions when she had done something fearless, something courageous. She focused on the feelings that these occasions elicited, and brought bravery into her body. You could tell when she "got it"—her shoulders broadened and her face changed. She told us she was ready.

Patti needed to make a space inside of her to receive bravery. If she was filled with fear, there would be no place for the bravery to live. She closed her eyes and imagined fear exiting from her.

Vickie and Carol stood facing each other. Vickie put her hand on her heart and said, "I own bravery. I give some to you, Carol." Carol opened her hand and received the bravery. She put her hand to her heart and placed Vickie's gift within. She faced us and said, "I own bravery now too." There is an unlimited supply of these "natural resources"—wisdom, courage, bravery, peacefulness, caring, self-respect. As long as we own them and give them away, there is a boundless granary. We are on this planet to assist each other; to help each other to be whole.

It Takes Two

One area where healing is often needed is between couples. I receive many letters and calls from women whose poor birth experiences have caused tears in the fabric of relationships. There are a myriad of books and seminars and programs on marriage and intimacy for those of you who are interested. Sometimes, just a walk together is all you need to "clear the air" or to feel closer.

Momdads have told me time and time again that they feel closer to each other during the time they are attending my classes. This may have little to do with the classes per se and more to do with the time commitment the two have obviously made for each other and their baby. On the other hand, I know that the classes are nurturing and that they are, above anything else, about loving.

Sometimes I just ask the couples to talk to each other—or to the group— about how they met. Sometimes, I'll slip a "homeplay" "assignment" into the hand of one of each set of momdads: "If you want to, plan a really romantic night for your partner this week with all the trimmings!" So many little, inexpensive things can be done to increase loving and to let someone know they are important to you.

But when people are angry at each other, or there are undercurrents, it is hard to let the loving out. That black ball of yarn clogs the heart this time, making it hard to give or receive love. Without giving, there is no receiving, and vice versa.

When I was pregnant with Andrea, I wanted to clean out any "debris" that I knew might prevent me on a psychological level from opening up and giving birth. I do not believe that this is necessary or right or even good for everyone; I listened to my own inner voice and knew it was right for me. I called Mary and said, "Got any new stuff to teach me?"

Mary remembered that on my list of people that I was angry with was my husband, Paul. "Bring him in," she said. "We'll clean out any cobwebs between you two." Paul's an incredible man. Did I dare bring him into this lioness's den?

Since we were planning a homebirth and I had once had a cesarean, Paul and I were both open to doing whatever came our way to get ready for the birth. When we arrived, Mary said to Paul, "Betcha didn't know that Nancy's been holding a grudge against you for quite some time. Eight years, to be exact." "Now, Mary, that's an exaggeration!" I said. I looked at Paul. "Nothing important, really. Just a few minor things." I looked at Mary. What a troublemaker and instigator, I thought.

Mary asked us to look at each other. She wanted us to maintain eye contact for several minutes without turning away. We couldn't do it! We'd look, avert our eyes, look again, start to laugh. Once, I could feel tears welling up, but they didn't amount to anything worth discussing.

"Just as I thought!" Mary said. I had no idea what that meant, and frankly, I didn't care to know. I found her to be flip, arrogant, and snitty that day, and I told her so. "Well, you must have had personal experience being flip, arrogant and snitty, yourself." she said. "Otherwise you wouldn't be able to see it in me. One has to know a quality before one can identify it, and the only way to know it is to have experienced it within." What was this crazy woman saying? And who cared anyway? Her pseudopsychological mumble-jumble was too much. I had to be equally nuts to be wasting a perfectly good afternoon unburying petty annoyances from the past.

Mary gave us each a piece of paper and a pencil. She said, "I know that both of you are still holding on to some anger or upset about the cesarean. I am talking now specifically about any upset that you feel towards each other. I want you to list any of those things that you are still upset about, so that you will be able to love unencumbered for the next birth."

Paul and I had been married for a number of years. We had a good relationship. But I had listed him among the people I was upset with at the birth. So, I began writing.

Paul watched me put a few things down on my paper. He picked up his pencil, scratched his head, and then put the pencil in his teeth. I could see that he was thinking. After a moment, he started to write. I looked over at him. What could he *possibly* be writing? What in the world was he angry at *me* for? I must say, that spurred me on for a bit. I added two other things to my list.

Mary said, "Look, you guys, you aren't going to share these lists with each other. This is just an opportunity to get anything out of your body that might interfere with labor. If you put the words on paper, they aren't inside of you any more. There's more room, so to speak." She'd said the secret word. What woman does not want more room to birth her baby when she is in labor. Well, I did at least. I started writing. All the big and little things that had gotten my goat. You might have thought Paul was an ogre, the way I wrote, instead of the gem that he is. I filled up one whole side of the page and a quarter of the next.

"Okay, put your pencils down," Mary instructed. I felt as if I was taking my SATs. "Okay, now who wants to share their list first?" Share the list? "Mary," I said, "you told us we weren't going to share the lists." "I lied," she said.

Great. I get the one therapist in the city who doesn't care if she lies. "Nancy, you go first," she said. Mentally, I had already decided which of my entries I was going to read. "Okay," I cleared my throat. "Well, Paul, I was angry at you because you didn't stay home from school the day I went to my doctor's appointment." Mary instructed me to use the present tense. She then instructed Paul to sit with his knees facing mine in an "open-bodied" position (legs uncrossed, arms unfolded, palms facing upward, fingers unclenched). I was to look him in the eyes as I read my list, and he was to look back. He wasn't to make comments or sly remarks: all he had to do was listen, and after I had completed each listing, to say, "Thank you for telling me that. Not knowing it is not between us anymore. I feel closer to you now."

He felt ridiculous. So did I.

I read the next thing on my list. "I am angry because when we left the apartment there was garbage in a big bag and I asked you to take it out and you said, 'Not now, later. I'll do it before you get home with the baby.' " I couldn't believe I was telling him this. But I remember that I had cleaned the apartment, and I didn't want garbage to sit around while I was in the hospital. Paul practically fell over. "You are angry about that?" he said. Mary looked at him. "Follow the instructions, please," she said. "Thank you for telling me that," Paul said, and I was sure I detected a note of something in his voice, although Mary didn't seem to detect it.

I went over my list, reading some of the things I had written. I said I was done. We switched places. Paul read his list to me. Nothing major. I thanked him. Can't say that my thank-yous were of the heartfelt type, but I thanked him. To tell you the truth, I didn't feel any closer to him, but I figured some days you're lucky just to break even.

When we were done, Mary looked at us. She said, "I love you both. I'd like to offer you an opportunity to read your lists again, this time sharing the things on the list that you deliberately avoided and have decided never to reveal. It's your choice. You can keep that stuff inside or get it out." I thought of the little balls of yarn. I didn't want yarn in my body when I went into labor this time! I had enough for my first labor (end result: cesarean) and my second (end result: epidural and forceps) to knit matching sweaters for Rosie Greer and Roseanne Barr.

I began to share with Paul the things that were on my list, the big things. I told him about feelings of rejection and abandonment. I was no longer reading off my list. I told him about my sexual feelings and my feelings of fear. I told him that I had been angry because I had wanted him to save me from the section instead of agreeing to it with the doctor. I had wanted him to fight his way into the operating room, but he had passively accepted the situation and left me to find out which of the doctors preferred "La Maison de Robert" and which recommended "Chez Moi." Each time I spoke, Paul thanked me. This time, he was really paying attention. He was looking at me clearly and directly. I felt understood and listened to.

Paul shared the rest of the things of his list. He told me how hard it had been to be in school and be 100 percent excited about the pregnancy. He told me that I had been so involved in childbirth that he didn't know where he fit in. He told me about his feelings of rejection and "scarcity." Mary did not intervene. Perhaps she might have if there had been a need, but there wasn't. She observed, and she trusted that we'd get through. Initially, she acted as a safety gauge. In time, her presence became less and less important. She suggested that we spend some time not talking, but just looking at each other. This time, it was much easier.

Later, Mary asked me to list the qualities about Paul that I most loved. She asked me to name the ones that had first drawn me to him. Without hesitation, I told her that the thing that had impressed me the most was his quiet, unassuming way. I realized that I was being unrealistic by expecting Paul to barge in on my cesarean or to "fight" with my obstetrician; these actions were not in character with the person he was. I had assigned him a role for which he was unsuited. Mary invited me to begin to appreciate the things about Paul that had been so appealing when we first met. He had done nothing wrong; he had just been himself. My heart opened to this gentle, sweet, peace-loving man who doesn't fight battles, wage wars, or interfere in cesarean sections.

Moving Through

Over the years I have found that, unless I am careful, I absorb the pain of the grieving women around me. In order for me to be as effective as I can possibly be, I must keep my channel open. When it is, the pain flows through me, so that I can feel your sadness and empathize with you, but does not settle inside of me. I want to help you with your pain, not absorb it or own it as my own.

Surround yourself with loving, supportive people who can provide a hammock for you as you swing gently from one place to the next. Remember that you are not alone: I have thousands and thousands of letters and have met equally as many women across the country who would understand and would be happy to be your friend. As Jeannine Parvati says, "The sooner a mother is willing to feel the pain of her loss and the insult upon her body, the better. However, we can't push a river. When she is able, she will experience her grief . . . and be open to healing. . . ."[16]

Healer Cathy Romeo reminds us that birth is a *passage*. It is a powerful, transformative, life-giving passage, but still a passage. What comes *after* the passage—the myriad of choices, changes, commitments—are the moments and hours and days of existence. ALL count. "Perhaps our birth passages will be more clear and free and healed when we can look *through* the passage, not just *to*, and envision the spectrum of moments that may come afterward."

There is a quote tacked up in my little office that says: "Be gentle with all that is unresolved in your heart and try to love the questions themselves."[17] When I do this, the answers, the healing, usually begin. So, be gentle with yourself. Survive . . . Grow . . . Learn . . . Love. None of us needs to be cast in Margaret Mitchell's sequel.

12 *Learning as We Live! Childbirth Classes in the 90s*

Did anyone ever have to teach you how to blink your eyes? Scratch an itch? Smile? No one has to teach you how to have a baby either.

If your labor were to begin this very minute and you didn't have a chance to read one more word of this book or any other book, or attend one more class, you would still be able to have your baby. "Women going through extensive training to learn how to give birth naturally—there's something wrong with that thinking!"[1] The word "education" comes from the Latin word "educare"—to bring out that which is within. Everything you need to know is within.

In the years since prepared childbirth has become "the way to go," the cesarean rate, the rate of drug-taking, and interventions have continued to climb. In *Silent Knife*, we talked about some of the problems with prepared childbirth classes—why most of them don't work and why so many people who take them and "graduate" are still seemingly "unable" to have their babies. For all the good that childbirth classes set out to do, few have done much, and much of what has changed has been for the worse.

It is discouraging, isn't it? I believe there is hope. But before we get to that, there are other things to talk about.

Classes That Don't Teach

I do not recommend that anyone ever take a hospital class. I know that isn't going to endear me to a number of really good childbirth educators who teach at hospitals. I know there are people who think you can, or have to, "work within the system." Whose system? Why? I receive enough letters and phone calls and have met enough hospital-"educated" parents to know that childbirth classes conducted in institutions established for the injured and the sick do not work. Conducted: that's one of the problems. The classes are often conducted like lectures.

Throw out all those charts of the insides and cross sections of people's inner organs. No one ever needs to see all the muscles and tissues and ligaments and bones inside the body in order to have a baby. This is not a biology lesson or an anatomy lesson, although sadly, in most classes, you would never know it. Scientific understanding, medical terminology, and classroom lectures have little place, if any, at a birth class.

One hospital pamphlet boasts about their epidural refresher classes. If I taught epidural classes, very few people would have one, guaranteed. We'd be talking about the fear of childbirth that leads a woman to chose an epidural and how to get through it. We'd be learning about the dangers of anesthesia to the baby. We'd be turning chickens into eagles.

Ah, how could I forget cesarean classes. Teaching women how to get open, mostly unnecessarily. Very few women need a cesarean section. Why not take a tomato, a juicy one, and slice it open with a small, newly sharpened paring knife. Lift the knife ever so slightly to the ceiling light; let everyone see how shiny and clean it is. Before the knife is inserted, there are a few things you must do: Hook the tomato up to an IV (a medicine dropper turned upside down with a piece of yarn will bring this all down to size) and a heart monitor (I use a walkman); String a needle onto the end of a cooked piece of spaghetti to use as a catheter; cover the lower portion of the tomato with a small, white linen napkin and place it directly in the center of a cutting board; Borrow several Ken dolls and dress them in greens: place them around the table, heads rotated slightly downward. Voila! A cesarean section that can be observed, discussed, and prepared for.

I learned a lot from my cesarean; who am I to prevent others from learning via that route? However, lying on a table without "trying" to birth is defeat, not empowerment: The women I teach who have had cesareans are disappointed, of course, but they feel strong and empowered nonetheless for having located places of strength they never knew they had and for "going for it." A "good" cesarean—one in which the mother has no responsibility except to learn how to take a spinal without complaining or wincing (although I suppose one could feel good about that, too)—is a sad way to grasp "empowerment."

I have asked cesarean instructors what they do when someone who is in the class is clearly in a situation that does not call for a cesarean. Do you tell them your opinion? "I am not the doctor." Do you tell them to call other people who had a similar situation and had a natural birth? "Not usually." Do you bring in couples who have had awful c-sections? "No." A couple who had a "good" experience was invited. I don't have to tell you again that if a cesarean is necessary, it should be an experience that supports and honors the mother, father, and baby, but to sit a group of people in front of you and tell them how to get cut open unnecessarily is disgusting. Who pays the instructor in these classes? The hospital. Who sends the couples to the classes? The doctors. If you encourage these people to seek other opinions, have VBACs, and so on, where would you be? Without a job.

"F" for "You Flunked"

Peggy wrote to me about her classes.

> I went to classes at the local hospital. We saw lots of movies. I came away more frightened than when I began. I hadn't been particularly concerned about pain— my mother had easy births and I felt I could do it. So I tried to visualize myself birthing and tried to imagine the worst pain I could endure. Once I squeezed combs in my hand, and the instructor said, "Oh, Peggy! It's *way* worse than that. You can't even *imagine* the kind of pain!" I came away thinking this ain't gonna be no piece of cake, after all, and I began to have trouble sleeping. I wondered if all the other people in my class felt the same anxieties, but everyone looked okay. Out of seven couples, though, five had sections, me included. I guess I shouldn't blame the instructor, but in a way I do.

Women come out of classes often feeling anxious and stupid. They are so full of terminology. They can't remember all the words and the places those words are supposed to go on the charts. I get many an eleventh-hour call—the couple who has finished their classes and feels overwhelmed and unable. Someone has given my name as someone who can help "undo" the damage.

A familiar scenario among these women is one in which they are pregnant and being tested in front of a board of medical examiners. "What are the ischial spines?" Let's see, they're the, the . . . um . . . things . . . that stick out in the front—or is it the back? "One wrong!" yells an examiner. "Spell coccyx!" c-o (now where does that "x" go?) x-y-ccyx. "INCORRECT!" the examiner bellows. And before the women have time to rub their symphysis pubis, the examiners lift them onto their tables, and begin to operate.

War Cries

In reviewing brochures for childbirth classes and workshops held all over the country, I am struck by the wars we seem to be fighting. I am reminded of the black and white World War II movies that are only shown at 2:00 A.M. these days. The rows of men seated in front of a gigantic map of the world. Pins represent submarines, and little flags on toothpicks represent battleships. Little metal airplanes, like the ones you can use for your "piece" in the game of Monopoly (only these are fighter planes) are movable by way of little magnets, glued to the bottom of the "aircraft" (the wall to which the map is attached is

Participatory Conception Class: A.D. 2089

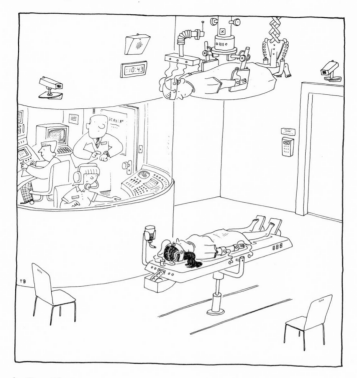

Illustration by Tom Bloom

magnetic). The general is in full uniform, medals shimmering in the lights, and announces, "Now hear this. This is The Plan."

We offer classes for childbirth educators on the "detection" of postpartum depression. We "evaluate outcomes" and are encouraged to check "alternative policies" available. We are shown "tactics" for being on the "offense." There are "multidimensional strategies" for pregnancy and birth and "combative techniques" for postpartum "isolation." We teach "proper" and "improper" "applications" of teaching "aids." We learn "theories" of teaching and learning, and we are concerned with "implementing" programs in teaching "facilities." This is all for natural ("natural") childbirth. What I keep learning is that when a war is fought, in truth, no one ever really "wins." It is time for diplomacy, détente, glasnost. Mostly, it is time to get off of the battlefield and out of the war.

Of course, one of the ways to do that is to take childbirth classes out of the hospital. Afraid to do that, you say? You want the couples to be "comfortable" with that setting, so that when they go there in labor, when they are at a vulnerable place, they'll feel relaxed and at ease? Is a goldfish supposed to feel comfortable in a house full of cats?

Best-Laid Plans

In childbirth classes couples are encouraged to make a "birth plan." Years ago I thought this was a good idea; I think we even included one in *Silent Knife*. It was an opportunity to zero in on (another war term) the things that were important at birth and to discuss with one's "caregiver" different points and options. It was a way to protect our interests—kind of like a prenuptial agreement. But we all know now that birth plans are mostly a waste of time. Even if the doctor reads it, agrees to it, and signs it, he can take that back at anytime during the birth if, in his judgment, that option would not be in the best interests of you or the baby. "Yes, Mrs. Jones, I know I said that you didn't have to have the monitor on the whole time, but I need to know how this baby is doing, you know"; "Seems as if your body just doesn't know how to stretch enough, Mrs. Gleason, looks like we'll have to do a little cut here"—even when he assured you that he never does episiotomies and knows what to do to assist the mother's body at the time of delivery. Birth plans are, in my opinion, not only unnecessary and a waste of time but completely ineffective. They're only a piece of paper, and all your options go up in smoke when something is "amiss" in the doctor's eyes during labor.

Birth plans inherently smack of a level of mistrust between the two parties involved. Instead of being a springboard from which a discussion of birth philosophy can arise, and a determination made as to whether your philosophies "fit," the list of options becomes a merit badge for OBs—if he signs it, of course he is one of the good scouts. Or is he? Since "natural" birth is fashionable these days and all OBs want to be considered flexible, they almost always sign on the dotted line. Just remember that technology has also given us erasable pens. And if you really trusted someone, you wouldn't be going through all these shenanigans just to ensure that your requests were understood and would be met: you would just know that they were/would be.

We are told that one good reason to have a birth plan is that doctors forget which woman wants which option. "Suzi Q." doesn't care if she has an episiotomy, so why not do one? "Nellie O." is going to bottlefeed, so it doesn't matter if her baby gets sugar-water. When the day comes that we all believe that no woman really wants to get cut and that all babies deserve to be given mother's milk, then we will dispense with "birth plans." The only plans will be those in our heart that know instinctively what is supposed to happen at birth—what "options" make for the very best, most natural experience. When we begin to honor and value human life, and the process by which that life "arrives" here, we will not have to make lists that tell others "we want complete rooming-in." The birth plans I have seen usually begin with, "Unless there is an extenuating circumstance." Seen through the eyes of most OBs in this country today, *most* births find themselves in the midst of "extenuating circumstances"—at which point "The Plan" might just as well be down the tube. In fact, in a cartoon sent to me, a doctor is seen folding a birth plan into a paper airplane as the couple is leaving his office.

Where Did We Go Wrong?

One Wisconsin birth activist writes about the classes in her city.

This area is still doing some very bizarre things to birthing women and those of us outside the system are really having a hard time getting the message across. I cannot figure out the mentality here, not of the instructors who are teaching such absolute nonsense, nor of the women who are listening to it. Last year there were four separate sets of classes in which *one hundred* percent of the couples had c-sections—and these were not cesarean classes! The instructor just goes on her merry way . . . and people keep signing up either because they don't know how bad it is or they feel they have no place else to go. The hospital teaches a VBAC class, which of course are always full since everyone was sectioned the first time around. It's like a conspiracy . . . The VBAC class is one two-hour session of telling mothers how high risk they are and what their statistical chances [of having a VBAC] are. The primary rate of cesareans here is 45%. The only accepted form of antenatal class is the hospital-run Lamaze course. The hospital has developed their own labor assistant's program using people only from their staff. I don't have to tell you where that is headed. Oh well, at least this state has great cheese.

I have heard Sheila Kitzinger speak many times.[2] She tells us that in most classes, women are taught to compromise, to ask for things tactfully, not to have preconceived ideas about what they want the birth to be, and to avoid setting their sights too high. She says they are being conditioned into submission and are being taught compliance. She says women are taught to exert self-discipline—not to cry out, to be nice to the nurse and doctor, to obey instructions—even to wait to push until you have been given permission! She believes that dependency is fostered in classes. I agree: "Ask your doctor about this"; "Make sure you have your doctor's permission to do that"; "Have you checked with your OB?" are commonplace evocations at most childbirth classes.

We treat women as irresponsible and selfish. We are not treated as adults and as a result often do not behave as adults. We are simply sucked into the system. We teach parents that they share the responsibility for their births with professional experts, and then we wonder why we see so many anxious mothers who are unable to make decisions and who look to the "experts" for advice. She calls it "meticulously conditioned helplessness."

In many classes women are told not how to avoid problems, but who will be there to help when they encounter any one of a dozen things that can occur during the course of a normal labor. Some childbirth educators won't recommend a book or show a particular film (on homebirth, for example) because the material is "too radical" or it has not yet been approved by the hospital staff. They should be shown anyway to expose people to different alternatives.

Many instructors haven't had a natural birth themselves and cannot understand what all the fuss is about a little demerol or nicentil. Many educators pay their allegiance as a member of the staff of the hospital for which they work, and are committed to maintaining the status quo rather than to altering the system.

As I travel around the country, I am greeted by hundreds of caring, well-intentioned childbirth teachers who are afraid of teaching anything that would alienate the physicians whose referrals are so important to them. They are very concerned about the number of unnatural births, complications, and cesarean sections that are occurring but don't know how to help alleviate those situations. I meet hundreds of instructors who want to teach a comprehensive, inspiring, exciting series of classes, something that will bring birth back to its rightful source. They know that even their own classes promote obstetrical technology, greedy institutions, and insensitive doctors. Childbirth education meant well, but it's been a farce.

Summa Cum Laude

Still, we have reason to be optimistic. More and more childbirth teachers are teaching in their homes, or at libraries, or in churches, where they don't have to be the least bit concerned about whether the hospital sanctions or censors the material. One woman, who left the hospital scene said,

> What a difference! I used to teach only what the obstetrical staff would allow, i.e., only what the doctors wanted them to know. I'd slip in a few things every now and then, but usually there was a doctor on staff "visiting"—to add credibility, I guess to what I was saying. Even when there were no OBs at the class, I felt like "Big Brother" was watching: what if one of the couples went back and told their doctor what I had said? Now I teach what I want them to know—what I wish I had known! I feel so much better, and I can tell real easy that they do, too: they aren't all out there recovering from sections and episiotomies anymore.

Today the Cesarean Prevention Movement sponsors a program called "Birthworks." In addition, midwives also teach classes as do individuals through NAPSAC, AAHCC, La Leche League, homebirth organizations, and spiritual groups. Many of us have "taught" childbirth by telephone or in a single evening in our homes. Some women who have been inspired by their own wonderful births find themselves "teaching" in their kitchens informally or at a playgroup meetings. Must we all be "accredited" in order to teach what we already know inside?

Goals

A while back, I jotted down a list of my goals for my childbirth classes. It reminds me where I want to go with these classes and helps me decide how I want to take myself there. If you are a childbirth educator, your goals may be different. If you are a pregnant woman, you may need something different from what I have to offer.

Goals:

To provide classes that are totally consumer oriented.

To create an understanding of birth as a significant life event for the entire family, the effects of which are immeasurable.

To help women understand the importance of taking responsibility for their births— and their lives.

To help each woman find her own strengths and potential.

To educate in a practical fashion by increasing the awareness of birth as a natural, safe, and normal occurrence.

To help women feel trusting and loving of their bodies and confident about labor and delivery.

To teach the concerns, dangers or potential consequences of unnecessary interventions into the birth process.

To stimulate concern for the alarming rate of cesarean sections and unpure births in this country.

To examine some of the psychological, emotional, sexual, and spiritual aspects of birth and how each of these relates to safe and satisfying birthing.

To help those with feelings of disappointment, sadness, confusion, fear, and anger—from their past birth experience or in anticipation of their first birth—to acknowledge, address, express, release or heal these feelings (if they so choose)— so that they can bring an integrated and peaceful mind-body to their experience.

To provide an experience of support, caring, enthusiasm, energy, and safety that can serve as a model for birthing.

To continue to examine my own beliefs about birth and the issues surrounding birth so that I can teach with as much clarity and effectiveness as possible. To continue to heal and grow on my own, to listen well, to teach enthusiastically and with confidence, and to have a whole lot of fun!

To learn as I teach: to keep the well full at all times.

To feel a sense of connectedness, respect, and appreciation for each and every one of the people who have entrusted themselves—or have been entrusted—to me. To remember that this work is a privilege.

To be true to myself. To live in my heart and to teach from it as well.

To LOVE.

Classes

My classes are from one hour to twelve weeks (2 1/2–3 hours each) long, depending on a whole lot of different factors.

The first task that has to be "addressed" in any childbirth class, I think, is to find a way for each person in that class to create "spaces" to receive the information that will be shared. If everyone is filled with fear, then confidence or determination, for example, will have no place to go inside of that body. Almost the very moment that I begin a class, just after I have said, "Hi! I'm really glad you are here!" I look around the room and ask, *"Okay, so what are you scared of? What are you scared about?"* I explain about the spaces they can "free up," and we go from there. As one person shares something that she's afraid about, others are nodding their heads: "Oh, so you've thought about that too? I thought I was the only one."

This usually takes some time, depending on how many people are in the room. The more we talk about what we are afraid of, the more peaceful and relaxed the room becomes. I'm afraid I won't be able to "do it"; I'm afraid if I have another cesarean, I'll crack up: I'm afraid of the pain of labor; I'm afraid my doctor will be on vacation; I'm afraid I won't love this baby as much as my first or that something will be wrong with it; I'm worried that we don't have enough money/time/energy for twins. On and on and on and on. We talk about these concerns, and we talk some more. We haven't even introduced ourselves, and we're talking openly and honestly and preparing for birth.

The next things I always say are

Why are you here? Some of you aren't the least bit sure why you are here! Some of you fathers probably wish you were at a basketball game or even home mowing the lawn! I hope that by the end of these classes, no, even by the end of this class, you'll be really glad that you are/were here. It's probably hard to believe, but once someone actually *gave away* his Celtics tickets and came here instead, even though his wife told him it was okay to miss that class! I hope this is a place that you really, really look forward to being at every week—a haven in an otherwise nutsy existence, whatever. I hope that in a short time you really FEEL how appreciative I am that you are here. I don't think I'll ever really know for certain why, but I feel so drawn to birth, it's so important to me: at some point during these next weeks, you are going to know inside your heart that that is true, and when you do, you will know how much I honor and appreciate that you are here, how grateful I am to you. . . . But for now, why are you here?

They come because they're going to have a baby. They come because they took childbirth classes last time and they didn't work. They come because somebody told them that this radical little lady had some information that would help them. They come because all their friends had c-sections and they want to avoid one. They come for a whole lot of reasons.

The next question: *"What do you need from being here?"* is a big one. If women/couples can get in touch with what they need, learn to put it out into the universe, and find ways to get it, they may find birthing that much easier. How many of you knew you needed something at birth—love, support, music, a back rub, something to eat, to take a walk outside, to get out of the hospital— but didn't follow those instincts and ask for what it was you wanted? In a childbirth workshop that I attended years ago, Claudia Panuthos asked women how long it was from the time they knew they had to urinate to the time they actually did. Some women said it took them five minutes, others twenty, still others said that they sometimes 'held it' all afternoon. Not one said that they went the moment their body told them they needed to. Our bodies are so wise, and yet we often ignore the messages that they are giving us or delay responding to them. This is true when we have feelings, as well. We suppress them, or judge them, or try to make them go away.

One woman told me that she was freezing cold throughout her labor. She'd had a jonnie on; I asked her if she had asked for more blankets or a sweater or had asked them to turn the heat up. She knew what she needed, but she didn't want to be a bother to the nurses. Sadly, she's no exception; many women become childlike and unassertive in labor. Even if you know what you need, if you can't put it out into the universe loud and clear, there's a lot less chance you will get it. Of course you can always wait for someone to notice that you are cold, but they themselves might be warm and not even think to ask.

We talk about how to get results. If you put something out into the universe, how long do you wait to see if it will come to you? How do you set things in motion so that you get what you need? This and other issues become the central themes of the classes.

My next question is: *What does support look like? What does it feel like? How do you know that you are being supported?* And so we begin to think about support. It feels warm and safe. It feels trusting. It feels like you don't have to be on guard. It's like wearing soft, bunny slippers. It's a touch and genuine caring. I ask: if you felt as if the people in this room were supporting you 100 percent, how would you know? They'd listen when I talked. They'd make eye contact. They'd not make judgments. It'd be okay to cry. I would know that what I said was confidential. I'd feel cared about. And then I ask: *How many of you would like to feel that kind of support here?* They all do. *How many are willing to give that kind of support?* They all are. I explain I want them to have an experience of total support and safety in these classes. If they know they can just be who they are and think what they think without fear of criticism or judgment, they'll begin to feel safe. If they feel warmth and affection, they'll begin to feel support. The classes become a model for supported birthing: we create a safe and wonderful space. If women have never really, truly felt total support, how will they know if they have it at birth? Feeling—knowing—what support "looks" like, what it feels like, and how to create it are extremely important issues for birth and can be experienced and emphasized throughout the classes.

Throughout the classes we talk a lot about setting limits and boundaries. Generally, people tend to gravitate to the same spot in the room each week, creatures of habit that we are. Once they get comfortable in that spot, we try out different places. At first, it throws them off a little. Jean, you sit over there. Carl, I want you to sit by the window this week. This is helpful in learning how to "stay centered." I've had two couples who have planned homebirths who transferred to the hospital, and both had VBACs. Both said that this little exercise helped them to stay relaxed in spite of a different surrounding. We do a lot— A LOT—with holding hands—feet massage, etc. to figure out what is okay with us in terms of other people 'encroaching on our space' (both physical and emotional space) and what isn't. We learn to check inside to see if it feels okay to be touched, and how to say NO when it doesn't feel alright. We learn that you do not have to allow anyone to touch you if you don't want to during labors.

In one class, there were two men who couldn't understand what was so awful about a cesarean. The following week, an idea popped into my head. I conducted the class with their pregnant wives sitting on them. For more than two hours, the men lay on the floor with their wives seated on their bellies. At first, Peter and Mark were amused. After a while, they became tired of it all. "Too bad, you guys, the cesarean isn't over. You can't move yet. You are still anesthetized." When an hour had passed, they both had had "enough of this!" Peter said, "Okay, Nancy, you have made your point!" I said to his wife, Ellen, "Is the cesarean over?" And she said, quietly, "No, not yet." Mark's wife, Michelle, said "Absolutely not!"

I told Peter and Mark they represented the men everywhere who just didn't understand what it was like to be sectioned—who thought that being tied down, unable to move, was "okay." For three hours, they remained supine. During refreshment time, their wives, Ellen and Michelle, were served a refreshing glass of juice and some wholesome, delicious snacks. Peter and Mark were given nothing. I wanted to do anything I could to help these men understand their wives' pain.

Near the end of the class, we formed a circle around Ellen and Peter and Michelle and Mark. I asked both women if they would be willing to tell their husbands one more time, in front of us, what it felt like to have a cesarean. Peter and Mark listened as their wives told them, for perhaps the twentieth time in two years, what they had been feeling. Both men, stiff, tired, and hungry, listened. Peter buried his hands in his face. He said to Ellen, "I'm getting it. In fact, I hated to see them cut you open. I thought I was going to lose you and I couldn't handle that so I distracted myself by seeing how many of the muscles and bones inside I could still name, after all these years out of anatomy class."

The women thanked the men for what they had done.

Everyone stayed very late that night. They all said they didn't want to leave to go home. But I had to set MY "boundaries and limits," and close to midnight I kicked them all out! Peter and Ellen both thanked me and went out with their arms around each other. Mark hadn't said very much, but that week, he left a note to Michelle on their kitchen table telling her he'd support her in a home birth.

Another night, there was a feeling inside of me that this was the night to dance. So I got some great music and put it on full volume. I mean, if you are too inhibited to let people see you dance, are you going to be able to let them see you give birth?[3] Is there even a correlation at all? I haven't the foggiest idea. I just knew that this was how I had to "conduct" that particular class. I hadn't known it until I did it. We even got the decided nondancers to join us. It was great fun and since then dancing has been a part of my curriculum.

I play lots of music in my classes. Once I wasn't really in the mood to talk a lot. It felt like a quiet, reflective evening. So I put on a tape of really beautiful music, lit a candle and turned off the lights. For almost an hour, we just listened to the music. Then, we ended up talking about quiet things, and the things that relaxed and soothed us, and about babies. I always play "Welcome to the World, Dear Child," "If You Want Me to Grow" (what a little baby might say to its parents if it could talk the moment it was born) "The Tears are the Healing," "River," and "Lady Without Fear."

We've sung nursery rhymes in class, and we have colored (if I am in the mood to let others use my 64-pack of Crayolas. Sometimes I just don't want to share.) Sometimes we color while we are doing nursery rhymes. We light candles. I once asked all the women to wear their sexiest nightgowns—over their clothes— and we talked about the sexuality of birth. We have even acted out our rendition of a Southern Revival Meeting: "You think *your* cesarean was bad, sister? Well, let me tell you about *mine*! Do you think *you* have suffered? NO! Not on your life have *you* suffered as *I* have suffered! Do you want me to tell you how much I have suffered? I will TELL you how much I have suffered! You had twenty four-hours of labor? I had *thirty-four* hours of labor, sisters and brothers, count-them, yes, M'am, thirty-four! *Oh how I have suffered!*" followed by the next person who is certain she has suffered far more. This has brought up much laughter and many tears as well.

I used to do a healing circle in the classes. Anyone who had had a particularly bad day, or week, could get into the circle and we'd sit around them and beam them some "good vibes." At first, the circle was empty; everyone would look around and giggle a little or look bored. So I got into the middle. I said, "Well, if none of you need any extra love and good feelings sent to you, that's great, but I can always use a little more." Then we had our talk about "needs," and the next week three people decided they needed to be in the middle. By the fourth week, the middle of the circle was crowded, and by the fifth, there was more middle than outer. At that point, we simply turned the circle inside out!

If someone has an "anatomy" question, I ask them to close their eyes. "See your pelvis?" (nods) "Okay, well see, there are two ligaments that cradle the uterus, one on each side, can you see that also?" Almost always, they "see." Later, when we do some things about birth, I ask them if they can "see" the birth canal and the baby coming through. We use visualization to see how the cervix opens up, how the baby descends, and how the hormones change and soften everything up. Each woman visualizes in her own way. Some of the women have written letters to their pelvis, or to the placenta, for example. We become well acquainted and very good friends with our bodies, indeed.

Once I brought down a can of tomato juice and poured it into a bowl so we could decide how much blood it would be okay to lose at birth. I didn't plan that one either. If I didn't have tomato juice in the house, I suppose I would have brought down the grapefruit juice and we could measure urine output like they do in the hospital. We do silly things and fun things and spontaneous things. More than once we have taken a walk at the end of class. Yes, we also talk about interventions and the place of birth, and labor and the baby, all in good time.

I want to tell you about one more experience that I had in class. It happened when I was talking about vaginal exams. I took out a pair of sterile gloves (still packaged) and held them up. As I was talking about how totally unnecessary most vaginal exams are, I ripped open the package so I could put them on. Laura was sitting in the corner. I heard her gasp. I looked over at her, and said, "Laura, what was that?" She said, "What was what?" I said to her that I thought I had heard her gasp. She said, "It wasn't me." A few minutes later, I took out another pair of gloves. I opened them, and was certain, this time, that Laura had made some sound. Others had heard it, too. I went over to Laura and asked her how she was feeling. She said that in fact, she had started to feel sick a few minutes earlier but didn't want to leave the class and miss anything.

She'd been feeling fine until I started talking about vaginal exams. I went back over to her and quickly opened up another package of gloves—right next to her face this time, and with very little warning. She gasped again, and this time, she heard it herself. "What's this about, Laura?" I asked. I was putting on a glove now and I was holding my hand up, as if I was just waiting to give an internal.

We found out in the next few minutes what the gasps were about. Laura had given birth at a big teaching hospital in another state. She had had a thirty-four-hour labor that resulted in a cesarean section. During her thirty hours in the hospital, people came in almost every twenty minutes, she said, to "check her." We calculated that she had had at least ninety vaginal exams before she was given a cesarean: we figured there must have been at least once or twice when somebody forgot or took a lunch break. I asked her why she didn't object, and she said that she thought twenty-minute checks during labor were routine. She said her vagina hurt for a month after her cesarean.

So what did we do? I didn't have ninety gloves. So we got paper and pens and each traced our hands several times on paper, making the tracings larger than our hands. I gave each person in the class one real glove, and along with our paper gloves, we went outside into my driveway. I got a trash can and matches. We handed Laura gloves, one at a time, and, one at a time she burned them and put them in the trash can. It was quite a ceremony, symbolic and all that. How many vaginal exams do you think Laura had during the rest of this pregnancy and her entire labor and delivery? If you guessed one, you guessed too many. She'd paid her dues. She figures if she has twenty-five or thirty kids, she'll bring the average number of exams per child down to a reasonable number.

We never introduce ourselves in my classes, but we get to know one another very well. Most of the classes "vote" to go an extra few weeks. Most continue to meet on their own, for a long while after the babies are born. People from the classes often attend each other's births. After a class is over, a grieving takes place for each of us, I think. I don't start another class right away. I wait a few weeks because I need a little time to rest and reflect. I miss them all for a long time after the classes are over, but I am filled with the love and energy that was given and received during the weeks we were together.

"Tuesday nights will never be the same," one father wrote me after the classes were over. One mother wrote,

> Every single week, I have gained more insight and understanding about myself. Because of the classes, I have begun to search within—a journey I should have taken long ago. My husband and I have opened the lines of communication—it is so much easier now! The little "birth parasites" that I had inside have moved residence. I am looking forward to this birth with more excitement and joy than I ever thought possible. I no longer "blame" myself for the cesarean—I use it as a learning experience. I feel a sense of self-confidence that I have never felt before. I learned these weeks that there are limits and boundaries that I can set—and that gives me a sense of freedom and well-being. There are no limits or boundaries to the love that I have, however, and that is sent to you in this envelope along with these words.

Another person said, "You teach a vision of childbirth. These classes are not just for birth, they are classes for living."

There are many effective ways to teach, and many different styles; mine is just one among many. I have learned so much from so many people. These classes are not just mine: they are the best of what so many people have taught me thus far. They feel good. They feel right. I wish that I could have taken something like them when I was pregnant with our first. Instead, I learned about hospital policy, the signs and symptoms of pregnancy, and of course, most importantly, how to breathe. Good thing, too. I found out that I hadn't been breathing right my whole life long.

13 *Birth!*

PART I BELIEFS!

If you don't change your direction, you'll end up where you are headed.

—Chinese proverb

Linda Goodman writes that medicine slowly but surely grew into the status of almost a religion, "supported by congregations of patients in awe of its white-coated high priests, who would not tolerate the slightest criticism of themselves or their new profession, and, in fact, demanded a kind of respect that nearly amounted to worship. . . . Enter the physicians—genuflect, please."[1]

If you are one of those people who believes that doctors know it all and that birth is a medical situation, you may very well find yourself on an operating table, ready to let them demonstrate their vast amount of knowledge by making a cut into your abdomen. The fact that you are in the hospital for birth makes it fairly easy to deduce that you do not believe birth is "safe." If you believed it was, you wouldn't need to surround yourself with emergency equipment and medically trained people. If you continue to believe that birth is unsafe, you may find it difficult to relax, release, let go, open up, and let your baby be born.

According to Alan Watts,[2] belief is the insistence that the truth is what one would like it or wish it to be. The believer opens his or her mind to the truth on the condition that it fits with preconceived ideas or wishes. (Faith, he says, is an unreserved opening of the mind to the truth, whatever it may turn out to be. "Belief clings; faith lets go.")

Mind and Body, Body and Mind

What we think influences what we do, and our experiences then influence our thoughts. We are like scientists, experimenting and calculating whether the results "fit" our lives. Scientists have proven that energy and matter are inter-changeable. Our thoughts affect our bodies and our bodies affect our thoughts. The mind and body are each an expression of the other. There is no separation of the two. They are inextricably bound together. "The slightest deviation from perfect health provides valid data to explore one's overall growth process [and feelings]."[3]

David Cayley tells us that the success of the obstetrical system is measured in mortality statistics. The quality of the experience is considered an extra. He says that it is not uncommon to hear OBs accusing women who want a homebirth or a purebirth of self-indulgence, "as if the feelings of the mother and the outcome of the birth had nothing to do with one another. The separation of birth as a physical event from the birth as a psychological event is an expression of the mind-body split which has characterized our culture generally."[4]

Energy moves from the body to the mind and the mind to the body, sort of like a figure eight. If we are afraid, for example, it will show, at some point, in our bodies. Goodman cautions us that fear is a powerful faith, "capable of changing the law of physics. Fear is faith in the negative, and strong faith manifests its images as swiftly and surely when projected by negative current as by positive." She says that a foundation beneath a process must be strong or supportive, "or it will fail, just as a house will fall down if the foundation crumbles." The foundation for birth, she says, "is absolute confidence." Some people, she says, long for something, but instead of bringing it into existence to make it a reality in their lives, they "bring about the opposite and blame it on some Deity, on 'fate', or on destiny."[5]

We have all heard that as ye sow so shall ye reap. Goodman says, "You are the Producer and the Director of the drama of your life. You cast all the characters in it, who mingle and act with you. . . . Because you are also the star of the show, it is sometimes difficult for you to realize how many 'hats you wear' in the production. If you did, you would know that you can change any scene, any time you wish." She believes that you can tune into the "Puppeteer" or the Higher Self or the Spirit, and ordain a "script change—perhaps even replacing one of the players or rewriting the scene." This is not done by wishing or hoping; it is accomplished by "ordering, commanding, ordaining."[6]

Our thoughts are incredibly powerful: "We are what we think, having become what we thought"; "Thoughts produce results"; "We can if we believe we can: Not because belief makes it so, but because we can, and belief lets our power manifest"; "We have the ability to project our thoughts outward into physical form and thus create our own reality"; "Thoughts persisted in produce states of consciousness which if persisted in produce physical realities."[7]

Hi, Cuz . . .

I love kaleidoscopes. Last year, I went into a new little gift shop in my hometown and immediately fell in love with one of the most beautiful kaleidoscopes I had ever seen. When I found out the price, my heart dropped. There was no way I could justify spending that much money on something that was definitely not a necessity in our lives. I went back to the store twice that week, and once a few weeks later, hoping that the kaleidoscope would be on sale—and secretly hoping that it would have been sold so that I could mourn it and get on with my life. It wasn't on sale, it wasn't going to be on sale, and it wasn't sold. I thought about that kaleidoscope often over the next few weeks.

A month later, my family took a trip to New York City. We were doing some shopping, and I ducked into a book store. Out of the side of one eye, I saw it: in an enclosed glass counter near the front of the store was "my" kaleidoscope. My heart leaped—and then fell again—as I saw the price tag—five dollars more than what it had been selling for back home. (A bargain, perhaps, considering we had just come out of F.A.O. Schwartz and I had seen the most wonderful stuffed animal moose for a mere $12,000.)

A few days later, we arrived home from New York. The screen door was held slightly ajar by a package on the doorstep addressed to me. I ripped it open and to my complete shock and delight, there was the kaleidoscope, shimmering royal blue with gold and green. I ran to my husband to thank him: "You bought it after all! You had it sent!" "I didn't buy that thing for you," he said. "You know me well enough to know I wouldn't spend money on something like that." "Yea, I guess you're right," I said.

The kaleidoscope had been sent from a cousin of mine in California that I had only seen three times in my entire life. We had been extremely close as teenagers, continued to write on occasion, and I had seen her three years earlier when I was out west. But it had been almost a year since our last contact. The note read: "I was shopping in Beverly Hills last week. While I was in a particular store, I started thinking about you. When I walked by the enclosed gift, I actually heard a voice that said your name! You are going to think I am crazy for sending such a silly thing, but I hope you like it anyway."

Are we connected, or what? What a lesson for me. What we put out loud and clear into the universe often manifests. Those of you who have dreams and desires about birth, begin manifesting!

In the chapter on homebirth, I told you about the phone call I received a few hours after I had "lost" the midwife who was going to attend me at my birth. I didn't even realize that I was putting out "vibes" then, but my tears were so pure and so loud that perhaps on some level, "the word" got out very quickly indeed. I believe that my letting go (physically by crying, and emotionally by beginning to understand, possibly for the very first time, that I—not a midwife—was responsible for the birth of this child) created the open pathway needed so that someone could hear my call.

What You "See" May Be What You Get

Ilya Prigogine states that in a paradigm shift, it is always more important to have a change of vision than to have a sense of small new ideas. "Without the statement of a new dominant paradigm, new insights will *never* [emphasis his] gain a foothold. The reason, once seen, is overwhelming: The ideas supporting a new paradigm cannot even be explained or articulated in the language of the old paradigm." You may need your own new 'paradigm shift' in order to birth normally. Expect some "turbulence," he says, as you change your belief system as you un-indoctrinate, untangle yourself from the web of the present American birth paradigm.

If only I had known Prigogine years back, I could have relaxed. All the "turbulence" in my life after the cesarean was just me, jumping to a higher order, that's all. All the nights I would wake up and think, "You are going to stay at home and have a baby. You are really off the wall. What is the matter with you?!" Nothing was "the matter"; I was shifting my paradigm, changing my belief system, that's all.

There have been a number of interesting "belief changes" among the women who have contacted me. One was a woman whose religion told her that she had to obey her clergyman. She went to him asking for a blessing to have her fourth child naturally after three cesareans. He told her that for her own safety, she needed to see a doctor and follow his advice. When she went to the doctor, he vehemently opposed the idea of a VBAC in her situation. She called me, pretty much resigned to another c-section, and said that in her heart, she knew she needed to listen to her religious leader. I asked her what he said. She told me: "To listen to the doctor." I said, "Follow his advice! In this country, the doctor is God. Have you listened yet to God?" She had a VBAC at home. She had to shift her belief system in some way in order to do so. Her clergyman later said that he fully expected her to follow the doctor's orders; in other words, to have the baby by cesarean in the hospital.

Virginia Sandlin asks,[8] "What do I want to be? The curious part is that the question is languaged as a future possibility. Of course, the reality is that I am being now; therefore, perhaps I should be considering the inquiry, 'What am I being now, and is that a support system for producing the results I want to produce? Is the way I am being now consistent with who I am or the statement I want to make in the world?' " Another way of putting this: Act "as if" you are already where you want to be. Act "as if" you have already had your natural childbirth, or your VBAC.

When some women write to me, it seems reasonable to conclude that their belief system is "iffy" as it relates to purebirth or VBAC. You can tell this either by their language or by the way they are setting things up. One woman wrote, "I am working hard toward this birth, but I feel the odds are against me. . . . I have asked a friend to be with me in labor. She is not especially knowledgeable about birth, but she is very metaphysical. . . . The things that concern me about her being the 'right' person are: she has had two cesareans herself and I don't think she likes my husband. He bears no negativity towards her, but I wonder if the chemistry is 'right.' I really can't find anyone else who would be a better choice, though. I do have second thoughts every now and again." Another woman wrote, "I don't think I can get a perfect situation. We can't get everything we want, and must make do with what we have. My midwife agrees that a heparin lock is unnecessary, but it's hospital policy. Actually, my own body seems to be the greatest hindrance—I think the baby is breech." A third woman said: "Oh, I knew pitocin was a drug and that any way of inducing labor before the body's ready would be asking for trouble, but by the time my body's ready, it's bad for the baby. . . . Maybe the second abruption was a result of the pit—or—maybe it would have happened anyway and it's a good thing we got the baby out on time." I want you to know that I have no judgments about either of these women—only an observation about their thought processes and beliefs.

Kimberly Wulfert, a psychotherapist in California remarks that new information (such as that received in childbirth classes) is "not taken as virgin material, but is carved by the perceptions and prejudices of the mind receiving it. A woman giving birth is inherently limited by her perceptual framework, so to speak." The woman enters the experience with a set of preconceived beliefs of what it will be like, "and it is these beliefs, more than the sensations or events that will define and interpret her experience." If this is so, Kim says, understanding beliefs would increase the reliability of predicting the outcome of her delivery. "This is important because the beliefs can be used in the prenatal months as a focal point in a therapy setting."[9]

Shirley Luthman has written a number of books on positive energy and personal power. She tells us that if we have to explain or convince anyone about our values, or belief system, then "we are not operating on the same plane." She says that we do not get respect or confirmation that our system is "right" by explaining or demanding. We get respect and confirmation by respecting ourselves and by taking responsibility.[10]

Balancing

As you have read, each of us has male and female energy internally. The feminine is intuitive feelings, perceptions, images, fantasies; the masculine is aggression, action-oriented, intellectual. Luthman says that "concept" is androgynous: men are as intuitive as women and women are as powerful as men. In our culture, "we have made the male form embody the masculine. The male principle without the female is violent and empty. The male principle is driving, logical, controlling—without the female, it will destroy you." In the feminine principle, power is depreciated. "Women look for men to assert for them so they will not look powerful or unfeminine, and men look to women to nurture them (without having to ask for it) so they will not appear weak or "unmasculine." As a result, she says, there is a tremendous power struggle between them: "When I give you power to do something for me that I cannot do for myself, I resent you even though there may be a lot between us that is positive. With that thread of resentment, there is an element of anger, distance, and distrust."[11]

Luthman says that the shift of women to places of logic, protection, and aggression and of men to trust, intuition, receptivity, and nurturance is difficult. People feel as though they are threatening their survival, sexuality, and identity by trusting that part of themselves that does not fit the cultural view of male/female. However, for those whose belief systems are not conducive to normal births, it may be important to push through the difficulty and to find "qualities" on the "other side" that allow for a new paradigm to develop. We are told that nothing external ever ensures security. It is that which we have adopted and embraced on the inside that allows us feelings of peace.[12]

The intuitive, spiritual, feminine aspect of individuals has not been incorporated into the fabric of our society because our culture has been based in the male process. We have only trusted what we can see and feel, not the intangible. The intuitive has been labeled capricious and hysterical as opposed to the logical, calm, stable male. If our belief system is based on the intuitive, we may have difficulty accepting it, owning it, and honoring it. We may fight to change it, or disallow it, replacing it with a more "acceptable" set of beliefs such as "doctors know best" or "hospitals are the safest place to birth a baby" or "women's bodies need help at birth." Shirley says that when we find a balance between the feminine and masculine, and our belief systems are based on that balance, then we're headed in the right direction. For example: "Assertion means letting your words, behavior, and expressions follow the flow of feeling . . . respect your feeling. It means, every moment in time, doing what you want to do and not doing what you don't want to do." It doesn't mean bullying someone, or ignoring someone else. It does, however, mean listening "from a higher place—and not the head." Once a belief system is formed, you must continue to be "assertive": "How can you expect large [steps] to work successfully when you do not take small [steps] to follow your feelings?"[13]

Many people have a belief system that says that the teacher teaches and the student learns. "The teacher ostensibly has all the answers and the students, like baby birds, wait, open-mouthed, for pearls of wisdom to drop into their beaks." Most of us support this arrangement in childbirth classes, "because it seems to reduce our anxieties, make us feel more secure, and keeps us from taking risks. It also keeps us infantile and our learning on a primitive level. . . . If we give up such a [belief], we have to trust our intuition—that the answers we need are inside each of us."[14] If we have the belief that others know better than we do, then instead of focusing on our own understandings and awarenesses, we assess others' reactions and gauge our behavior accordingly. Most of us, Luthman says, have developed our rational, logical minds way out of proportion because our education focuses on that. "The ability to be logical and rational is commendable and valuable, but sometimes logic gets in the way. We don't need to discard it or jump impulsively, but we must learn to trust our feelings."[15] She says that as we give ourselves more and more power to direct us, intellect becomes the follower—so often we sacrifice ourselves! As we become more trusting of our own intuitive process, we learn that it assists us in understanding. We can let go of external supports without fear of destruction or loss. "As I trust me . . . I . . . focus less energy on protecting me from you."[16]

Meditation speeds up the opening of channels between the intuitive level of consciousness and the cognitive level.[17] For one of my birthdays, a friend bought me everything anybody could possibly need to meditate, including a small rug that had been blessed by at least two gurus and a swami. I got up faithfully three mornings in a row and proceeded to (a) fall back to sleep (morning one); (b) count the threads running horizontally in the guru rug (morning two); and (c) mentally alphabetize my marketing list for that day (morning three). I personally "meditate" more easily by taking a walk, listening to music, taking a bath, and swimming. Some people paint, run, make bread, or garden.

As we begin to be more intuitive, we get our own sonar or radar—we get vibrations—long before we reach the danger point. So many women say, "How will I know if I am that small percent of women who needs an intervention?" According to Luthman, if you are intuitive, the amount of energy available to you increases, and you will know. "As you begin to make decisions . . . *trust* [emphasis in original] that this expanded level of consciousness will not betray you no matter what the current external reality appears to be." She writes:

> I assert in the direction of getting something I want, but if my assertions get blocked, I stop and take stock. Perhaps I am going the wrong way for me, perhaps the timing is off and I need to wait a while, or there may be another way of accomplishing the same thing. . . . If I am in a situation in which there seems to be no avenue open to me, I let go and trust my intuitive process to give me the answer when I need it. Again, my timing may be off. Other events that I do not know about may be developing and will change my course of action. . . . There may be something I need to learn by staying in an immobilized state. . . . Face your pain, cry your tears, rage at circumstances or people—whatever clears your consciousness and spends your feelings. However, at that point, consider that something inside of you is always pulling you in a positive direction. . . . Once it happens to you, it belongs to your past. Learn from it.[18]

Luthman says that it is not her intention that we become obsessive about everything that has happened to us until we figure it out. Instead, she encourages us to open ourselves to whatever meaning may be within our experience to know. If no answer comes, "simply file the data away, and trust that it will, in time."[19]

Mehl and Peterson remind us not to blame ourselves if things do not go well. "To believe that personal responsibility for health means that the person is 'choosing' ill health [or a bad birth] from a position of total freedom of choice, would imply a degree of control that none of us experiences in our lives. Herein lies an aspect of holistic health so misunderstood in present-day society. While it is true that the client is choosing from those choices available at the time, the choice itself arises from a position of compromised freedom. Complication represents a movement toward resolution within the client's experience of limited options. The human organism naturally works toward resolution of stress; the degree of 'choice' involved is experientially far from what the client desires."

Decision making, they say, is inherently nonrational; "Eventually, we must act, not on facts, but upon our feelings after weighing the facts." They remind us that in a holistic approach, "we are interested in anything that works, even if we can't explain how or why it works."[20] And, of course, the decision not to choose is one choice and may be the choice that we decide to live with.

If we assume that there is a "center of consciousness inside each of us that knows all the answers and is unerring in its direction of the evolution of ourselves," then we can relax and just "do" our births. If we know that even "limiting, unpleasant, or even destructive" processes are providing learning, then we can just "be." If we consider everything that happens to us "in the light of what the more expanded aspect of my consciousness is trying to teach me—when I stop fighting myself—then the war is over."[21]

"I Birth Joyfully and Easily"

Many women seem to believe that "birth will be difficult" or that "the pain will be insurmountable." Luthman remarks that we often function on the belief that a particular outcome is desirable or worthwhile only if it is difficult to come by. We feel virtuous when we have had to put ourselves through a wringer to accomplish something. She says that perhaps we set up painful circumstances in order to learn something vital and imperative on our journeys. We can fight and kick our heels and scream, or give up in despair, but we come back to the truth—that each of us is in charge of us. She suggests that we let go of old beliefs that do not serve us and create new ones. That which is most beneficial, most productive in aliveness and growth, is accomplished smoothly and easily; when an outcome evolves with ease and fluidity, the satisfaction I receive is deeper, truer, and lasting; as I let go of my need for limits, the possibilities open to me are truly beyond my wildest dreams.

In *Birth Reborn*, midwife Dominique Pourre talks about her change in beliefs.[22] It began when she birthed her own child. Until then, she believed that it was important for a mother to place her trust in doctors' and midwives' hands. "I could no longer be the first to touch the baby. I would not, any more, whisk the baby into another room, for some mysterious reason I've long forgotten. I would no longer wear rubber gloves, so that the infant's first contact would be with human skin. . . . It wasn't easy. . . . I would say to the mother, "You can deliver the baby yourself. Reach out and grasp those tiny arms, they are reaching for you. Don't be afraid, you can do it. It's your baby."

> You don't give up the professionally sanctioned role of "baby-snatcher" without a great deal of self denial. When I was the official "snatcher," I was so relieved by the sight of the baby; I would think "That's it, a baby boy, here he is, alive! I can hold him, I have the right. Oh, I was so scared he might not exist. Yes, just like you, the mother. I had the same feelings, the same anxiety. And now, I'll give

you a present: your child. But first, I have to examine him, bathe him, weigh him, dress him."

As Dominique changed her beliefs about who the baby belonged to and about birth as a dangerous event, she began to stand back. She writes a beautiful passage: "I hear her as she cries out, and I no longer try to quiet her. She becomes my teacher. I listen to her, I study her lessons. I myself am also pregnant, pregnant with her words, her pains, her strange cries which even she does not recognize as her own. I am overcome. There is nothing to teach her." Later, Dominique says, "I leave the room, exhausted, full of her emotions, her joy. . . . I have been taught: where women are free, we will learn how they give girth best. They will show us. They will trust us. Look at them. Listen closely."

Ah, Yes, I Remember it Well

We all have beliefs about birth that we carry on a cellular level from our own entrances into the world. Babies are fully conscious beings, and their experiences in utero, during birth, and postnatally produce basic belief structures about the world in general—even though most people have no conscious memories of those experiences.[23]

A midwife whom I met many years ago told me about a birth she had attended. The baby was born, healthy and strong. She was put to breast and spent quite a bit of time nursing contentedly. Two hours later, the placenta had not separated, and the decision was made to meet a supportive doctor at the hospital for assistance. The mother did not want to subject her newborn to the noises, bright lights, and germs of the hospital, and made the decision to go with her husband and the second midwife—leaving the baby at home with the first midwife. The placenta separated on the way to the hospital and the parents were only gone from their home about an hour. However, only moments after they had left the house, the baby had started to cry pitifully. The midwife rocked the baby, sang to it, and swaddled it, but nothing helped. She then offered the baby her breast for soothing. Within minutes, the baby had fallen asleep; the midwife put the baby in the cradle, and straightened up the room.

Almost four years passed, and the same woman became pregnant and called the midwife. At the home visit prior to the birth, the midwife was sitting on the living room couch. The almost four-year-old little girl woke up from her nap and walked into the living room. She went over to the midwife and said, "I remember you! You gave me 'nursies' when momma went in the car!"

Baby Talk

Another midwife told me about a precipitous labor during which the fetal heart tones were lost. The baby was coming too fast for transfer. Just as the midwife instructed her assistant to call an ambulance, she heard the baby say, "I'm alive!" so loudly and emphatically that she was certain everyone in the room had heard. In fact, one of the other people in the room did hear it (out of four others). This midwife has since "communicated" with a number of babies in utero, as have a number of others.

Mothers themselves, of course, communicate with their babies on so many different levels. When a Momdad asks a question in my class, I'll often tell her to ask the baby and see what s/he thinks. In labor once, a woman asked for "something to take the edge off." I asked her to check this out with her baby— to ask the baby what IT wanted. She started laughing—"It wants a sliced turkey on rye with lettuce and tomato—hold the mayo!" We got her the sandwich, which she wolfed down, and that was the last we heard about pain medication.

A technique called "rebirthing" may result in memories long since forgotten. Rebirthing advocates believe that since we form impressions about the world from our earliest times (the moment of conception) we can recall what we learned, embrace it if it is positive, or release or exchange it if it hinders our growth or prevents us from living well. "The thoughts we have are personal laws, and we operate upon them until they are unravelled and reversed. Feelings of being stuck, or 'not ready' (premature) can originate during birth."[24]

Beliefs

At the beginning of my workshops, and during the first weeks of my classes, I spell out a series of beliefs or philosophies. Everything I say or write about birth is based on these beliefs. So, here are some (not all) of my basic beliefs about birth. You may not agree with all of them, and some of them you have heard already, but knowing them will help you to understand why I say some of the things that I do in *Open Season*. They are listed in no particular order.

Birth is a normal physiological process that does not require tools, tubes, chemicals, drugs, machines or doctors.

Women and babies are designed to experience childbirth; they are designed to come through the experience safely and unharmed.

The pain of childbirth is healthy, normal, appropriate pain.

The spiritual, emotional, psychological and sexual environments in which a woman births are as important as other considerations—such as the size of her pelvis or the size of the baby—as a matter of fact, more important.

The attitude in our country that doctors deliver babies—rather than the belief that women give birth—perpetuates the high rate of unnatural births (including cesarean sections). Political and economic incentives also perpetuate the problem.

Any intervention into the birth process can (and most likely will) confuse the body and upset the process. This is true whether the interference is medical, physiological, or emotional.

Birth is a significant life experience. Its effects are long-lasting. It must be an experience which honors women, babies, families, and society at large.

Women are capable, strong human beings who are fully able to meet the challenges of giving birth—especially if they have information and support—but even without these.

There are very few reasons for intervention, and very few reasons for a cesarean section. These should be reserved for the rare occasions when Mother Nature needs a bit of assistance, not as routine procedures to "get the baby out."

If a woman with a previous cesarean does not feel that her body is healed, she will not allow a subsequent labor to become strong enough to birth the baby; No woman will continue to labor if she believes that the labor will harm her or her baby. For a woman to feel physically healed, emotional healing is usually necessary.

If the people who attend women at birth have upset, unfinished business, or fear about birth, or if their belief systems are not conducive to normal birthing, these thoughts may affect the birthing woman. We must all work to heal on psychological and spiritual levels about birth.

Good nutrition is essential for pregnancy and birth. Most doctors know beans about the vital role that nutrition plays and often harm women with their diets and recommendations.

Maternal well-being, the healthy integration of the birth experience, is of paramount importance. (Panuthos)

If you really don't want an episiotomy, or a forceps delivery, or a cesarean section, for example, you simply make certain that when you are in labor you have chosen a place where these procedures are unable to be performed. It is as simple as that.

It is the woman's responsibility to birth her baby and to make the decisions leading to this time in her life. It is not the doctor's or the institution's or the midwife's decision.

The caring fathers of the soon-to-be-born babies are extremely vulnerable in the hospital setting. They often become the doctor's cohort, with the woman and baby the pawns. Fathers are birthing, too, and together with the woman they deserve and need support and reassurance.

Each of us is either an advocate for birth or for the system. At this point in time, the two are mutually exclusive. We cannot be both. The system is not an advocate for women or babies or birth.

Women get to choose who—and how many people—they want at birth. They get to kick out anybody they don't want/like.

Love helps a baby get born.

PART II   SPIRIT!

It is not the man in the moon at all. It is not His face, but a faint echo of Her tender, maternal and nurturing image on the surface of the Moon, as gazed upon from Earth. . . . If you'd like to [see] for yourself, when the Moon is full—or near full—when it is

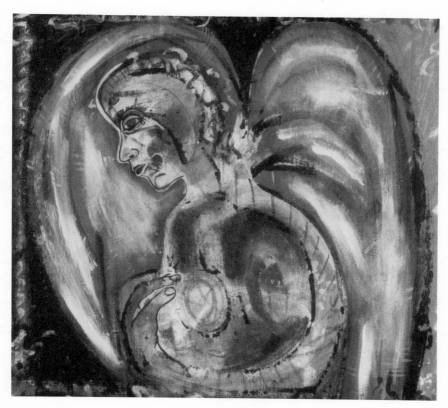

round in shape, not crescent—here is what to look for: The supremely feminine, cameolike face is seen in profile, facing toward the left. . . . Once the image springs into clarity for you . . . it's unmistakenly the profile of a woman of "unearthly" beauty. . . . It's a moving experience, and once you've seen it clearly, you will always see it clearly, each night when you look into the sky. [25]

Womanplace

Each of us has a "womanplace," the place inside that knows how to conceive the baby, nourish it, and, when the time is right, to birth it. It is not a place apart from us; it is within us. When it is acknowledged, encouraged to become more fully alive and present for us, and then experienced, our minds clear, our eyes sparkle, our confidence is bolstered, and our hearts are peaceful.

Whenever a pregnant woman asks me "What should I do?" I ask her to access her womanplace. The wisdom that she needs is right there for her to behold. The answers are all inside of her. The womanplace knows about pregnancy and labor and birth. It is a spring of information and resource. It is the place from which we bring forth new life.

Because I feel my own womanplace in my heart, I assumed that all women did. As I was talking about the womanplace in class one evening, one woman exclaimed, "Oh! I know where my womanplace is! It's in my fingertips." I found out a few minutes later that this woman was a pianist. She expressed her creativity, joy, and aliveness through her fingers. Through them, she felt confident, free, uninhibited, giving. Another woman said that her womanplace was at the soles of her feet. She spent the whole summer barefoot—mostly gardening. She loved the feel of the soil; it was how she felt most connected to the earth and to her own spirit and soul.

Some women feel their womanplace in their womb. Some behind their eyes. One woman knew that her womanplace was in or near her vocal chords—she had a beautiful voice and loved to sing. Almost as soon as I begin to talk about the womanplace, the energy in class begins to change. We feel wise, peaceful, and knowing. We feel loving and connected.

Nourishing the womanplace helps babies to be born. We find ways to remind us of that place inside—different ways for each of us. Fresh flowers; music; crystals or gemstones; a bath by candlelight; a certain piece of clothing; certain books; a painting; laughter; a garden salad. As the womanplace grows, it begins to fill us up inside, and the more it does so the more we seem to instinctively "know" about labor and birth. Fear begins to subside and is replaced with calm energy and excitement, together.

The womanplace is an eager participant in each pregnancy and birth. However, she must be invited to the "home" in which she already resides. She must be called forth, as it were. It's as if she "rents" a room within; in order to be with her, you must open the adjoining door. She is always fully available. Occasionally, she unlocks the door from her side and appears "out-of-the-blue."

Elizabeth said that she became aware of the resident within at each of her visits to her doctor. "It was as if someone was tapping me lightly on the inside—and it wasn't the baby. I had lots and lots of Braxton-Hicks contractions—except when I was at my appointments with him, they stopped. I think I heard my womanplace tell me that my labor would stop with him, too. I switched to a midwife."

Some women have drawn pictures of their womanplace. We have experimented—drawing with our eyes closed, with our left hands instead of our right (or vice-versa). We have pretended that we are the "woman" who resides in the womanplace and have drawn from the "inside out." The pictures all differ, and they are all wonderful. They are all magnificent expressions of the beauty and uniqueness of womankind. Many of the pictures, I am told, were framed and displayed long after the birth was over.

When women ask their womanplace (WP) what they need to do in order to have a good birth, the replies vary: Eat better, change hospitals, stay at home, nothing at all—you are doing fine! Sue's WP told her to make a tape of her own voice. During labor, she listened to herself reading her favorite poems. "At first, I hated the sound of my own voice. But after a while, it was really powerful to hear me, supporting me!" The womanplace is described by others as the inner spirit, the Shakti (feminine) principle, the Divine Goddess within, the Medicine Woman, and many others. It really doesn't matter what you decide to call her—just know her, feel her energy, and be with her. Ina May says that birth can be an experience that enables each woman to expand her limits and transcend who she thought she was, or it can be an experience of separation and despair. She says that every woman is conscious of the "teeming potential of her inner space." She calls the pregnant inner space a "room, heavy with life."[26]

Womanplace to Womanplace

In *Listening to Our Bodies* and in many other books on women's spirituality, we learn that women have deep spiritual connections to and reverence for their bodies. To a woman, her body literally is "a temple that reflects or even *is* [emphasis hers] a sacred process."[27] This is one reason why cesarean section, episiotomy, and so many other violations at birth are often so hard to resolve. In *Mothers on Trial*, Phyllis Chesler remarks that spirit wounds are the keenest wounds that can be inflicted on women. "When a woman is brought before our man courts [or, for our purposes, returns to the obstetrician who cut her] and has no marks of violation upon her person [low horizontal incisions are often covered by the pubic hair; episiotomy scars are within the folds of the perineum], it is hard to realize that her whole physical system may be writhing in agony from spirit wrongs, such as can only be understood by her peers."[28] I have come to believe that many of the women who "love" their cesareans either deny or never came to know the womanplace inside of them. It is a stranger to them, or, for a variety of reasons, an unwelcome element within. The womanplace expects to bring forth a child naturally, purely—and it aches when this is denied. It is deeply confused and saddened by the intrusion of machinery and knives at birth, often enraged, and temporarily disoriented. Although it is always willing to be healed, the prerequisite if often difficult: the woman must be willing to "get conscious," that is, to acknowledge and feel the emotional/spiritual pain.

In *Wounded Woman*, it says that "Tears . . . can be congealed in icy form with the dagger-like points and edges of icicles. These frozen tears can turn a woman's heart to stone." Other tears are not redemptive, "because the growth of the soul is frozen in bitter resentment." Linda Leonard says that tears may also rush out in a torrential storm that floods the ground on which the woman stands. They can wash the ground right out from under the woman, "and in this muddied earth she can get stuck, unable to stand on her own. Flooding tears can drown the woman in a sea of sorrow that may turn into self-pity and deluge the soul." It is no wonder that some women refuse/are unable to address the painful issues that surround births-of-violation. However, "there are also tears that fall like fructifying rain which enable growth and spring's rebirth. This crying is both helpful and hopeful, for it breaks through defenses and acknowledges wounds—the wounds that must be accepted before healing can occur. These are tears of transformation."[29]

Again, we must remember that "we cannot affirm life without affirming women."[30] The first woman in most of our lives (forgetting the delivery room nurse) was our mother. Schaef says that many women refuse to claim their own lives because they are afraid of breaking the bond with their mothers.[31] As women reclaim themselves and begin to define themselves from within, they find new fulfillment and strength. They stand on their own. Schaef, Lerner, and others all tell us that this "emotional umbilicus" is often hard to sever, for we are afraid that we will lose our bond with our mothers if we are different or "apart from." I was once in a women's group where we did a visualization exercise in which we were asked to imagine our umbilical cords still attached to our mothers. "Now cut the cord, sever it," we were told. In my mind's eye, I took a pair of scissors, but they wouldn't cut through. Then I got a serrated kitchen knife, but it was too dull. I got a hack-saw, and that wouldn't do, either. Finally, I got a blow-torch and that did the trick. Rather than feel excited, I felt terrified. I had to learn that the aliveness that I feel "unattached" allows me to be a better daughter and to love more fully. Separation/connection is a big issue for women, for as we cut our own umbilical cords and then those of the children we carry we are also called on not to distance, to stay "in touch." In addition, it is vital that we stay in close communication with our Mother Earth.

Many times I have read that it is through suffering that we bond to other women. Indeed, I was extremely moved when I read an article entitled "Distant Voices: The Lives of African Women."[32] Twenty thousand women of color from all over the globe appeared in Kenya for a United Nations Forum to improve their condition. They "held out their hands to each other. Women came from both sides of the Atlantic at great sacrifice. Many American women took out mortgages on their homes; many of them walked long distances. The goals for some of the African women were lofty: to get pipes—water—into their villages." I cried as I read the article; my heart shouted out against injustice everywhere, and I felt a certain pride and kinship to each of the women there. We are all struggling; our struggles are different and they are the same.

For a long time, I felt closest to women who had had cesareans. They understood what I had been through. I felt an automatic bond with these women. I felt alienated from women who had birthed normally. Since then, I have received hundreds of letters from women who express those feelings. One says, "I did not feel normal. After my cesarean, I felt out-of-place and strange. No one I knew seemed to have those feelings because of their birth experience. I did everything I could to appear "normal" to my friends. I went places, I visited with people, I invited people over. When one relative offered to pick something up for me because, 'I know you can't bend over yet,' well, I bent right over for her of course! And I declared over and over, 'I don't feel any different than my friends who gave birth vaginally.' But my "normal" act covered up from most people the deepest anguish I have ever known. . . . Now that I have learned that what I am feeling is normal, I realize that I've always been normal! I had an abnormal experience, but I have reacted to it in a very normal way." This woman, and others like her, went on to start a cesarean support group. Their pain and desire to heal brought them together.

As women grow and heal, they give up their suffering. "This almost always causes a strain in relationships. If we give up our suffering, we lose . . . a bond" that we have with one another.[33] One cesarean support group leader said, "As I healed, I found that I didn't feel comfortable in cesarean groups where there seemed to be no real "reward" for healing—only jealousy or contempt. When I decided to leave my position, I wasn't cheered on. Women felt I was denying or sublimating. In fact, with their help, but mostly with a great deal of effort and determination on my own part, I had come to a place of acceptance and peace, and was ready to move on to other things in my life." We must value healing and learn to connect through joy. Our feelings of closeness to one another should not have to depend on the length of the incisions on our bodies.

The woman who said that no one she knew had bad feelings about their vaginal birth experience later realized that every one of her friends had painful memories of their births. "Not one can recall having their children without hurt feelings about what was done or not done. How horrifying that everyone is grieving. I was blind to that before." As we heal, we begin to see more clearly. This woman believed that only the spirits of cesarean women were wounded, and as we have already learned, that isn't so.

Luthman believes that we are beginning to let go of suffering as a way of learning. She says that we are developing a sensitivity to our connections with all of life.[34] Caroline Sufrin says that many of us are finally waking up from our own personal "nuclear winters." Ghandi says that it does not matter how small the beginning may seem to be: What is once well done is done forever.

Virginia Sandlin tells us that everyday we wake up a new person. Today is the day, she says, to fully participate in your life, in your healing, in your aliveness. "Let yourself out!" You are the person that you spend all of your life with. You get you. You're it! It is time to have an experience of you that feels wonderful. When you put 100 percent of you out into the world, others begin to mirror that 100 percent. Bring out the best in you, and the best will begin to reflect all around.[35] Elisabeth Kübler-Ross says that everything begins with loving ourselves and with a sense of peace within: "It is contagious! The ripple effects are beyond your imagination."[36]

In "The Spirit of Healing" we are told that healing is a process of becoming whole at a number of different levels and that love provides the optimum condition for healing.[37] "Confront the opposition with an enveloping love that will permit him to regain his capacity to trust and to love." The organization/move-ment Beyond War says that we must not see "oppositions." One of their basic tenets is as follows: I will not preoccupy myself with an enemy. I will resolve conflict: I will not use violence. I don't know if you are all going to lambaste me for writing all of this in a birthing book—but I know inside of me that I have to include all of this, that's all.

Potpourri

One of the spiritual concepts that I've heard from time to time is that we choose the people and events in our lives in order to work through particular issues or to learn certain lessons. If this is so, we choose our obstetricians and our OB scenes. Luthman says that it doesn't matter whether or not you believe this. Just pretend that you chose the doctor and situation to develop some aspect of your consciousness and then consider what that might be. "The minute you consider the possibility, even in pretense, you automatically take yourself out of the victim role. You utilize your experience to develop and understand parts of yourself."[38] She says that many people spend time learning to forgive. If we consider that we choose them, she asks, what is there to forgive? Obviously, we needed them to be exactly the way they were, with all their faults and assets, in order to learn what we needed to know. And, if they had not been available, we would have chosen others with the same or similar ways of being.

I went to a Blessing Way a few years back. Blessing Way is a ceremony used for any transition a person may experience (puberty, graduation, a certain birth-day, marriage, birth, moving to a new place, divorce, etc.). It is a celebration of the life process. Some say it originated with the Navajo Indians; others have different explanations. It is a heart-centered, fun and filling time. Birth Blessing Ways honor pregnant women or the new mother. They are an opportunity to "fill up the mother" (with love, poetry, music, symbolic gifts, food, etc.). As she "takes in" the abundance of love and good thoughts showered on her, her energy—and her ability to nurture—increase, and she has "more than enough" to give out at birth and to her new child.

Of Psychics and Airports

Evidently, many people believe in reincarnation, astrology, tarot, and so on. A woman from the Southwest, "by a vast divine coincidence," ended up on the phone with a spiritual healer who just happened to be visiting in her town. He did some readings for her and "unlocked" the key to a problem with her child. Another woman found answers to her child's difficult behavior: According to "a wonderful and talented" psychic, her son had been in several wars and had sustained multiple head injuries. For years, they had trudged from one doctor to the next, looking for help. Carla said an astrologer helped her with her pregnancy and birth. In this culture, we seem to overlook anything that isn't scientifically or medically proven. I was moved by the stories that these women and several others told me.

One thing that happened to me still astounds me. I was in Chicago where my plane had landed due to inclement weather. I had a seven-hour wait until I could get another plane home. I was tired and grumpy. I was approached by this strange-looking young man wearing a weird-looking necklace and a hat with feathers and rocks sewn on it. He asked me for $20. He said he had no money. He had his airplane ticket to Boston, but he had left his wallet at a friend's house back in California and would need the twenty to get from the airport in Boston to his sister's house. I told him I couldn't lend him the money. He said, "Look, I know you are going to lend me the money." I asked him how he knew that. He said that he just felt it. He said he had looked around the whole crowded airport and knew that I was the one. I asked him, "Where did you say your wallet was?" and he said, "At my friend's house in Sebastopol, California." My heart skipped a beat. I know *one* person in Sebastopol, California, my friend, midwife and author Nan Koehler. But I didn't say. He went on, "I stayed with my friends last night on their farm. She's a midwife. I left my wallet on their table." I said to him, nonchalantly, "I have a friend who is a midwife in Sebastopol." He said, "I'll bet it's Nan Koehler. She's my friend, too. My wallet is on her kitchen table!" Then, like a magician pulling something out of his hat, he reached into his pocket and said, "Since I was going to Boston, Nan asked me to call a friend for her who lives there named Nancy Wainer Cohen. She gave me this." In his hand was a brochure for *Silent Knife*. He looked at me and said, "Oh, my goodness. I'll bet that you are Nancy Cohen!" I said, "Here, I saved you a dime." I handed him $19.90. [Not twelve hours after I typed this story, I received a letter from Nan Koehler: "I saw Brant on Tuesday, and he still talks about meeting you at the airport!"]

Linda Goodman says that whether or not we realize it, we are all enrolled in a spiritual classroom.[39] A Course in Miracles says that we don't get to choose if we want to take the class—only "when." I have heard it said that coincidences are Spirit's way of letting you know Spirit is there.

Room for Spirit

Birth is nothing if not a spiritual experience—and an experience that in many ways embodies the essence of woman. There are many spiritual books which may help you with your birth, labor, or healing process. I have received a number of wonderful books as gifts from friends, each of whom found something of great value within their pages.

Judy Lockwood's book, *Rim of Fire: Meditations for the Modern Madonna*, addresses the challenge of finding spiritual strength for the awesome task of being a parent. During the birth process, when the largest part of the baby passes through the mother's birth canal, a point of maximum tension is reached. "Often the mother experiences an intense burning sensation, the 'rim of fire' after which the rest of the child's body can slip through the mother's own. It is my contention that this microcosmic rim of fire, is a metaphor. . . . If birth can be made more humane, loving, and spiritually centered, the result can only be good for all." Judy believes that we must reintroduce female sacred rites of passage of human life into our experience.[40]

Author Adrienne Rich portrays two aspects of feminine culture. One is an awareness of the women who have come before us—our "foremothers." The second is an attachment to the earth as a goddess form ("with an image similar to that of woman—walked on, unappreciated, freely exploited, but also strong and enduring"). Woman's spirituality focuses on the goddess, the female principle of creation. Until 5000 years ago, there were many goddess religions. The Divine was seen as female, God was female since life comes from the female. More and more, in letters I receive, women write to me about their connection with a goddess. Tina said, "When my first child was born, she looked up into my face as if she were seeing the face of God. I looked back at her, seeing the same, a feminine manifestation of Him. It was at that moment that I opened to a female deity." Caroline writes: "I prayed to the Goddess. I saw her in the full moon that greeted me as I went into labor. She was with me throughout the beautiful pains of birth."

I have experienced great joy with birthing women. I have heard it said that cosmic truth requires an eternity to be true in. What is cosmically true is the joy women feel when they give birth. A passage in *Ever Since Eve*: "The whole room actually turned pink. It was the dead of winter—still pitch dark outside, so it wasn't sunrise. The doctor noticed it too and he's straight as an arrow. . . . He didn't understand it either, this rose colored light absolutely filling the room."[41] Those kinds of things happen at birth a lot, ya know. . . . The less chrome and steel, the less interference, the more room there is for Spirit. . . . When women are 'put under' or 'drugged-up,' the "richness of the birth experience is stolen from them"; the ability to experience the spiritual tones of birth is denied them as well. It has been said that the mind is a maker and a fashioner of quite formidable proportions: the Spirit beats it by miles.

Spirit yields miracles. Birth is a miracle. Babies are miracles. Life is a miracle. And women are miracles. They are rainbows! Linda Leonard says, "The image that comes to me is a crystal. A crystal has different facets and when turned to the sun in different ways, it reveals unique forms of color and brilliance . . . Turn the crystal and allow the qualities to shine forth in strength."

Shine forth. That's what the moon does.

PART III   LABOR!

And the day came when the risk to remain closed in a bud became more painful than the risk it took to blossom.

—Unknown

Birth is not a disaster waiting to happen.

—Janet Leigh

(Pink and) Blueprints

I once heard it said that it is not truth but faith that keeps the world alive, and that if we lose faith the birds who now fly fearlessly across the earth would drop in terror, the fish would drown, and the whole world would probably lose its way.

Labor is a process by which a baby gets from here to there—that's all we know. We must forget everything that we've heard about labor and just "be"; we must be willing to "discover" and to just let the experience unfold. Like dying, there is a point at which we have to do it alone; there comes a time when the laboring woman goes, in essence, to a place where we cannot follow.

The above paragraph is derived from notes I took at a talk given by midwife Janet Leigh a number of years ago. Years before, when I had had my cesarean, and even my first vaginal birth, I had forgotten those things. I'd forgotten that babies are designed to be born, and that, in fact, they birth themselves. By the time I was ready to give birth to my third, I had remembered. There are women all over the world who have never forgotten, and women who are beginning to remember again.

Hi, Birthmate

One suggestion that many women have found helpful for labor is to close their eyes and think about a place in the world where there is no birth technology. A place where the women just know how to birth. There are no blood tests to determine if they are pregnant, and no ultrasound or amniocentesis to find out "what's happening" or the sex of the baby. There are no "due dates"; if the baby is born by this moon, fine. If not, then surely by the next.

Every woman chooses her own location in her mind's eye. Some women choose a warm climate, near water. Others go to a place that is snow covered, near mountains. It doesn't matter. Once they have found themselves in a culture, or a tribe, or among a group of people who view birth as the completely natural experience that it is, they "locate" a woman who is at the same point in their pregnancy as they are. Sometimes that woman appears instantly in their mind's eye; one woman in my class found herself walking through a village, until she came to a cottage. She knocked on the door, and found her birthmate.

Once you have found your own birthmate, let her guide you through this pregnancy and labor. She is not afraid. She holds birth inside of her as a part of her life experience. When the time arrives for her to birth her child, she will simply birth her child. This does not necessarily mean quickly or without effort. When the time is right, she simply will birth her baby.

My own birthmate is a woman from Africa. She has been with me for years now. She has beautiful, dark skin (no zits) and dark, sparkling eyes. I love her hands. We walk and talk, and she teaches me about birth her way. There is a passage in Isaiah: "I have called you by name, you are mine." She has a name. Sometimes we are like schoolgirls together, playing near the river. Always, the woman part of her is alive and strong. She is very excited about this new baby of hers, and yes, she will assist me as I birth as well.

When a woman in my classes has questions or concerns about labor, she often goes to her birthmate and quietly asks for an answer, or some help with her problem. "What would you do? Mari?" "How would you handle this, Tatiana?" the women ask. Invariably, gentle and wise council is returned. It is amazing how relaxed and calm most women become when they bring this friend into their being. Because we are "of like mind," because we are all from one source, because we are connected in spirit, we have access to information from our distant sisters. We can relearn and recapture what has seemed all but lost to us in this culture.

"When I got 'stuck' at seven centimeters, I didn't know what to do," said Barb. "I called you and you quickly explained about this helpmate, or birthsister, or whatever you call her. I got a picture of a woman in Peru. I don't know why it was Peru, but it was. She was at the same place in her labor as I was. Of course, she didn't know she was seven centimeters, and they didn't do a vaginal exam in the place where she lived. I asked her to help. I watched her walking and rocking her body. I did the same. I watched her squat, and I did that too. I tuned everyone out for a while. It was as if she was in the room with me, and we were laboring together; her presence was that strong! After a while the contractions became stronger. I started to feel scared, but I looked into her eyes and saw complete calm. When she pushed her baby out, I watched. I felt like pushing, too, and I followed her example. It was incredible. I know she was a part of me, a part I created, and I own that. Still, she was apart from me, too. Someday I am going to Peru."

Some women have difficulty picturing a woman from another land. They find it easier to bring a mammal into their minds. One woman chose a mother bear, another a deer. In each case, the women allowed their animal sisters to help them birth. (One had an 8 x 10 picture of a bear framed for her labor. She stayed at home and birthed not in the bedroom but in her den.) Another, having read that female elephants attend each other during birth, chose an elephant for her guide.

Aren't the fathers supposed to be the birthmates? you ask. Aren't they the ones who are supposed to "coach" the mother? A "coach," by the very definition of the word, knows the ins and outs of the games. He knows all the 'plays': he's had experience and he knows a number of creative and inventive 'solutions' to "the game." Fathers can't be coaches. They've never had babies before. In a very real sense, they are pregnant, too. Together, as a unit, I believe they should be supported. The more love and support the fathers get, the more they have to give out to their women. No, husbands are not coaches. When they tell you that you are doing fine, there is a part of you that wants to believe them. After all, it is with this person that the baby was conceived, and you are partners/ lovemates. But the womanplace inside of you rebels: How can he say everything is alright? He's never had a baby before!

You will not need to go to Africa or "deepest, darkest Peru" at all. Simply close your eyes. Standing all around you are women who provide you with strength, confidence, wisdom, and peace. Keep them with you as you birth. They are present-day women, as well as those who have come before us.

Moan, Groan, Complain, and Bellyache

According to Ivan Illich, culture makes pain tolerable by interpreting its necessity; only pain perceived as curable is intolerable.

> A myriad of virtues express the different aspects of fortitude that traditionally enabled people to recognize painful sensations as a challenge and to shape their own experience accordingly. Patience, forbearance, courage, resignation, self-control, perseverance, and meekness each express a different coloring of the responses with which pain sensations were accepted, transformed into the experience of suffering, and endured. Duty, love, fascination, routines, prayer and compassion were some of the means that enabled pain to be borne with dignity. . . . Pain was recognized as an inevitable part of the subjective reality of one's own body in which everyone constantly finds himself, and which is constantly being shaped by his conscious reactions to it.[42]

The idea that skill in the art of suffering might be the most effective and universally acceptable way of dealing with pain has been rendered either incomprehensible or shocking. Illich says that medicalization deprives any culture of the integration of its program for dealing with pain. The experience of pain, he says, depends on its quality and on genetic endowment and on at least four other factors other than its nature or intensity: culture, anxiety, attention, and interpretation. All these, he says, are shaped by social determinants, ideology, economic structure, and social character. "Culture decrees whether the mother or father or both will groan when the child is born."[43]

Soldiers who hoped their wounds would get them out of the army as heroes, Illich says, rejected morphine injections they would have considered absolutely necessary if similar injuries had been inflicted by the dentist or in the operating theater. In our society, pain calls for methods of control by the physician rather than an approach that might help the person in pain to take on responsibility for his experience.[44]

The Torah states that a woman will bear her children in pain. However, a more exact translation of the word "pain" is the word "sorrow." Childbirth educator Bruria Husarsky writes, "When we look forward with excitement to the event, we experience joy and pleasure—what then is the pain?" The pain of birth, she says, is not necessarily the physical pain of labor, but perhaps "the isolation and the humiliation and the lack of love in the birth environment— that is the pain. It behooves us and those around us to spare us the curse since it is not a command. It is our ambivalence and conflictedness—that is the pain." Sorrow.

Grantly Dick-Read remarked years ago that no greater curse could befall a laboring woman than isolation. Yet, some women choose to be alone to birth. I was at one birth where ten people encircled the laboring woman. She wanted each and every one of us there, and the circle around her was her protection. However, many women have told me that, in spite of a number of people at their births, they felt completely, totally, and hopelessly alone. Human bodies in and of themselves do not constitute support: there has to be a loving spirit inside and a willingness to give of it.

At another birth the woman asked everyone to leave. She listened to her inner-knowing, and she knew that she needed to do this on her own. She isolated herself. Janet Leigh talks about an altered state of consciousness that most women need to get to in order to birth. People who do not understand this often block the woman from "going there." At selected times, Janet says, it may be important to keep the connection with the birthing woman, and eye contact or direct communication may help. At other times, these become interferences that prevent the woman from getting to that altered state or to that instinctual place where she must be in order to birth. It may be hard for others to watch the woman "leave them" or to hear it. It is primal, she says, animalistic, sexual. It is other worldly. Michele Odent notes that the conditions that foster this altered state of mind are rarely present in hospitals. Jami Osborne says that women have to go "where the angels go," and Lynn Richards says that a woman must let herself float away into "laborland," past the point of no return. "If losing control is what she fears the most, then losing control is what she must do. For when she finally lets go, the baby will come."[45]

Caroline Sufrin from Ontario wrote the following after her homebirth after two cesareans: "I screamed. That *was* agony, that last primal scream that birthed our son. I will always hear it. I *want* to hear it again, again. It lifts me to greater heights than I have ever felt before. You see, it was a scream of triumph. Triumph of my body that functions as nature intended. Triumph of pain. A scream of love for the child thus born, for my man, and for my children and for me, yes for *me*, too. A scream in celebration of new life. In celebration of my womanhood."

Some months after I had finished teaching a set of classes, I was reading letters from some of the Momdads in that class. I opened up one letter that said, "The only criticism I have about the classes, Nancy, was that you didn't talk enough about *the pain*! It was really excruciating. I did it, and I'm proud. I just wish I'd have known sooner what I was going to have to deal with." The very next letter that I opened read, "I think you spend too much time on pain. The contractions, all the way through, weren't all that much worse than the ones I have endured for years with my menstrual cycle. From what you said, I thought that at any time they were going to 'take off' and I was going to be left at the start." I always tell my classes that you never know.

Some women describe labor as extremely painful and others as literally pain-less. Chris, a homebirth VBAC mom from Ohio, wrote that when the pain got really intense, she said to herself, "No one else can do it for you. You might as well get to it and get it over with!" Marie, a natural childbirth educator from California, said that she had an absolutely painless birth. "I never felt like 'this hurts'—only like 'I'm working.' " Marie got to the hospital very late in labor. She was put onto a gurney, pushed three times in the hall, and had her baby. She was a single mom and said, "I did this all by myself. No dad and no doctor kissing me all over the place. I took the baby immediately and stopped at MacDonald's for lunch on the way home." Other women find themselves ex-hausted and depleted after a painful delivery. It depends on so many things.

Dr. Anne Seiden once wrote that no one would expect a runner to finish a marathon without pain. But would anyone propose shooting him up with pain-killing medication? "Mastery of pain can be an important source of satisfaction and growth."[46] Leeann said she felt as if she had "won the baby by default" when she was given a spinal near the end of delivery.

Elizabeth Nobel says that the pain of birth is the pain of opening up. It involves the heart as well as the mind and the body. "The pain of letting go is the pain of letting go of control."

Most doctors are afraid of the pain of labor. It is foreign to them, being something they can never experience or control. In an effort to "help us out" they speed up our labors, shoot us with drugs, or anesthetize us for cesarean sections. It is also an attempt to anesthetize themselves from the pains they feel: fear, loss of control, and so on. By reducing or eliminating our painful sensations, they create a setting in which they no longer have to deal with their own issues. Ram Dass, a spiritual teacher, says that if you are freaked out of your skull about pain, you cannot do much except offer a drug. Stay centered, he says, and offer your *being*. One psychologist remarked that men may indeed be jealous. There is no experience in their own lives that even approximates birth. So they go out and build skyscrapers and wage wars and do whatever they can to feel creative and powerful.

Last year I viewed "The Birth Project," a collection of seventy magnificent works of art in needlecraft, conceived by Judy Chicago. It is a traveling exhibit on the subjects of birth and creation, and it truly gives us pause for thought about women and their own magnificence. Weavers and artisans from all over the country submitted their works to Judy Chicago and were selected to stitch her canvases. The patience and dedication it took to complete, stitch by stitch, these enormous and awesome pieces is mind-boggling. One piece is especially astonishing: reds and oranges and yellows all swirled (in embroidery yarns) into images of fire and flames. In Judy Chicago's words: "The feeling is not one of anguish. . . . The aura surrounding the figures seems to radiate the pain away from the feelings of it—transforming the heat of the pain into power."[47]

Trust

When we are just beginning to trust on an intuitive level, "energy is only beginning to get unblocked and is thus, easily drained or intruded upon in this embyonic stage."[48] As we progress the energy level reaches such an intensity that it forms a much more powerful defense than any rigid external structure or ways of being.

> As we get in touch with our own natural rhythm and a sense of how it meshes with the rhythm around us, we have our own built-in radar or sonar. We get vibrations, long before we reach a danger point, which tell us to change direction. As we tune into and trust the intuitive level, we become aware of the slightest nuance or clue that tells us we may be somewhat off the track. As the trust, based on rhythm, builds, we develop increased awareness about other aspects of our being. . . . With such expansion comes a strong sense of power and the gradual elimination of any fear or anxiety.[49]

The flow of energy through us becomes increasingly so powerful that not only does it eventually prevent the absorption of negative energy, but it also purifies other energy that comes into our atmosphere. "Thus, I feel that we can heal just by being in the same room with another person, without having to do or say anything. Have you ever been in a room with people who are high on life and expansive when you were depressed? After a while, you find that you either have to let go of your depression to be with them or leave them in order to hold onto your depression. You cannot maintain the depression in the face of their positive energy."[50]

Earlier, I said that sadly, most women become childlike and unassertive during labor. I want to qualify that sentence a bit. An article that I read recently says, "There is within each of us a child. A child who wants to be led, taken care of. That child feels that it is not in control of its life; he or she is the victim of power, forces and authorities which it cannot understand and which it cannot control. That same child, however, has another side to its personality—an exuberance, a vitality, optimism, creativity and enthusiasm. That child can have great trust in the world, as well as an implicit trust in his or her innate ability to deal with that world."[51] In fact, children are often extremely assertive; they know what they want and when they want it. When you allow the free child within you to be present at birth, her being will most certainly assist you.

How many hours in labor is enough? How many are too many? Some women's limits are defined after a few hours. Others labor for days and days until their babies are born. Some women push once and their babies are born; some push for hours. Birth is a physiological process. So is conception.[Sometimes it takes a man no time at all to ejaculate, other times it takes longer. Try wrapping a fetal monitor around the guy's penis while sticking a catheter up his urethra and poking him with an IV—then tell him if he doesn't get an erection and ejaculate within five minutes you are going make an incision in the scrotum to get the sperm out. See if that makes it easier for him. Tell him the tip of the penis isn't wide enough to get out all those millions of sperm, so you will just have to make a little cut into the tip to enlarge the opening and speed things up a little bit. While the analogy is certainly not perfect, both ejaculation and birth are totally natural expressions in the human experience and take place, when the circumstances are favorable, in their own time.]

The shortest labor among the women I have worked with is 30 minutes—start to finish. Pat had been having "mild cramps" for days, but nothing that prevented her from going about her daily routine. One evening, she felt as if she was coming down with the flu, so she got into a warm bath to relax. Her baby was born in the bathroom within just a few minutes. The longest was six full days of continual active labor. On the third day, the mother "gave up." But her husband and labor support people said "No way! Everything is fine, keep at it! You don't want another section, do you?" On the fourth day, the labor support people were feeling a little tentative. The mom screamed "what? after all this get cut open? Are you kidding? You want to go to the hospital, you go. But you'll have to go without me!" On day six, the mom had really had it. She was about to go into the hospital when she felt the urge to push. Her baby was born a few hours later. This woman told me that she had had two abortions years earlier, a miscarriage, and of course her cesarean. She now believes that she was laboring on a psychological level for each of the babies she had lost—one each day. The last day was really the labor for this baby. In that sense, the week-long struggle was a real catharsis, a real healing for her.

A physicist from Alabama tells us that part of Einstein's theory of relativity demonstrates that space shrinks as speed increases. This has been demonstrated by scientists, we are told, in various ways, and most of us have experienced this when we are driving on an interstate. As we increase our speed, the highway seems to get smaller, giving us less room to maneuver. According to the theory, the highway actually is smaller for the passengers in the speeding car than for a pedestrian observer. Elaine, also from Alabama, writes that this can be applied to childbirth. If doctors' effort to speed labor is successful, they would also succeed in making the pelvis smaller relative to the baby, though not of course to the doctors or to the x-ray machine—to whom the size of the pelvis remains the same. The baby may very well fit given the proper time, but not if you try to jam it into the pelvis and then out. Those of you who have watched my tiny little boot demonstration know this. When I take my time and change position, my foot goes into the boot. Both my foot and the rubber (the baby's head and the pelvis) are flexible. When I try to shove it in, or even just to quickly get it on, it gets stuck.)

Elaine goes on: "I think midwives understand this theory intuitively, perhaps because they also look at birth from the baby's point of view. As an aside, I didn't think my fast cesarean was better than my twenty-five hour VBAC labor and birth. And I can think of lots of other instances where faster is not better. I (like many women I know) prefer slower sex to faster sex and a leisurely meal to a burger and fries at the drive-thru. And faster is not better if it leads to an increase in the loss of life on the highway.

Maryah said that the doctors kept giving her more pitocin to speed things along. They told her it was dangerous for a baby if the woman was in labor for more than twelve hours. "I finally yelled at them, 'Why not just stick me and the kid in a microwave so we'll cook faster?' You know, I think they'd have considered it if I'd've fit."

Dr. DeLee, one of the most revered men in American obstetrics, stated that normal birth was pathologic and compared it to a baby's head getting caught in a door; Dr. Edward Hon, who developed the EFM, compared normal labor to a railroad crossing where cars get smashed up. In an article entitled, "Don't Tell *Me* What It's Like to Have a Baby!," the author writes, "And I still can't figure out what could have been the motivating force behind [someone] telling, "You know, the pain Dustin Hoffman went through in "Marathon Man" when Lawrence Olivier mercilessly drilled away at his open cavities. . . . Well—labor is worse. . . . [Someone else] told me, 'Wait until your doctor tells you to push— you'll feel like your insides are coming out!' " Mary writes that in her community, women still seem to like to tell their horror stories. "It sometimes seems like a contest to see who has had the most harrowing experience!" With images and stories like these, it's no wonder we are concerned about the amount of time it is going to take to put this event in our lives behind us.

The American Journal of Taking Baths

The medical literature on labor ranges from debates on which position is best for us for second stage to the lithotomy position and fetal descent. While some of the research articles have helped us all tremendously, I thumb through the obstetrical literature and want to cry. Numbers, statistics, graphs, and charts about our pregnant bodies and our fluids and our heartbeats. If only they could *really hear* what our cumulative heart is beating out to them.

I practically fell off my seat when I saw an article in a nursing journal a while back. It was entitled "Therapeutic Effects of Bathing During Labor." While I am sure the person who conducted the study was well meaning, and I imagine that this kind of article is the only thing that will convince some doctors that bathing in labor is okay, I just shook my head in disbelief. Bathing is referred to as "hydrotherapy" and we are given its definition: the external application of water to the body for therapeutic effects. We learn about "composition" and "molecules" and "conduction," and finally, "immersion temperature." After a lengthy "chat" on these and related matters, we are told that "Rather than interfering with labor, hydrotherapy seems to have the opposite effect." Labor sometimes progresses so quickly in the relaxed atmosphere of this technique, we are told, that thirty-eight babies were unintentionally born underwater at this clinic without reported adverse effects." We are even told what temperature the water should be, and if the bath lasts longer than 15–20 minutes, hot water should be added to maintain the bath water at a comfortable temperature and the water should cover the person's body completely."[52] I can't even comment.

Many spiritual books are available that can help you toward that (not so) faraway place that laboring women go. Read them if you like to read. Read them if you want suggestions. Above all, remember again, you never have to read another word in order to have a baby. If you check into your womanplace, you will quickly know which books are right for you, or how many you need to read (or whether you need to read at all!). "The bird does not consult a book in order to soar."[53] My African birthmate never read a book. She can't read. A little later in this chapter, I will offer some additional suggestions for labor: it is by no means complete but will perhaps assist you in some way. First, however, let's discuss labor support for a few minutes.

Labor Support

In conclusion, let me note that if I told you today about a new medication or a new electronic device that would reduce problems of fetal asphyxia by one-half, cut labor length by one-half, and enhance the mother-infant interaction after delivery, I expect that there would be a stampede to obtain this new medication or device in every ob unit in the United States, no matter what the cost. Just because the supportive companion makes good common sense does not decrease its importance. . . . It is safe . . . no purchase order is required, there is no need for approval from regional planning boards . . . no waits for FDA approval or long waits for repairs. . . . However, there is the real hazard that it will be considered unscientific and therefore less important than medical intervention.[54]

If the hospital that you are thinking about using does not encourage labor support, you've got the wrong hospital. If they limit the number of support people you are "allowed" to have, ditto. Hospitals these days want to be considered progressive, and they need money. Of course, it may be better to arrange things ahead of time. Birth, as we all know, is not a time to have to plead or battle. Some hospitals believe that the personnel they employ are all you need for "support." They still do not understand the intricate and delicate interactions among familiar faces and energies that can help to make the labor easier for the birthing woman. If the hospital is the least bit "iffy" about private labor support, I'd see that as another "red flag."

Marion says, "It is suicide not to bring a private labor support person to a hospital, any hospital. People there are often tired and just kinda hope the mother will precipitously 'drop the kid' the minute she arrives. Other times they are bored—it's been a 'slow night' and they stand over you like a bunch of vultures waiting for their evening meal." This will appear true to you, or extremely unfair—depending on your perception. Midwife Debbie Drexler says that a labor support person can help a couple stay at home for an extended period of time, provides continuity of care once they are in the hospital, and serves as an alternative source of information. Mary Jo writes that "on reviewing my own experience it becomes more and more apparent that such a person would have been invaluable to me to help me feel that what I was experiencing was within the realm of normal." Labor support person (LSP) Sally Kirwin writes, "She can say with great credibility, 'Yes, this is what labor is like.' "[55]

In some hospitals, LSPs have one foot in the door and one foot out. Coreen, an LSP from New Hampshire, said that she was "greeted" by one hospital with "scorns and scowls" and a warning: If you open your mouth, you're out of here. She said that another time, she was barred from a hospital because the doctor had forgotten to call ahead to tell them the parents were bringing support. Hospital protocol required this call; the doctor was away and could not be reached. Michelle wrote that she managed to get her second LSP into her room by "ignoring the looks we were getting and walking around as if we knew what we were doing."

One hospital in my area insists that the LSP sign a form stating that she will not interfere with medical or nursing functions necessary for maternal/fetal well-being. This form also says that if the LSP is detracting from the management of the labor, the physician and nurse will ask her to leave. I wonder if the physician and nurse were asked to leave by the LSP for distracting the mom, if they would be so gracious. An LSP from New Jersey wrote that the "Board of Nursing here seems to have the power to set us back by asserting that labor support is practicing nursing without a license. As far as I can see, nursing is practicing labor support without nary a clue as to how to do it."

In *Childbirth Wisdom* we learn a number of things about the kind of support that women receive at the time of birth. In some tribal cultures, the attendant is the woman's mother or women from her family. Birthing is among people she knows and trusts. In a number of tribes, it is assumed that the woman will do everything for herself. Friends of Midwives advocate Archie Brodsky writes "All the time and attention given a woman before and after delivery—are considered unnecessary in a country where women assume that they can give birth on their own."[56]

Support from Dads

Although I do not believe that fathers are supposed to be coaches—and there is even a growing voice inside of me that wonders if some of our childbirth classes might best be held with women only—I know that the love and support of partners is extremely important. Carl Jones has written a number of books on birth for fathers and has co-authored a "Labor Support Guide for Fathers, Family and Friends."[57]

Marilyn Moran writes, "It's her naked husband she needs, the feel of his skin, and the scent of his body. No holding back . . . she knows and trusts and enjoys his sexual touches and knows how to spontaneously yield to them. And that is what is needed during birth—no holding back."[58] I wonder how many fathers would feel comfortable being totally naked in a hospital setting, and yet this kind of skin-to-skin contact is so very vital to so many women at birth! Lisa said, "I said to my husband, 'Whip off your shirt!' which he did. It wasn't good enough. I didn't want to feel his T-shirt either. I wanted to lean against him and feel his chest against my back." Visually, your man's body may assist you in labor as well. Will the hospital you are considering feel comfortable when the two of you, stripped right down to your birthday suits, start cuddling and snuggling? Will *you?* Will they respect your privacy if you want to make love?

Marilyn, a staunch supporter of do-it-yourself homebirth, reminds us that birth is a sexual experience. "For no other reason," she says, "it should be an intimate husband/wife experience. For nine months; the birthing woman has been responding to her husband's genital stimulation, i.e. growing a child is a result of their contact."[59]

Caroline wrote:

> "Rock of Gibraltar" I named you when we first fell in love. The only man I have ever met who could put up with me twenty-four hours a day . . . You loved me for who I was. . . . You always supported me and my . . . uh, stubbornness (?) when you knew it was important . . . Breastfeed? Sure. Child-led weaning? You agreed. Tandem nursing? You defended me from criticism. Family bed? I know how you feel about it, yet you supported me . . . Vaginal birth after two cesareans? Okay by you. Then—the final bomb—at home? You hesitated, you agreed. Rock of Gibraltar, did you also hear my heart screaming for our birthright? Maybe yours was screaming, too.
>
> You gave me the will. You gave the pain its purpose. Your eyes burned me with love. I have never seen a man look at a woman with the love I saw in your eyes for those . . . hours of screaming. Not fear—love. I had no idea you loved me so much. I had no idea I loved you so much. And now, many, many days later,

it remains, and strengthens. We have given birth together you and I. We have looked at eternity together. Now I know I will always love you.

Dale said, "My husband's humor and wit carried us all. He even distracted the nurse with a few excellent lines, and she forgot all about the IV! He made me laugh! Afterwards, he said, 'That was fun! Let's do it again sometime!' and he meant it." Shirley Luthman says that laughter temporarily frees us of fear. On the energy level, the dissolution of fear always opens up the individual . . . humor clears the channels which fear and anxiety block.

A dear man named Fred took the time to write: "[Reading about labor support and birth] has taken me into a world I did not know. It has made me deeply sad and somewhat ashamed of my own lack of understanding and support of my wife at the birth of our two children and even more recently at births of my two grandchildren. I have already called my daughter and my former wife to talk to them about this. What I missed!"

Men. What do you think?

Some Suggestions for Labor Support

Wear something pretty. Eat something healthy. Smile, you're having a baby! Get love. Give love. Read a book. Write a book. Write in a journal. Try out some baby names. Take a walk. Pat your cat. Light a candle. Blow it out.

Get some suggestions from Sylvia Olkin's book, *Positive Pregnancy Fitness*; she has wonderful relaxation tapes and a lot of information about yoga, too. Dance!: Ann Cowlin, director of Dancing Through Pregnancy, remarks that in ten years and with over 1,500 participants in her program, the cesarean rate is half the national average. She believes dance is a tool for helping women become fit in mind and body, one that helps to develop a sense of well-being.[60] Rest: Katy didn't dilate for several hours. She asked everyone to leave her alone and she got into bed and willed herself to sleep. When she awoke, her labor picked up.

Sing!: Sarah Benson, a music and imagery counselor, uses sound and breath to help eliminate stress, increase energy, reduce pain, and facilitate the process of birth. Each of us has sounds—birth music—that become our own "instruments" to bear our children. Midwife Heather Laier remarks that ancient civilizations in Rome, Athens, Egypt, India, China, and Tibet were very much aware of the power of sound in influencing matter and in healing. She says that sound is vibrational energy and vibrations are the fundamental creative force of our universe.

I will forever remember a friend of mine who soothed me at a very difficult time in my life. I couldn't stop crying, and she started singing, "Tender Shepherd"—my favorite childhood song. I stopped crying immediately to listen. To this day, just the memory of her voice heals.

Jasmine Miller uses acupressure (acupuncture without needles) to relieve pain and to assist slow labors.[61] Barbara Soderberg, a monitrice from Connecticut, uses shiatsu, a form of ancient Oriental healing that also helps ease pain and promotes relaxation. Some women have chiropractic adjustments during labor. Some take homeopathic remedies, some herbs, some flower essences.

Some women go to their sanctuary—a place they have created inside of their minds—to rest and relax. Some women read poetry. Others talk to themselves in the mirror. Be your own best friend; tell yourself all the things that you would tell your friend if she needed a pat on the back!

Put some color into your space! Every color has a different vibrational energy of sorts, too. As long as three thousand years ago, the therapeutic effect of colors on soul, spirit, and body were known and practiced. Extended observation of blue or black will lower blood pressure; yellow and red are invigorating. Several books describe the healing effects of sound and color. Yellow is glowing, freeing, illuminating; orange, invigorating, energizing, positive, festive; red, energizing, vital, expanding; purple, deepening, mystic, introverted; blue, quiet, spiritual, wide; green, soothing, passive, calming. Brown, stabilizing.[62] I have been very much aware of colors and their effect on my feelings and emotions since I was quite young.

Linda Goodman makes some interesting statements about color and sound. She tells us that the singing of birds sets up a particular sound vibration that promotes the growth of the young leaves of trees, plants, and flowers, so that the birdsong is fairly constant all day long in the spring, while the new growth is occurring. But birdsong ceases during the summer months, except at dawn and twilight, and sometimes, if not quite all the leaves are full, during the early morning hours. "Isn't it lovely to know that the birds tell the grass, plants, trees, and flowers when to grow? . . . How can anyone think that birds lead lazy, useless lives? . . . [63] The word NATURE contains the word 'tune'. . . . Everything in Nature and in human nature," she says, "is composed of Color and Sound. These are the forgotten rainbows and the forgotten melodies of universal harmony."[64] And what are the colors associated with birth in hospitals? Three that are considered devitalizing—the white of the uniforms, the black of unconsciousness (the numbing anesthesia), and the gray slate institutions.

Love yourself—love womankind! Think "open!" Heal a hurt. Laugh! Judith Goldstein tells us that in several tribes worldwide childbirth is a time of great merriment. In other cultures it is time for storytelling, singing, and chanting.[65] Get a massage. Do a puzzle. Picture your baby.

Take responsibility. Lynn Richards says that doing so is the most difficult task we are given in life: "Why should it be easy in birth?" Peggy said, "I came to realize that I didn't want to be held responsible for any misfortune, so I thought of the doctors as an insurance policy or guarantee for security and safety. If anything happened I wanted someone else to be held responsible. By the time my labor started, I was ready to accept full responsibility for whatever happened in birth. I felt I couldn't trust a doctor's way over and above my own. I couldn't let anyone else do my labor for me."

A Few More Words

Childbirth Wisdom asks: Are easy, natural births limited to tribal women? The answer: Something in the lifestyle of the woman giving birth makes the important difference. "Easier birth is made possible by the attitudes, way of life, and other intrinsic practices of the materially minimal lifestyle, and not by the physical (racial) character of non-Western women." Women who have a "strong, splendid body and a lack of inhibition" find birth a part of their feminine life cycle, and not the horrendous physical assault that we in this country so often find it to be.[66]

We needn't fear labor. Fear is "courage turned inside out,"[67] or "faith in the negative."[68] As you labor and birth, that which has been inside you becomes visible to the world. As one woman said, "I labored for myself and also for my friend who had four cesareans. When we labor for and with each other, it gets easier." Perhaps Ardean Orr, a woman from New York who had four cesareans, felt another woman laboring for her in the little corners of her heart. Perhaps she wanted to pass the gift along: she had her fifth child at home. She sums up her feelings about labor as follows: "No thank you, Dr. Lamaze. I'll coach myself, Dr. Bradley." Sonya Peterson agrees. "I know that my body will get out anything that it got in."

PART IV   BABY!

"My birth was like a log flume ride—wheeee! Ohhhh Lord! I got a little wet but it was incredibly exciting and I wanted to jump on and go again!"

—Gary Shandling

My ideas about birth were formed when I was around eight or nine years old. I was growing up on a small farm in central North Dakota. My father raised registered Hampshire hogs and he taught me to care for them when they were farrowing. I was instructed to be very quiet, slow, and gentle in my actions and to do nothing that would disturb or bother the sow. If I did not follow these simple instructions and upset her, the sow could become violent and hurt me, turn on her newborn young and trample or even kill them, and if the birth of the rest of the litter was delayed because she had become so upset and agitated, they could be born dead. Since the goal of raising pigs is to have large, healthy litters, I was entrusted with a great responsibility. I was told that if the sow was upset during her farrowing, it could cause her to be uninterested in the care and feeding of her little pigs and neglectful of their needs. Sows are very good mothers unless they are harassed, upset or mismanaged. All they need is food, water, and shelter, and they produce a good litter that they care for well. If an eight year old can quickly and easily learn what to do and what not to do to help a sow produce a good litter, why can't our meddlesome maternity care system see what effect their "care" is having on today's mothers? and their babies"

—Jody McLaughlin, Minot, N.D.

Oh there are so many miracles of life
that I can't fathom at all,
like being born . . . —
and when it's time,
an ancient river of blood
will flow on through me,
when it comes time to see this child free;
just like the river that opens to the sea,
I'm gonna let this child flow right out of me . . .

—Linda Arnold, "River"[69]

She looked around her on a crowded street and said to herself, "Every single one of these people was born." Pregnancy—the whole process seemed to her half miraculous and the other half preposterous.

—Laurie Colwin, *Another Marvelous Thing*

Simmerin'

It's worth it. It hurts but it ain't sufferin.' It is not sufferin.' It's pain, but it ain't the sufferin' kind. It's a good hurt.

—from *Motherwit*, Onnie Lee Logan

So it is your due season. No more due "dates"—they just make us crazy. Less than 5 percent of all women deliver on their "due date," yet most—especially first-time mothers—look to that date as if it were sacred. The normal due time may range from thirty-seven to forty-two weeks—and beyond. But, astonishingly, I recently read an article in a popular woman's magazine that said, "At 42 1/2 weeks, your doctor will decide whether to induce labor or deliver the baby by cesarean section." He will, will he? The prediction of the actual date of birth is of great concern to modern urban dwellers, "whose lives are complicated by schedules and commitments and the belief that a multitude of preparation is necessary for a smooth delivery. In contrast, traditional women do little, if anything, to prepare for an oncoming birth."[70]

Birth is instinctual—something for which a woman needs no preparation: "On the contrary, a woman must unlearn what her conscious mind has acquired." Bringing birth back to women is no small ambition. "The history of obstetrics is largely the history of the gradual exclusion of mothers from the birth process."[71] The mother knows fully well what to do and needs no instruction because she is so in tune with her own body and with the energy that is rushing through it. Yet women end up "like tethered cows in an electronic space age milking parlor, taking up the minimum space, making the minimum fuss.[72] Even some women who had no intention whatever of breastfeeding have been known to start to nurse their babies right after birth, "not remembering until some hours later" that they had planned to bottle feed.[73]

Sylvia Klein Olkin calls the preparation for birth "inner bonding." Others call it "conscious gestation." The nice thing about it is that it is done automatically. Even though people call a woman a mother-to-be, she is already a mother in pregnancy. She mothers the baby from the very beginning. When babies look at their mothers for the first time, they know her.[74] Birth is an experience that a mother and her child share, regardless of how they feel "intellectually" about it, and prenatally there is conversation, dialogue. These talks, discussions, or little chats are part of the bonding process. However, according to Virginia Lubell, "people still see this process as occurring after birth. Woman can't be much more 'bonded' than growing a baby inside of them." The last weeks of pregnancy is a particularly good time to sit down with the baby, "get comfy, put your hands around your baby, greet her/him, give a hug, get quiet . . . and listen in return." You can say anything at all to your unborn child, you can explain anything, and "in the privacy of your communication with your child you can say things you might not even be able to say to anyone else. Babies understand.[75]

As always, someone is always there to capitalize on something that is natural. According to a recent article, we can "Build better babies through fetal education at Prenatal U." One of the classes at this institution of "lower learning" gives the mothers megaphones and has them speak vowel sounds into them. Certain vocabulary words are repeated over and over again (such as ice cream, powder, yawn, and throw-up).[76] In the novel by Laurie Colwin entitled *Another Marvelous Thing* the pregnant dad learns that the educational process can begin before birth. "He thought he might try to teach the unborn to count. 'Why stop there?' Billie said. 'Teach it fractions.' "[77] On the other hand, an awareness of how bright babies are prenatally may help us all to make better decisions about their births.

Mothers who seem very well connected to their babies in utero do not always seem to have the same connections with their newborn. Apparently, they do not transfer the information they have gathered and experienced with their unborn child to this newborn baby before them.[78] According to birth psychologist David Cayley, the disconnection arises in part from our language. We talk about the "new" baby, when in fact, this baby has been with us for three-quarters of a year. It also arises from the way we program childbirth—as a potentially "painful, fearful and dangerous experience for which one needs to be institutionalized. This pattern separates us from both the primal and sacred dimensions of birth. We lose connections with our babies and ourselves."[79]

Connecting with ourselves requires, among other things, an appreciation of our feminine bodies. We have a menstrual cycle, which is not a "curse." It is a cycle in time, an affirmation of a system that *works*. Our bodies grow babies, they are not inefficient "incubators"; they produce milk—not a "drink" or a "liquid" or a "beverage" but a complete food, a total diet, for our young. We have birth canals, moist, yielding, warm. Our bodies are wondrous.

Hot 'n' Sexy

Birth is no more "dangerous" than conception, although you might never know it listening to obstetrical voices. It may be more painful than conception, but, in most situations, it can be just as pleasurable. Many women describe the descent of the baby into the birth canal in deeply sensual terms. The sounds women make during uninhibited labor are often similar to those made during lovemaking. In fact, Michele Odent tells us that the right environment for birth is exactly the same as the environment in which to make love.[80]

Tina Raymond, a childbirth educator from Mississippi wrote a wonderful spoof entitled, "Participatory Conception Class, AD 2089."[81] Since women want a healthy baby, they must prepare carefully, right from the first step, she says.

> You have chosen the preparatory coitus method of conception. . . . Because of that, the hospital requires you to take this class. Our special conception program is designed to allow prospective parents to experience the complete reproductive cycle without worrying about medical complications. Perhaps you have read the possible benefits of unmedicated participatory conception and are hoping you will be able to enjoy such an experience. . . . By practicing the techniques [which I will present], some couples find they can experience unmedicated coitus. . . .

The birth canal is not a dirty place. Doctors, however, generally believe that females "always have a certain amount of infection in their vaginas."[82] According to "Hostile Womb" our uterus may be the site of an "immunological siege."[83] One woman said, "If they think they are so dirty, why are they always clamoring to get their fingers—and anything else—in?" Women often remark that their babies "just had to be cleaned off" before they were allowed to hold them. Why not just throw them both in the sterilizer with the rest of the instruments?

It Begins . . .

So, labor begins. So what do you do? You labor. It's that simple. Or, even easier, you get out of your own way and let your body labor.

Alan Watts writes,

> For it is a way of thinking which divides a person from [herself] at the very moment when she needs to "get with herself." That is to say, that when the will is struggling with itself and is in conflict with itself it is paralyzed, like a person trying to walk in two opposite directions at once. At such moments the will has to be released from its paralysis in rather the same way that one turns the front wheel of a bicycle in the direction in which one is falling. Surprisingly, to the beginner, one does

not lose control but regains it. . . . The same is true in sailing, for when you want to sail against the direction of the wind, you do not invite conflict by turning straight into the wind. You tack against the wind, keeping the wind in your sails. So, also, in order to recover . . . the automobile driver must turn in the direction of the skid. . . . The problem is to overcome the ingrained disbelief in the power of winning by love, in the gentle way of turning with the skid, of controlling ourselves by co-operating with ourselves.[84]

Women must create a climate in which they can "forget" themselves.[85] In so doing, they *remember* how to birth.

Some women begin their labors with a prayer or a nursery rhyme, or decorating the room with balloons, or with a song, walk, bath, or phone call. Some bake cookies; others go back to sleep.

Obviously, not all women can finish painting the baby furniture or keep appointments during labor. Each of our labors is different, and each of our responses to the labor is different.

Let me take a minute to remind you that we've been the victims of another obstetrical hype. Until recently, we were supposed to believe that if you were over thirty-five, you might as well forget about pregnancy and normal labor because you were too old. Now, however, "they" are finding that women over thirty-five are still capable of delivering healthy babies—that the risks aren't nearly as high as "they" originally thought. In fact, one article tells us that "biological clock-watchers got reassuring news from a study of nearly 4,000 pregnancies: Delaying a first child until the 30s or even 40s does not result in worse outcomes."[86] Of course, older women have twice the number of cesarean sections, the study found, "which may reflect the greater vigilance and more conservative treatment of older women."

As labor progresses, women's reactions vary. Eileen said that she handled her blossoming very well but felt sad. She loved being pregnant and didn't want it to end. Mary couldn't wait to get the baby out. Some women labor easily, and some don't. Odent reminds us that ultimately, when a woman's labor is difficult, she must use all the strength she has to bring her child into the world, she must trust her own capabilities and potential during labor. Elizabeth Noble says that anyone who works with childbearing women must be careful not to set themselves up as experts, because "however much we may know about birth in general, we know nothing about a particular birth. We must let it unfold with its own uniqueness."[87]

In *Silent Knife* we talked about purebirth, a term that some people loved and others hated. But the term "natural" is still a joke when it comes to most births in this country. Births that are passed off as natural are anything but. The new definition of natural childbirth has expanded to include "a birth in which the mother is awake and delivers vaginally," regardless of how many drugs or interventions there have been.[88] (As we learned in *Silent Knife*, there are "natural cesareans" too).

The term "purebirth" isn't about failure or success, nor is it about value judgment. It is a way to define what birth really is, free from interventions, interference, and institutionalization, even without complete "perfection." As Lynn Richards states: "To seek a pure birth may be a path through which we learn to recognize our own needs. But to require a 'pure' birth is only a set-up for failure. Life is not ideal, nor is it pure. . . . I have rarely known women who had a "pure" birth—a birth that measured up completely to their ideals. Yet, every birth is perfect. Every birth teaches us the perfect lesson."[89]

Elizabeth Davis, author of *Heart and Hands*, a wonderful midwifery guide, writes, ". . . Obviously, birth is part of a larger configuration, beyond the comprehension of friends or attendants. Birth is a pinnacle atop a lifetime of conditioning, relationship dynamics, sexual encounters, family interactions, and one's own experience of being born . . . To attempt to reduce or formulate a woman's birth experience presents a set-up for frustration, a betrayal of her humanity, and a limitation on her perceived potential for growth and change." She says that "birth . . . reminds one of the greatest mysteries of all . . . we [cannot] judge different experiences and choices. Instead, we must . . . validate and humanize those experiences—in and out of hospital."[90]

Our foremothers had purebirths, and all of them took place out of hospital. They weren't always easy, but that isn't the point. The point is that they had their own labors, not a doctor's or a machine's. Peg wrote, "I wish I could have seen my great grandmother in labor, birthing naturally, or hear them tell, in their own words, about the time in their lives. I could have gained so much from them. As an heirloom, the art of birthing passed down from one generation to another is a legacy worth more than all the gold in the world to me."

You can bring your foremothers to your births with you. On both a spiritual and a physical plane, you can bring in anybody, or dismiss anybody, that you want. You can invite elves, fairies and angels. You are the Queen. As midwife Jami Osborne has said, "Everyone else is a 'lady in waiting' to the Queen (even though the Queen herself may be waiting!) There is a sense of honor and respect for this royal woman. She is a goddess." True. This is your show.

You don't have to show anybody anything if you don't want to. You can play to a packed house or do a solo or a duet. Birth can be as social or as secluded as you choose; nudity is private but does not mean shame. "Modesty means not having to be poked and prodded while you are naked, and in front of seven residents and four interns," says Jane. Cats and dogs generally go to a quiet, comfortable place, away from intrusion.

Beth asked one of the midwives at the hospital to leave her birth. "She was newly hired, and eager to be helpful, I am sure, but she was cloyingly attentive, massaging my legs without asking and telling Ted what to do when he knew better than she did. The other midwife was a power-tripper, constantly saying things like, 'If you don't have this baby soon, I'm going to put you on pit.' I wanted to tell her to butt out, but I politely told her to leave, also. I was getting a reputation, but I was taking care of myself." Another woman didn't care for any of three midwives that the hospital employed. Her husband wrote to the hospital, which did not allow private labor support, and said, "All you get around here is your pick of a poor litter. . . . In addition, we did not appreciate the anesthesiologist coming in when my wife was in hard labor to tell us about the options that were available—epidurals, spinals, etc. Next time, if we want him, we'll call him: don't have him call on us." Toxic people are those with a "vacuum cleaner" effect: "they seem to suck the energy out of you—someone who leaves you drained and depressed even though you felt fine to begin with and nothing particular happened during your time together to annoy or upset you. . . . This happens with people who are angry or annoyed themselves but who act nice and polite."

Musings

Serendipity means "happening upon or making fortunate discoveries when not searching for them." Once when I was walking near a lake, I found a Mickey Mouse pin. I love Mickey Mouse! Finding it was serendipitous. I learned that the word comes from the Island of Ceylon, the "aisle of silk"—where adventures take place. Birth is a big adventure! Joseph Campbell says that the adventure we are ready for is the one we get. He also says that in order to be a heroine, we must give life to something bigger than, or other than, ourselves.[91] All birthing mothers are heroines. Campbell also says that we must listen to our hearts or we will become schizophrenic. No wonder so many laboring women in this country "lose it." They are listening to obstetricians and to the beat-beat-beat of the fetal monitors. He says that each of our brains must serve "the humanity of the body. The brain is not the primary organ; the heart is." The fear that we have inside is our Dragon. How do we slay it? We listen to our hearts. "Find your bliss and follow it."[92] When you do, you come alive. Drugged women in labor are not fully alive. You cannot be fully conscious when you are drugged: you will never slay your dragon. Consciousness, Campbell says, means turning toward the sun. (By the way, he reminds us that the whole vegetable world is conscious!)

Pickin' up

Soon, the baby will come through, too. How soon? Who knows? It doesn't really matter. When it's time.

Men Applause

Women have four directions, or characters, or archetypes. The north direction is Mother—nurturing, generous, giving; south is Hetaera—our sexual aspect—

beautiful, desirable, sensual; east is Amazon—our strong, independent, self-sufficient, courageous nature; and west is Medial Woman—the intuitive, creative, wise, spiritual aspect. When the most positive aspects of each of these archetypes is present, we may be in a position to birth more easily and more fully.

Purebirth, natural birth, changes a woman. She learns about strengths she wasn't certain she had. She has feelings of fulfillment and pride and confidence that may have been there all the while, but are now brought to the forefront. It is possible to feel these changes, even with a medicated birth—depending on the amount of decision making, participation, and control a woman has felt. Some people feel threatened by this "move" to a stronger, more independent place. "Whereas husband and wife may have fit together like two pieces of a puzzle," the woman's new shape (figuratively and literally) may not fit as easily. "Will he change along with her so they can continue to fit together?"[93] Some men know intuitively that the experience of birth may alter the woman's perception of herself, and if they aren't in a framework to be able to accept that change, conflicts may occur. While the vast number of couples I have worked with grow closer during pregnancy and birth, some relationships may find themselves in choppy waters during labor and birth.

One woman wrote, "The truth? I didn't need my husband much at all. Don't get me wrong. I love him. But he could have taken an extra hour to get the pizza—I really needed—wanted—the midwife, more." Another woman said, "The more I said, 'Let's go!', the more fearful he became. He kept telling me that he didn't want me in pain. I finally shouted, 'Well, one of us better want some pain or we will never have a baby!' " Jeanine said her husband opposed her the whole nine months. "It became a battle of wills. He refused to consider a labor assistant. His lack of understanding and refusal to budge made me feel as if I could not trust him. That's one of the reasons, I think, I stayed out of his view during most of labor. Perhaps acting calm when I really needed to cry out was partly responsible for the long, difficult labor—but I could not let him see how bad it was. He would have thought I was 'rubbing it in his face'—that he wasn't 'enough' or whatever. When it was time to 'turn myself in' [go to the hospital] I was angry with him and with myself that we had no one with us for labor support."

Anne wrote, "My husband pretty much thought I was a mental case about wanting a VBAC. He expected a cesarean with no labor and had no reservations about it. He expected me to follow the doctor's instructions. He viewed VBAC as a "woman's lib" thing and believed I was brainwashed by all my reading on the subject. When he finally understood that I was going to go into labor, he saw nothing wrong with medical interventions. He expected to take photos and didn't want to have to support me through what he said was going to be 'hell.' I know he was frightened, but I couldn't reach in to the fear—instead, it was all defense, denial, and distance. We had a rough time of it, neither one of us able to see it differently."

In "Deliver us from the Delivery," one father writes:

Let's take a look at the history of baby-having . . . Primitive woman would go off into primitive huts and groan and wail and sweat while other women hovered around. Primitive man stayed outside doing manly things, such as lifting heavy objects and spitting.

When the baby was born, the women would clean it off as best they could and show it to the men, who would spit appreciatively and head off to the forest to throw sharp sticks at small animals. If you had suggested to primitive man that they should actually watch women have babies, they would have laughed at you and probably tortured you for three or four days. They were real men.

. . . At the beginning of the twentieth century, women started having babies in hospitals . . . The men who were present . . . were professional doctors who were paid large sums of money and wore masks. Normal civilian males . . . remained in waiting rooms reading old copies of Field and Stream—an activity that is less manly than lifting heavy objects, but still reasonably manly.

. . . Now women expect men to watch them have babies. This is part of the experience of "natural childbirth," which is one of those terms that everyone uses but that nobody really understands. Another one is "pH balanced."[94]

Glenna and her husband got along fine; it was her sister that she had problems with during her pregnancy. Other women have found that their desire for a natural birth—and their growth in the process of going for one—alienates them from friends, relatives, and neighbors. Most of the women found ways to have their births and keep the relationships civil (Sometimes the only way to do this was to "not talk about the birth at all!").

Medium High

Things are moving along now. Breathe! A nice big breath. This is hard work. When you breathe deeply you feel more alive, energized. You can go outside if you like, or a warm bath might be nice now; what do you think?

In The *Wisdom of Insecurity*, Alan Watts says, "I have always been fascinated by the law of reversed effort. Sometimes I call it the 'backwards law.' When you try to stay on the surface of the water, you sink, but when you try to sink, you float."[95] In *Other Women*, Lisa Alther says that "the secret" is learning to surf— the waves keep rolling in, each different from the last, and you have to ride them "instead of getting pounded to bits."[96] It's time for some laughter, too, for birth is a time of joy. Laughter opens us all up, connects us, lightens everyone. It's relaxing, it's healing. It doesn't cost anything. On an energy level, laughter can change our perceptions and help us to see alternative choices. "When one can see the ludicrous aspects of a dilemma, she is temporarily free of fear. The dissolution of fear opens up that part of the individual which has the answers on an intuitive level. Humor clears channels which fear and anxiety block."[97]

What is funny to one person isn't to another. A number of years ago, when Michel Odent first came to Boston to talk about the birthing center in France, he spoke at Harvard Medical School. A group of childbirth educators and midwives were on one side of the room, and the doctors and medical students were on the other. Michel showed slides of women sitting in little wading pools, laboring and giving birth right in the water, even when their water had broken. One of the doctors said, "How do you keep the water sterile? Do you put anything in the water to keep it clean?" And Michel said, "Only my socks." You can guess which side of the room laughed and which side coughed and looked aghast. Birth, after all, is serious business.

When you want something to happen, Goodman says to focus. You can begin early on to bring that which you want closer to you. "Desire, genuine desire. Desire, when it stems from the heart and the spirit, when it is pure and intense, possesses awesome electromagnetic energy. Released into the ethers each night as the mind falls into the sleep state . . . and each morning as it returns to the conscious state . . . it will surely manifest that which has been imagined."[98] Continue to focus. It's sometimes easy to "forget" that there is a baby amidst all these sensations, all this activity, all the pain. This kind of focusing is not a tight, rigid, blinders-on kind of focusing. It is an imaging that assists you as you let go, open, and bloom. The commitment to birth doesn't come from the head; it comes from the heart. True commitments always come from the heart.

When mothers of young children are on the telephone, they generally allow their little ones to do almost anything that would not be acceptable under other circumstances. They can pull out the pots and pans, dump out the crayons, and make designs out of mayonnaise on the kitchen wall. Anything, as long as mommy gets to talk for a few, precious, uninterrupted moments. Right? Then, when they get off the phone, they look around and could kick themselves for what they allowed. For some women in labor; it's the same way. They beg for drugs—"Do anything! Just take this pain away!"—and they later wish they had thought twice about what they had agreed to.

Song Sung (Baby) Blue and (Pastel) Pink

Birthing women do not make "noise." Every woman has her own, unique, birth music. Although there comes a point during many births where the "music" has a universal sound, each woman also has her own song. We all have eyes, noses, and mouths, but our faces are all different. According to a number of sources, sound is capable of molding the ethers into shapes and, through these shapes, to make an impression on physical matter.[99] We actually influence our uterus with our sounds. Yet, most hospitals are still uncomfortable with women's birth vocalizations; they perceive them as unpleasant, unnecessary "noises." In fact, there is a difference between the terror-filled shrieks and cries of an unsupported mother and the cries and expressions of a woman who, in freedom, calls out her labor to the world. A woman must be in a place where she feels comfortable enough to express the sensations and pain of her labor, or to go within and say nothing at all. Women are told, "If you make noise, you'll push wrong," or "Don't make noise, you'll get a sore throat."

One of the women in my classes sounded like a fire engine siren. She started out soft, then got really loud, only to get softer again: Ooooooooooooooo-AAAAAHHHHHHHHHHHHHHHHHHhhhhhooooooooooooo! Another, sounded like she was rehearsing for the lead in a melodramatic play: "Help me! Somebody help me! Please! I know I am going to die! Won't somebody help me, please?!" She did not want a medicated birth—only the opportunity to cry out when so moved. Katie whispered the word "baby, baby, baby" for hours. Roberta said nothing at all, not one word during her whole labor. In Suzanne Arms' "Five Women, Five Births,"[100] one woman says, "I screamed and I swore . . . but when I went with that fully, I felt no pain."

More

There is a whole generation of young women who are terrified of birth and who want to be drugged. Betty Friedan writes that "the promise of empowerment of women that enabled so many of us to change our own lives is being betrayed by our failure to mobilize the next generation to move beyond us." She warns that we must begin a new round of consciousness raising.[101] I have spoken to a number of women in their early twenties who have just begun exciting, challenging careers; they are all strong, committed, and hard-working women. But when they talk about birth, they are frightened and want anesthesia. Birth is one area inherent in women's lives that is biologically ordained to provide them with an experience of unmatched empowerment, and yet many cower in fear and feel unsuited to meet its challenge. Birth is a microcosm and a metaphor. When the "task" is "accomplished," there isn't anything in the world that you can't do.

Cookin' on High

Those of you who are staying home to have this baby, isn't it nice to be?! Those of you who are thinking about going to the hospital, perhaps it's time to think about heading down there soon.

And More Again

Carol, from New Jersey, met her doctor at the hospital. She had thought about switching but decided that she was strong enough to teach him some things, since he was flexible enough to learn. "If a care provider is at least somewhat open and reasonable, I feel that continuing to work with him/her will do more to help further the goals on cesarean prevention and natural birth than to keep searching for the ideal which doesn't exist. My doctor turned out to be great—a diamond in the rough." Sharon said, "I avoided confrontation by responding to my doctor's suggestions for intervention by saying things like, 'You may be right. I'll consider that,' and 'I hear that you want me to have a monitor strip. I'm not ready for one yet. You can ask me again in an hour,' and 'I have taken your viewpoint into account. It was very well-stated.' I wasn't selling out or kissing face: I was laboring fight-free."

OBs may sometimes be motivated by a need to protect themselves against their own unwelcome feelings. Tom Verny believes that their own birth memories—unconscious though they may be—may get triggered "and each finds a way of defending himself against the anxiety that those memories elicit." Sondra Ray says that just because we cannot consciously remember something does not mean it was not recorded or does not affect us constantly. Alan Watts says that men often huddle together, "shouting to give themselves courage in the dark." As you have read in *Silent Knife,* and in a number of other places, for sure, when a woman is opening to give birth, she is in an open state psychically, too. In that state, she often receives "vibes" that would normally be inaccessible to her. If there is fear in the room, the birthing woman may pick it up and incorporate it as her own. Choose your birthing people carefully!

In my classes, I do a birth visualization that is actually quite realistic. Women often call me after their births and tell me that because of that visualization, they felt somewhat familiar with labor fairly quickly, as if they had "already done this before." We go through the blooming together, with each "blossom" (Sondra Ray calls them "expansions")[102] getting progressively stronger. And I tell them: "All you have to do is breathe—that's all—just breathe—and let your body do its work. Just breathe—and smile—'cause you're havin' a baby!" I remind them to think about the baby, or about their strength, about the people they love and the people who love them. They imagine themselves eating, walking, or relaxing in a warm tub. They get to "try out" the birthplace—to see if they have chosen a place that feels right for them, and to check out the people in that scene, too. They get to "feel" their hormones, the ones that will be helping to open their bodies when the time is right. They think about the qualities in their partner that they love, and they remember a time in their lives when they felt most receptive and desirous sexually, and they allow those warm, opening feelings to be in their body. They think about opening, and releasing, and giving birth. By the time they have "pushed" (in their mind's eye) their babies into the world, they feel many of the feelings that are present at the real birth—exhaustion, exhilaration, pride. They really feel as if they have just had a baby. This visualization has also been helpful for some women who have never had babies, or who have had only cesarean sections, to give them an experience of what birth might be or would have been like. Since there is a "collective consciousness," women know about birth on a cellular level. This process just wakes that level up for a bit. Fear is greatly reduced and replaced by eager anticipation.

Perception/Surrender

Women who are filled with fear about the birth experience are generally unable to experience the blossoming as anything but body-shattering. Women who see the pain of childbirth as the healthy activity of a soon-to-birth body perceive the blossoms much differently: they are equal in intensity—just as powerful—but they are "do-able." One woman likened her labor to a gale-force storm wind, with her holding onto a palm tree and swaying in the storm. "But my grip was tight, and in the midst of all of it, I was still in awe of Mother Nature and even her ability to produce such monumental 'gusts'! I allowed the winds to kind of blow 'through' me—and I wasn't afraid of the storm anymore. I just had to trust that it would be over—and wait for that time." Another described blooming as the womanplace inside of her expanding until it filled every available bit of space inside of her. Many women feel the birth in images of the ocean's waves, ebbing and flowing: Marianne, more "businesslike," said, "It hurts like hell, but I'm doing them, one at a time, until they are done. Period. End of sentence. There will be no more cesareans for me." And there weren't.

Your attitude will have a lot to do with how you "take on" your blossoms. Just "allow" them, and in time, you will learn what your labor is. It is wonderful to feel the point at which a woman stops fighting her labor and just begins to accept it: As she accepts it, she begins to get into the rhythm of it and to be with it, instead of away from it.

I rarely show movies or slides any more because, first, they aren't generally necessary and, second, sometimes they're damaging. The birth visualization seems to be the best "movie," for it is screenplayed and directed individually and produces wonderful scenes in technicolor.

Speaking of Push!

Well now, I can hear you beginning to push! Pat had a precipitous birth. She was alone at home and knew the baby was coming. She said, "I realized when I began pushing that I felt no fear. I knew exactly what to do. If the common cat could waddle into the linen closet and hatch nine or ten on your brand new Fieldcrest towels, I ought to be able to do one. I even knew that if I pushed too hard, I would rip. I'm thinking to myself I'm going to have to wash the Laura Ashley sheets—so I got off the bed. I started to laugh, just thinking

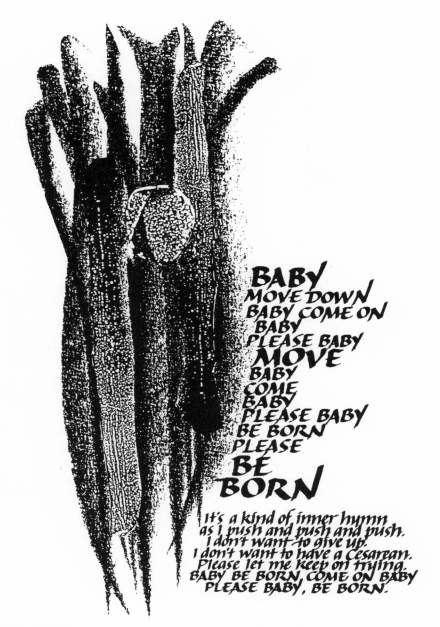

BABY
MOVE DOWN
BABY COME ON
BABY
PLEASE BABY
MOVE
BABY
COME
BABY
PLEASE BABY
BE BORN
PLEASE
BE
BORN

It's a kind of inner hymn
as I push and push and push.
I don't want to give up.
I don't want to have a Cesarean.
Please let me keep on trying.
BABY BE BORN, COME ON BABY
PLEASE BABY, BE BORN.

about the sheets—and the baby crowned. . . . After Rosie was born, I got out my best Waterford crystal and had a glass of Perrier."

Not all women birth that quickly, and some feel that pushing is the hardest part. You just never know.

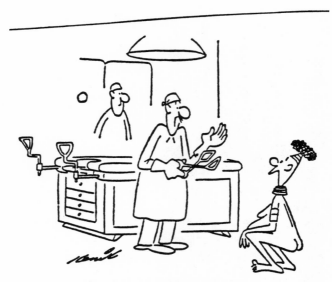

"All right, then, have it *your* way!"[1]

From *Birth Reborn*:

They say that during the last hours before birth you lose contact with the outside world.

This was true for me. I found myself "in another universe on a distant planet, drifting in a sea of sensations."[103]
Caroline writes,

Forty hours of bearable contractions. And then . . . unbearable. . . . Two minutes apart? One minute apart? Who knows? A sea of pain. At the start of each, I swear to request transfer to hospital. I scream through it. At the end I decide, okay, JUST ONE MORE. God, for an epidural? Maybe cesareans are easier? WHY AM I DOING THIS? Doctor's daughter, come to your senses! Use modern medicine! NO!!!! Four hours later. . . . I can't take it anymore, that's what I tell them. So, does she produce an epidural or something sensible, that midwife? No, more voodoo—she lays beside me, comforts me, screams with me. It feels good."
    Forty-five hours after rupture of membranes. I HAVE to push. Scream. Hauled up to squat by him and the second midwife. Again . . . again . . . again . . . again, no end. Will I really give birth vaginally? Is that really a head? They are excited, amused at my disbelief. My soaking forehead against his neck, his arms around me, a last scream of agony. My child is born. Pink, bloody, vernixy, gugly, ugly, beautiful. It is not possible. . . . Sea of confusion replaces sea of pain. IT IS NOT POSSIBLE. Sea of confusion: Why did I do that to myself? Why did I allow that to happen to me? Why did I take that pain? Why? HOW? So I'm not intelligent but I AM sensible . . . or have I lost my senses TOO? The hospital, relief was only a few minutes away, why in the name of God did I go through that? Why?. . . . Love. Love. Sea of confusion is calming. . . . LOVE.

Baby!

The baby! Lift your baby!! Look at your baby!!!! Congratulations!

OB Gerald Bullock says that he has never seen a baby be born cold. "Babies get cold away from their mothers—and then, when their body heat goes down (from being bathed, or unwrapped and diapered), they can't be with their mothers because they have to "be in a warmer." They get cold because we fail to protect them properly by taking them away from the world's best warmer—a mother's warm bare breasts, her body, and a warm blanket around them both. Hence, my heretic comment: " 'I want the baby kept with the mother to protect it from the nursery!' You can imagine the anger from highly trained nursery nurses the first few times I made that comment in public. . . . No one should take that baby away from the mother without asking permission from the mother."[104]

Research at the University of Colorado in Boulder revealed that infants separated from mothers (monkeys) showed immunosuppression which lasted even after the mothers were returned; maternal deprivation causes a lower immune response.[105] According to Odent, the infant's need to be with his or her mother is impossible to satisfy in most hospitals. The child, being cared for by so many, becomes confused. Breastfeeding, he says, remains the only way to reduce the ill effects of "neonatal kidnapping" committed in technologically advanced maternity units.[106]

Dr. Robert Howard writes that the Golden Rule applies even to babies. He says that the baby belongs to its mother and father and that germs and hypothermia are false issues.[107] And for the most part, so is everything else: putting drops in the babies' eyes, shooting them up with synthetic vitamins, putting them under bili-lights, giving them sugar water, sticking them in isolettes, basinettes, cribs, chopping off their foreskins—anywhere but in the mother's arms, twenty-four hours a day from the moment they are born. Imagine! Having to *footprint* babies in order to identify them. According to Sondra Ray, a baby should not be removed from its mother for any reason for at least the first week of life. She says that in Bali, babies are not removed from their parents' presence for six months; they are not even allowed to touch the ground for that time. Then there is a spiritual "grounding ceremony." She said that Bali children grow up to be superior adults; in the many months she was living there, she never saw fear, anger, or conflict. When babies are held for as long as they wish, this takes away negative feelings of abandonment "and separation, and the torment of longing to be held."[108]

One way to create better beings is to create better birth—safe, sane and humane births,[109] and one way to create better birth is to create more confident, empowered (and willing-to-be empowered) and delighted women. Louise said, "This was it. The ultimate. If I live to be a hundred, I don't know that it will ever feel quite like this again. But you know something? It won't matter. This will be with me, living inside of me every single minute for the rest of my life."

Leeann wrote, "I have really been through the medical mill. Yet on the other hand, I am amazed by my own resilience and by the strength of my determination I never knew I possessed. This was my baby's gift to me, a gift of myself."

Johnette wrote, "I kept thinking that everything was due to my childbirth teacher's positive encouragement and support. But this morning, all of a sudden, it came to me, that it was also because of ME—that another person would have responded differently to the same set of circumstances, but I took hold and it was my decisions and my innate person that had shaped those events as much as anyone else. It seemed so foreign to me to think of being that strong, that I feel as if it has touched me to the core."

There is an ancient Sanskrit poem that reads

> Look to this day—for it is life,
> the very life of life:
> In its brief course lie all
> the realities and truths of existence:
> the joy of growth,
> the splendor of action,
> the glory of power.
> For yesterday is but a memory
> and tomorrow only a vision.
> But today, well lived,
> makes every yesterday a memory
> of happiness,
> and every tomorrow a vision of hope—
> Look well, therefore, to this day!

No After Pains

A woman I know had a VBAC after a long labor. It was to have been a homebirth, but after a number of hours, the decision was made to go to the hospital. Of course, her midwife Ilene accompanied her. The midwife on call at the hospital was Jenna. Over the years, Jenna and Ilene had had a number of philosophical as well as personal differences. Their efforts to heal their hurt had only resulted in more pain and had caused a rift between them. Both realized that, in order to help the mother, they had to put aside their feelings and work together. This was difficult at first, but the labor was incredibly intense, and they turned their attention to giving the best possible love and care that they could. "In the sharing of this woman's most victorious and triumphant moments of giving birth," Ilene says, "we began singing songs, and crying, and hugging each other. We both walked away from this birth feeling at peace and loving towards each other, and as though a weight had been lifted. There was no need for words, explanations, or confrontation about the past—all was healed." The

The Unwritten Commandment

I am bound
by a law
created
before
Fire
before
The Flood
The Wheel
The Age of Bronze

Like Eve I was cast
in the beginning
of things
on molten sands
on beaches
on fire and
volcanic rock.

I fantasied
believed I could
break free
but the cry I follow
is an ancient one
buried deep
in me.

This unseen canon
links me
resisting anvil
and hammer

I have no choice
but to go
where woman
has always gone
and answer
the needs of
my child.

     Jean B. Laier

healing that took place was a rebirth for these two midwives—a new beginning for them.

If you birthed at home, you don't have to go anywhere. If you are in the hospital, you may want to gather your things and take your baby home. The paradigm is changing. I've even seen articles in women's magazines that say that there is no reason to stay in the hospital more than a few hours after birth. Next time, you may want simply to birth at home and eliminate the hospital altogether.

One woman wrote, "I created an affirmation for myself. Over and over, I repeated: I am protected. I am creating. I am strong. I am safe. I am at the ocean. I am talking to dolphins! I am free. I'm at Mardi Gras! I am peaceful. I am connected. I WILL birth this 'child.' I WILL! I WILL! I WILL!" I changed it to: "I AM birthing this child. I AM." And I did.

14 *Not for VBACs Only*

And they thought that I should have had another cesarean? That experience, that momentous, miraculous event that should have stopped the world, they thought I shouldn't mind missing?

Not bloomin' likely.

—C. L.[1]

> I pushed him out
> myself
>   after 2 cesareans he was born at home
>   I pushed him out
> myself
>   he wasn't cut out of me like the first two
>   I pushed him out
> myself
>   and, in that magnificent act of painful surrender
>   called birth
>   I started to understand
> myself

—Caroline Sufrin[2]

There is a poster that has been hanging up on my wall since my early VBAC days that says, "Those who say it can't be done are usually interrupted by others doing it."

We all know now that repeat cesarean is a lie perpetrated on the trusting North American woman. When you think about all the cesareans that didn't have to be done and all the unnecessary pain, misery, and suffering that could have been prevented, it boggles the mind. I have learned never to trust the

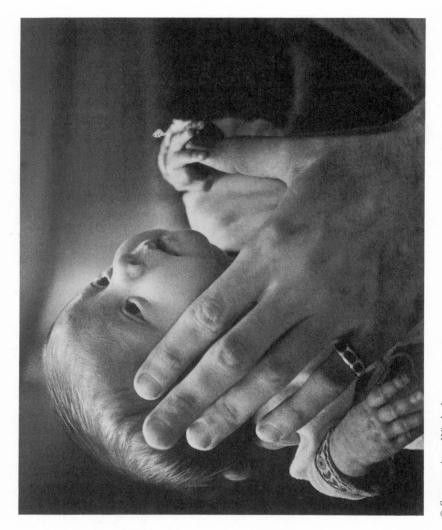

medical profession in matters of birth, ever again. I find it interesting that the almighty benevolent ACOG has allowed the general public to believe that VBAC was their idea. They would have kept cutting us forever if not for the strong-willed, determined, angry women who kept having VBACs in spite of all their scare tactics. After a while, they began to look really stupid. They kept telling us we were going to rupture and die, that what we were doing was foolish, insane, life-threatening. Rather than apologize, they had been fifteen years behind the times, they devised a strategy to get them out of their mess: Why not make the VBAC *their* idea?

Treading Cautiously

Thousands of women had VBACs before studies were published substantiating their safety. We knew they were safe and didn't need studies to tell us so. But the doctors did need the studies, and they started flying out of the OB journals left and right. Some of the studies questioned the "efficacy" of cesarean section or discussed the "risks vs. benefits" of VBAC over repeat section. The risks are that everyone will find out that there is almost no risk with VBAC and that hospitals in this country are going to have trouble booking their ORs on "repeat c-section" surgery day. In actual fact, most medical providers would rather do a repeat section any day. Why should they hang around for several hours waiting for the baby to come out when they can do a section, get paid well, and be out of the hospital in forty-five minutes or so? Most medical providers have refused to do, argued against, balked at, and then finally given into VBAC.

Article after article has come out in favor of VBAC, although not all of them with the enthusiasm we would have liked to have seen: "From our data, vaginal birth after cesarean appears to be safe if conducted in a carefully selected population that is closely monitored in a prospective manner"[3]; "there is no evidence that VBAC has a negative effect on maternal or child health"[4]; "In a proper clinical setting a TOL [trial of labor—a term we don't use anymore. It isn't a trial. It's a labor. Just a labor] can be expected to reduce intra- and postpartum complications, febrile morbidity, blood transfusions and antibiotic therapy. . . . Our study suggests that TOL not only is a safe procedure but also is associated with an overall reduction in maternal mortality."[5] "Exclusion of patients from a TOL after a previous C/S for CPD or FTP does not appear to be justified,"[6] "Large numbers of selected and motivated women can be expected to undergo vaginal deliveries after cesarean section in a safe manner."[7] "[VBAC] can be accomplished with low mortality and morbidity rates, and a good fetal salvage in carefully selected cases."[8] Fetal salvage. We are barbarians. Other articles say a more liberal policy on VBAC is "warranted"[9] and that it seems "reasonable" to consider the policy of once a cesarean. Translation, for those of you who do not speak medicalese: VBAC is safe.

They should have said it this way: VBAC is safe. We don't have to cut women anymore! We shouldn't have been re-sectioning them in the first place! We have been doing a blankload of unnecessary C-Sections, and we'd better stop. But you see, to make such an enthusiastic statement would have been an admission that they were wrong, and as we learned in Chapter 7, men don't like to admit they made a mistake. By being "conservative," by making it look as if it really isn't so safe, but just a little safe, they can save face. Robert Mendelsohn states that doctors are egotistical and paranoid; he suggests we deal with them first by dealing with the paranoia and then by trying to get around their egos.[10]

Gaining Confidence

Many articles tell us that VBAC has significantly fewer complications, and that even with multiple cesareans, the risk is less than that of repeat cesarean. Phelan et al. states, "The policy of 'once a cesarean, always a cesarean' should be abandoned."[11] Another study states that "The number of previous cesareans, the existence of previous, unknown kinds of scars, and infant birth weight appear to have little, if any, prognostic significance for uterine rupture."[12] An article by Graham states: "Continued accumulation of cases showing the efficacy of post-cesarean section trial of labor should encourage a reassessment of the continuing practice of elective repeat cesarean section."[13] We are told that "women who have had their first cesarean section for failure to progress or 'cpd' should be given the opportunity to have a vaginal delivery in their next term pregnancy and that a previous cesarean section in itself is rarely an indication for elective repeat cesarean."[14] It goes on to say that the persistence of elective repeat cesarean is based on philosophic, rather than scientific, reasons. Better change your philosophy, guys. One article states that a 73% VBAC rate should be possible: "This is encouraging news . . . [women] can anticipate the probability of cesarean section to be about 25%, a rate not much different than that in the general population. . . . " A 25% c/section rate is horrendous. A 73% VBAC rate is, too. Goal: a 97% VBAC rate—nothing less; a 3–5% cesarean section rate—nothing more. Almost all the articles say that *a previous cesarean is no reason for a subsequent elective repeat section*! [Some studies have shown VBAC rates to be as high as 85–89%.]

Richard Porreco and Paul Meier tell us that "Because CS involves maternal trauma, possible neonatal respiratory morbidity, and other drawbacks, interest has grown in [VBAC]. . . . Since many patients unfortunately have been taught to fear vaginal birth after cesarean, psychological aspects of management are particularly vital." They go so far as to state that the use of a birthing room is "an appropriate setting" for VBAC; "there is no need for restriction to standard delivery rooms." Even if the woman is "overdue," there is no justification for routine repeat cesarean section: "Again, we feel that patients with a prior CS should be managed exactly as other patients." Although many doctors recommend that VBAC mothers arrive at the hospital in early labor, they feel this is unnecessary. "Having them under intensive surveillance in labor and delivery can needlessly alarm attendants and lead to harmful intervention that may result in a repeat cesarean."[15]

ACOG—A Cog in Our Wheels

So, after one article upon another had appeared favoring VBAC, ACOG (the American College of Obstetricians and Gynecologists) could remain silent no longer: it issued VBAC Guidelines.[16] Everyone was so excited that ACOG had supported VBAC. However, the doctors who insisted that their VBAC mothers follow ACOG's guidelines usually found that the women did not have VBACs. But instead of concluding that ACOG's guidelines made it very difficult for a woman's body to birth normally and abandoning the guidelines, they often concluded that VBAC just didn't "work." And if it wasn't going to work in most instances, why bother putting a woman through labor—only to have her end up on an operating table? Indeed, one article states that "a practical reason to continue the practice of elective repeat cesarean section relates to the time requirements of allowing a patient a trial of labor. To pursue the natural course of labor predestines many patients to arrive at the hospital unexpectedly. . . . This can interrupt the physician's schedule and alter the plans for support mechanisms in the patient's family. Scheduled deliveries are the most efficient for all concerned."[17] In a "round table" discussion on cesarean section and VBAC, one doctor said, "A major unspoken issue of the increasing use of cesarean section is time: the physician's time, the scheduling time, and the interruption of office hours. The other unspoken issue is compensation (versus fee for vaginal delivery), which is rarely mentioned."[18] I'll mention it in a few minutes, I promise.

When ACOG issued its guidelines for VBAC, I issued my own. Each was in response to an ACOG statement I didn't agree with. If you want to have a VBAC, do not follow any of ACOG's guidelines; You do not need to discuss VBAC with a doctor; You do not need to have a low segment transverse incision; If you had a cesarean for CPD, you not only have a good chance for a VBAC, but a GREAT chance, even if this baby is larger than the last. You can have a VBAC with a ten, eleven, or twelve pound baby, or with a breach presentation, or with twins, or with triplets; You do not need to be in the hospital early in labor—in fact, the earlier you go, the greater your chances for ending up with a repeat section; you do not need a fetal monitor—in fact, electronic monitoring triples the chances that you'll end up with an unnecessary section; You do not need to dilate a certain amount each hour—you can dilate in your own, sweet, merry time!; You do not need to be in a facility with an operating room, anesthesiologist and pediatrician on call—stay home, relax, have a good time. None of the women whom I had taught or counseled followed ACOG's guidelines, and almost all of them had vaginal deliveries. No one I know follows the guidelines to this day, and with rare exception, they all have VBACs.

Many doctors, though nervous and resistant, agree to VBAC under some circumstances. However, many automatically screen out anyone who has had more than one cesarean. Meanwhile, women with two, three, four, and even five and six c-sections have had their babies naturally, and many of them stayed at home. This made the doctors look dumb again, and so out came more studies to back up one by Meier and Porreco, who a number of years earlier had stated that "a more liberal policy regarding patients with two or more previous low transverse sections also seems warranted.[19] One article stated that a commonly held concept was that the risk of uterine rupture increases according to the number of sections: "However, even with four previous cesareans" there seemed to be no higher increase in risk.[20] Another study remarks that there is "little evidence to support the concept that multiple uterine scars increase the risk of uterine rupture."[21] Dr. Irwin Kaiser, who had attended VBACs for many years, wrote, "It is my impression . . . that each section heals by itself without reference to the number of previous sections."[22] More and more studies, more and more data—and they all came to the same conclusion: a vaginal delivery after more than one section was safer than another operation. The risk of uterine rupture was virtually nonexistent.

Now we know that it is okay to have a natural birth even after several cesareans. But some doctors caution that if a woman has a classical incision, then she can't have a VBAC. But of course, women who have had classical incisions are capable of having their babies vaginally, some at home. One woman wrote, "My doctor told me that when a vertical scar ruptures, the babies just pop out and die. Nothing happened to my scar. My baby popped out—vaginally—very much alive and kicking." Many women with T incisions have their babies vaginally, as well.

When I think back to the first twelve years of my VBAC teaching career—and the hours I used to spend in class dispelling the myth of uterine separation—I could faint. As the years progressed, I spent less and less time on it. For the past three years, I have not spent *one minute* on the subject in any class; it rarely even comes up any more. Uterine "Rupture"—is at last a nonissue. The doctor who continues to bring it up still has a "rupture mentality," and there is no room for that at a VBAC birth.

For those of you who need more information on this subject, check *Silent Knife*, the C/SEC and CPM newsletters, and Lynn Richards' book on VBAC. The risk factor is less than that of abruptio placentae or shoulder dystocia, or cord prolapse. So there is no reason to allow the possibility of uterine rupture to deter your plans for a natural birth. By the way, as childbirth educator Jane Szczepaniak has said, you can only have one VBAC per cesarean per lifetime!: "Once there has been a vaginal birth, all subsequent uninterrupted vaginal births are only normal vaginal births." Also, there is no limit to the number of subsequent vaginal deliveries a woman can have, either.[23] And one more thing—no one should be examining scars anymore.

The Nonissue

VBAC educator Laurie Brant writes that because the incidence of uterine rupture is so low, it is hard to get information on the subject. Laurie attended a birth in which there was a uterine rupture; both mother and baby are fine. There has never been a maternal or fetal death associated with a low-segment incision. The incidents where there were serious ruptures were on uteri that had never been sectioned—and pitocin was generally responsible for these situations. One woman who had never had a cesarean wrote, "If I had a minute of your time, I would tell you that I was one of the women that allowed herself to be induced. Mothers and babies can die or become brain damaged as a result of these drugs that begin or "augment" labor. I lost my uterus, practically lost my own life and my baby. If I had a minute of your time, I'd tell you to think for more than a minute if someone wants to induce you."

Beth Shearer remarks that in most cesareans done for "suspected scar rupture," the scar turns out to be intact after all. "When it does occur, it is an entirely different event from a classical scar or an unscarred uterus. With immediate transport . . . a suspected rupture of a low transverse scar may in fact be more easily controlled at home than a placental abruption or cord problem." Beth attended a birth at which there was a rupture. Transport to the hospital took about twenty minutes and was at 6 cm for "failure to progress and because the mother demanded it." Upon her arrival to the hospital, the monitor showed a normal contraction pattern and fetal heart tones. The mother's vital signs were all normal. An IV was inserted, an epidural given, and an hour or more after the arrival, the cesarean was performed. A partial separation of the uterine scar was discovered, with a slow internal bleed. Total blood loss was estimated at two units, so there was no need for transfusion. Beth said that the mother clearly needed transport and a cesarean and would have been in trouble somewhere down the road, but at no point was she or her undiagnosed twins in danger; the baby underneath was pushing the upper baby up, which is what caused the separation and the lack of progress in labor. One lesson she said that she learned was the importance of listening to the mother (who felt she needed to go to the hospital) "but I also lost my fear of a low-transverse scar being a sudden dire life-threatening emergency."[24]

Alive and Kickin'

There have been *no* maternal deaths associated with VBAC in all the literature—ever. Several articles state that mortality fears for mother and infant in VBAC are completely unsubstantiated.[25] In contrast a number of maternal deaths are associated with elective repeat cesarean section. We can only wonder why these women did not go into labor and have a VBAC. In one case a woman wanted a VBAC but was discouraged by a number of scare tactics and decided to have a repeat cesarean after all. She died of an embolism. We all know that elective repeat cesarean delivery poses considerable risk for both mother and fetus (morbidity is 100 percent for mothers and high for babies, too). "In comparing the best results achieved by elective repeat cesarean section with the worst results of patients undergoing a trial of labor, it has been pointed out that "the risk of maternal death secondary to a trial of labor with scar rupture was one-fortieth that of a maternal death at the time of an elective repeat cesarean section. The risk of perinatal death in the same situation was one-quarter to one-fifth that of a perinatal death resulting from an elective cesarean section."[26]

Choosing: Lie Down or Stand on Your Own Two Feet

Women sometimes choose to have a repeat cesarean based on their past childbirth experience.[27] If their labors were long and difficult, they might "prefer" a section: their cesareans were "salvation from a painful labor which they have no desire to repeat." They are frightened to go into labor again. They are frightened to be in labor. "What do [women] learn from their physicians about trial of labor, how does physician communication affect their choice, and how important is medical information when compared with other motives for choosing VBAC or repeat cesarean?"[28] In my experience, most of the women who remained fearful also had fearful physicians; the woman's decision to have surgery was met with relief on the part of the OB. "It was her choice, I gave her the options," the doctor will say. I'd have liked to have been a fly on the wall to see how the "options" were presented.

"Is a practice justified only on the basis of the patient's fear? If a practice is associated with greater risks to the both mother and fetus, can it be justified on the basis of the patient's preference alone? Fear . . . is not justification for cesarean section."[29] Healing of the previous experience (including information about any interventions or factors that might have influenced the length and severity of the labor), reassurance, and support may help the woman choose a vaginal delivery. Unfortunately, it is far too easy these days to find a doctor willing to schedule a repeat cesarean. All those task forces and consensus development conferences—even many doctors admit: they were a waste of time, a failure.

One woman said that her doctor mentioned VBAC to her at the end of her first prenatal.

> My reply was that I had never met a woman who had had a vaginal delivery after a section. I told him I would go for a repeat cesarean. He replied, 'Am I ever glad you said that, they're tricky things.' I opted for a repeat because I was afraid. I was afraid to be told at the last minute, 'Sorry, but we've decided on a cesarean after all,' like so many other women I had talked with. I didn't think that I could cope

with that again. I was really afraid for my sanity. All those feelings from my first baby's birth kept rushing back. I was afraid of them.

Another factor that seems to contribute to a woman's opting for a repeat section is convenience. Some women feel that knowing that their doctor will be available (if they scheduled a repeat cesarean) or that their mother will be in town to help with the children justifies scheduling a section. "Convenience for patient or physician, fear of failure, and supposed risks related to uterine rupture are not sufficient reasons to perpetuate the practice of elective repeat cesarean deliveries."[30]

According to Carol Shepherd McClain, women who can visualize a different (better) outcome the next time around opt for vaginal births. One woman that McClain interviewed had had an emergency cesarean that was "frightening, painful and demoralizing." She and her husband became estranged several months after the operation, and she was depressed for over a year. She later reconciled with her husband, and became pregnant, choosing VBAC "to avoid the physical and emotional hardships she associated with her cesarean." Another woman chose VBAC because she felt "curious" about birth and did not want to be incapacitated afterward. McClain says that women who opt for cesarean section do not recall their previous surgery as having prolonged their recoveries or upset their lives. "These women constructed scripts in which the previous labor was a totally negative experience (painful, exhausting, frightening, even threatening to the [baby]) and in which the decision to perform a cesarean was greeted with relief.[31] Margaret Catanese writes that any actions designed to help a woman choose VBAC over a scheduled c-section are worth the effort. Opting for a VBAC, she says, "provides maintenance of individual integrity and homeostasis by avoiding unnecessary surgical intervention. . . . Repeat cesarean sections are in many cases unnecessary surgery, and the avoidance of such lends itself to maintaining wholeness of the individual."[32]

Mint Green

If the 500,000 repeat c-sections that were done between 1980 and 1985 were VBACs, surgical fees and costs for 1.2 million days of hospital stay would have been averted. Since VBAC has yet to gain a firm hold in the United States, you can see that hospitals in this country are making a killing out of repeat cesareans. It makes more sense economically for doctors and hospitals to keep us under the knife.[33] There are hundreds of studies out, but still, women are being cut. Beguin says that perhaps "in the near future, it may be that third-party providers will require a trial of vaginal delivery before reimbursement for repeat cesarean birth unless there is an absolute medical indication for a repeat procedure."[34]

**The Medical Misogynists Guide
to Malevolent Maternity Care**

1. Size them up.
2. Butter them up.
3. Wind them up.
4. Work them up.
5. Shut them up.
6. Feel them up.
7. Hook them up.
8. Shoot them up.
9. Rough them up.
10. Tie them up.
11. Cut them up.
12. Wake them up.
13. Lock them up.
14. Hush them up.
15. $Hold them up$.

Jody McLaughlin

Hi Gerry!

Dr. Gerald Bullock says that he can *guarantee* a failed VBAC. Just follow his advice

Doctors: . . . be noncommittal enough in the early interviews: the issues won't come up again until later in the pregnancy. It is the rare patient indeed who has the presence of mind and strength of conviction to change doctors late in pregnancy.
. . . During the pregnancy, be sure to add to the mystique of the previous cesarean by ordering several ultrasounds and suggesting an amniocentesis, so the mother will understand how different and potentially dangerous her situation is. Never mind informing her that the risk of amniocentesis [is] higher to the baby than the risk of VBAC . . .

If by chance the mother hears about cesarean prevention classes or VBAC group meetings, tell her they are a bunch of crazy radicals who have only their own crosses to burn and do not have her best interests in mind.

Be sure to spell out whatever criteria you have in considering VBAC for them. Tell them that the baby must . . . not weigh more than whatever is your own limit (never mind that your guess at the weight is often as much as two pounds off). Give her your own personal allowances for the amount of time you feel is safe for her to labor. . . . Make her understand that she will be laboring against a deadline.

If you are not successful in getting the patient to consent to a repeat cesarean . . . early in labor, do not despair; all is not lost. There are several ways still in which you can get her to give up the notion of VBAC. Make sure she remembers what a high-risk patient she is, and keep an ever constant vigil for "catastro-phe"... Don't give in to the frivolous request to ambulate. It is imperative that you know exactly what the contraction pattern is . . . she must therefore be confined to bed from the time of arrival to the time of delivery. Have the perseverance to insist upon monitoring. . . . Be kind and considerate, and apologize for not being able to allow her more flexibility. . . . Say things like, "Of course, your baby's safety is our primary concern."

. . . When the patient arrives early in labor, look at her critically and say some-thing like, "Do you really think that you are going to have that big thing from below?" . . . A note from anesthesiologists: Be sure that you come in fairly early to do your "routine preoperative history review." If you do it right, you can leave the impression that almost all VBAC mothers eventually go ahead with a repeat ce-sarean. Then return to her room frequently to check her progress . . . Explain what will happen "while" she has her cesarean, not "if" she has it. . . . If you are not trained in conduction anesthesia, explain to her why general anesthesia is safer for her and the baby. . . . Finally [for other staff members standing outside the door], you might say something like, "Is that blood ready? Get it stat! What if she ruptures?"[35]

Another Tootsie

One Tootsie says that a woman wanting a VBAC must unfortunately prepare for the possibility of a repeat "failure," regardless of her best try. This doctor from the south writes, "It has been my experience that the woman feels much better about the situation if she finishes her labor with the feeling that she was given every possible chance and all the support that anyone could muster." He remarks that his clients who had surgical deliveries, however, invariably came back later saying they were glad for the chance to give it all they had and that even though they were perhaps exhausted, they felt better for having been given all the time they needed for a thorough attempt.

My "management" of VBACs was the chief reason I was suspended from the hospital here, despite the fact that over the past ten years, I have had more personal experience with VBAC than probably anyone else in the state, and also despite the fact that I have never had a complication related to the prior c-section.

One major charge is that I allow my patients to make their own decisions rather than making them myself. Isn't that the way it is supposed to be? Shouldn't we explain the pros and cons, to the best of our ability, and leave the final decision to the mothers involved? I am told that I should tell mothers what they should do, and refuse to take care of them if they refuse. Many of the people who come to me have consulted other physicians who have made autocratic rules they have refused to follow. Then the physician tells them to go somewhere else. So they come to my office, and those same physicians expel me from their society for offering the flexibility they were unable to tolerate. Perhaps it boils down to a difference of opinion regarding patients' rights.

Sign on the Dotted Line—Then Perforate

I received a letter from a woman in Pennsylvania who ultimately decided to have her VBAC at home. She had heard about a group practice in her area that was supposedly "liberal" about VBAC. When she read the form they wanted her to sign, she decided she'd be better off as far away from their office as possible. The form read:

> You are requested to sign the following form. It gives your legal permission for Dr. V. or Dr. H. to deliver your infant either by Vaginal delivery or by Cesarean delivery. . . . Most of us visualize our birth experience in the new labor and birthing suites, the lights lowered . . . a feeling of reverence, contentment, satisfaction encompasses all. But should we plan only for our births with this image in mind? Will we feel disappointed, guilty, disillusioned—a failure—if circumstances beyond our control dictate a cesarean birth? . . . Rather than taking even the smallest risk of having an unfavorable outcome with a vaginal delivery, the doctor may opt for the surgical delivery. . . . [As for VBAC], many patients will automatically choose a repeat cesarean because of the convenience of scheduling the delivery, the avoidance of painful labor, fear of complications, or lack of support of . . . family for a vaginal delivery attempt.

This outrageous piece of propaganda goes on to list a number of "dangerous conditions" that can occur and reasons why cesareans are performed. "Few physicians or patients can control the size of the prospective mother's pelvis, the position of the baby, or the main causes of fetal distress in labor. . . . Emotionally, the mother should prepare for either type of birth—vaginal or cesarean. By doing so, the patient will hopefully avoid feelings of inadequacy and disappointment about her mode of delivery."

Eileen, from Washington, said, "My doctor kept telling me how dangerous this VBAC was. I asked him for articles and books that proved c-sections were safer. He said he didn't have it in black and white, but no logical person who cared for the well-being of his or her child would consider such a thing." Jill, from Florida, writes, "VBAC gives power back to the women, so most of the physicians here are unenthusiastic about it. They still do not bring it up unless the woman herself does. When I said this to one doctor here, he said, 'I know, I know.' And he wouldn't condemn them for this? You are right: the buddy system is strong. I am scared for all pregnant women today!"

One doctor in Florida charges several thousand dollars "up front" and then an extra few thousand once the VBAC was "finished." He will not file an insurance claim for VBACs. Melissa, also from Florida, wrote, "My doctors let me do it because our persistence and determination would permit nothing else. In this area, the only women who have VBACs are the ones coming in crowning. I think if the doctors could, they'd push the babies back in even then. Two friends of mine had repeat sections after they were fully dilated and only pushing for an hour; the doctor said that was 'enough of that'."

In one hospital, it is okay to have a VBAC if it has been five years or less since your last delivery. If it has been six years or more, the woman is scheduled for a repeat cesarean. Who sets these arbitrary numbers and who in her right mind would adhere to them? In Mississippi a woman had a VBAC without any intervention, only because she arrived at the hospital too late for them to hook her up to anything: her doctor arrived after the fact. "I had spent nine months negotiating a purebirth—but they had insisted on the whole nine yards. I just kept stalling at home."

Bernice lives in Massachusetts. She had taken my classes before she became pregnant, so it had been some time since we had talked. She "forgot" that vaginal exams weren't necessary in the ninth month. She had been examined that afternoon and was very upset. "I am three days overdue," she said, "and I just had a doctor's appointment. He told me not to get my hopes up. He said the baby was so high that he couldn't even reach it. He said he had never felt a baby that high before, and he said he thought we should schedule me for a cesarean." Bernice refused and had a seven-pound, fourteen-ounce VBAC son one week later. She said, "I think the baby was just trying to get away from his probing fingers."

Anne, from Connecticut, wrote, "The total feeling of achievement and elation of a VBAC is somewhat depressed after an invasive, intervention-filled birth. I was no match against an apprehensive, fear ridden hospital and OB staff, who felt I should be grateful just for letting me have a chance under any conditions, theirs. You do it their way, or no way."

Mara, from Illinois, wrote, "Now comes the point that the doctor walked back in and said to me: are you ready and have you decided. And I said yes we have, and I'm not having a Cesarean section without a second opinion so transfer me please. I transferred hospitals and doctors in the middle of my labor! We had to call an ambulance and transfer because the hospital would not take any responsibility to make arrangements. We arrived at the second hospital with Bill still attired in his first-hospital scrubs. Our VBAC baby was born 3 hours later."

In the Midwest, one group practice tells their VBAC mothers that they must have an ultrasound between 12 to 14 weeks. As to labor, VBAC women will be able to take ice chips and "for your well-being, IVs and fetal monitors will be used." We read on: "Your delivery will be done by your doctor. . . . Your hospital stay will be one to three days, depending upon the length of your labor and any complications that arise." This form reminds the woman that she can change her mind at any time during the VBAC labor and go for a c-section.

Felice said, "A pregnancy after a cesarean is stressful! You have to look for a doctor agreeable to VBAC—not in this community, the doctors always do repeat cesareans. When you finally find one 'out there,' you discover that you are 'high-risk.' You walk into the office feeling hopeful and excited, and you come out with a heavy heart."

Many women are told that they are "too small" to birth a baby. Illich says that a diagnosis—or label—by the physician can brand her forever with a permanent stigma. "Like ex-convicts, former mental patients, people with their first heart attack. . . . [people who are labeled] are transformed into outsiders for the rest of their lives. Professional suspicion alone is enough to legitimize the stigma even if the suspected condition never existed."[36] Thousands of women who were sectioned for CPD find that their babies are born vaginally. One woman, who was told she'd never even be able to have a "five pounder" had two vaginal deliveries after her two cesareans—one baby was nine pounds!—and she said that he came "sliding all the way!"

Of Course, You Can!

When a woman calls me and says, "Do you think I can have a VBAC?" my response is that it makes very little difference what *I* think; it matters what *she* thinks. I ask, How much does it mean to you? What steps are you willing to take to reach that goal? Are you willing to stay at home to have your baby, if necessary? Again, if you go into a place that has a 30 some-odd percent, or higher, rate of c-sections, you have automatically raised your chances for having one, just by virtue of walking through their front door. If you really don't want a c-section, don't put yourself in a place where they do them.

Birth/VBAC in Special Circumstances

Each of the following women had a VBAC. Each had her own unique situation, and now has her own story to tell.

CATHERINE (VBAC with bone spurs)
My first baby was born three years ago after a very long labor. It ended in a c-section because when I was fully dilated they discovered that I had bone spurs on my coccyx. The doctor said I could only have a vaginal delivery in the future if I wanted to have my tailbone broken surgically right then, which I did not, because he said it is very painful recovering from that, far more excruciating than another cesarean. I was resigned to another section. I thought that maybe I was one of those cases where a c-section is required. But then I heard about another woman who was scheduled for her second cesarean due to a similar situation and she went into labor before her surgery and delivered vaginally, a large baby, to the amazement of her doctor! So I realized that these things are not as certain as we are led to believe. . . . My VBAC daughter was born at home.

DOROTHY (VBAC—partial placental abruption)
After spending time taking VBAC classes and choosing a doctor, Gene and I made an effort to release the spinning thoughts—as well as fears—in our heads. Once major decisions concerning the birth were made, we felt we could let the rest go and proceeded to spend more time in meditation allowing for a greater power to take over.

In the thirty-second week of the [pregnancy], I started bleeding. Not a placenta praevia, I was informed, but a placental abruption (partial). A subsequent episode of bleeding was followed by a one-day stay at the hospital. Although Ritadrine was prescribed, I did not take it. Once again, the following week, the bleeding started and again I was hospitalized. . . . Three days later I went into labor and delivered vaginally in four hours. The birth was indeed an awesome, miraculous and joyful one for us . . . such a deep sense of satisfaction. . . . Our little son Gabriel weighed four pounds, 13 oz. and had absolutely no problems from being five weeks premature. He began breastfeeding within one hour after birth. We were able to use the birthing room and have our 4 year old son with us for the birth. The doctor we used had attended hundreds of VBACs and is such a supporter of trial of labor that he will not do a repeat section unless it is medically necessary. . . .

My older son was incredible during the delivery. His eyes like two silver dollars, he was both supportive and totally absorbed by the birth process. He stood right next to us the whole time and missed nothing. We all felt so very close. It was worth the seventy mile drive to be in such a supportive hospital. Our doctor was flexible and accessible, self-assured and experienced.

. . . The difference between the two births was greater than I ever could have imagined. Recovering from a cesarean was wrought with anxiety and depression. This time, we felt good. Although there is much to be criticized about hospitals, doctors, and western medicine, there are some benefits to the medical field that cannot be overlooked. We made our own choices within the context of our situation, and feel truly proud and blessed.

ELLEN (VBAC—meconium; Rh negative)

Labor was so much harder than I expected, overall the whole thing was more painful than the cesareans! However, so much more rewarding, fulfilling, exhilarating—to give birth, to watch it happen, the natural, right way! If I had been in the hospital I would have had a third cesarean. There was meconium in the water, and I know they would have whisked me right off to the OR. Also, I had the additional complication of being RH negative and I had to take and preserve "cord blood." I called the hospital lab the next morning—that told them that it was a homebirth—and I had to go in that day and give my blood for typing with the baby's blood. Baby positive. No antibodies. When I was sitting in the hospital, the nurse had to fill in the lab report form. She asked "Name of patient," and I replied, "There is none." So she asked, "Name of mother, name of baby," and I gladly gave that information to her.

BARBARA (VBAC—overweight mother)

My first baby was a vaginal birth. My second and third were both c-sections for "failure to progress." I am over forty years old, I'm short, and I weigh about two-hundred sixty-five pounds. My physician, who had consented to giving me a "trial of labor"—under extreme duress, I might add—was not on call. His partner would not hear of a vaginal birth. He wouldn't even come in to talk to me—he sent a message via the obstetrical resident that I would have to resign myself to a c-section. Well, he didn't know Barbara Jean M———!! I had a conference with every OB resident on the labor and delivery unit—stalling for time, of course. I convinced them to wait two hours. I would have stalled them again. At 7:29 P.M. I gave birth without anesthesia or c-section to a 9 lb. 10 oz, 22 inch, baby girl. I had only one small laceration. Everyone was completely astonished that I and my baby were fine. I am overjoyed and I am very proud of my persistence.

ETTA (VBAC after 2 cesareans:
one low transverse incision, one classical)

With my first cesarean, I had a low horizontal incision. My doctor was simply too inexperienced and too frightened to deliver a breech. I had major complications from the surgery. . . . Two years later I had a repeat cesarean. To add insult to injury, my second section was a classical incision. And guess what? I just had my third baby—a VBAC! It is definitely okay to congratulate me!

MARILYN (VBAC—mother with muscular dystrophy)

I have muscular dystrophy. I was told that my uterus, being a muscle, wouldn't work, so I had a cesarean. It was very hard for me afterwards. I had difficulty walking and my co-ordination in general became—and remained—markedly worse. When I became pregnant for the second time, I thought, if my uterus doesn't work, how did I get pregnant and grow a good healthy baby the first time? I was afraid that another cesarean and I'd be in a wheel-chair or bedridden for life. I was assured that a section couldn't have that kind of effect on my illness but I don't believe them.

In labor the nurses kept telling me I wasn't progressing and my contractions weren't productive. They were so discouraging. They all looked exhausted and angry with me for trying. But I hung in there, thanks to my husband and my LSP, and I am happy to tell others that my baby was born vaginally. No medication and no interventions. My doctor even got down on the floor and helped as I squatted. Because of my weak legs, I can't squat well generally, but during the birth I did!

DEBORAH (VBAC—diabetic mom)

My c-section left me devastated. I have always been in control of my life, except for those eleven days (three days before when my OB decided to do a section to eight days after it when I was finally released from the hospital). I still ask, "How did it happen? How did I lose control?"

My OB had called me "at-risk" but my pregnancy had progressed normally. I was confident that with proper care and close monitoring of my diabetes, I would have a healthy baby. I was also under the care of a diabetes specialist. I had always been able to manage my diabetes from age thirteen, when I was first diagnosed, through minor illnesses, living away at college and every challenge a diabetic faces daily! Frequently throughout my pregnancy, the specialist and I disagreed over what was best and who was in control. He had a set program he advised all of his diabetic pregnant mothers to follow which included a hospital stay some point mid-pregnancy. I could not understand the benefit of a 3–5 day hospital stay versus being an active working woman with a regular schedule. Neither of us was ever really satisfied with our visits, but my blood sugar was in control and my baby was growing.

I began to lose control in the decision making about a week before my due date. My OB had a consultation with a specialist and then called me at home and said he had scheduled a c-section for Tuesday morning, three days away. We asked about inducing labor, but the doctor was firmly set on a C-section. It was "the best way." We felt we had no options.

I became pregnant twenty-three months after my cesarean. During those months I dealt with a lot of anger, but fortunately I turned most of it into a determination not to lose control again. I had never used my diabetes as an excuse for anything and I wasn't about to let it become an excuse for another c-section. When I was thirteen, a nurse in the hospital told me diabetes was a handicap, not an illness or a disease. I had to overcome this handicap to live a normal life, but if I let it overcome me it would turn into an illness or a disease. With this in mind, I read everything I could find of Type I diabetes and pregnancy. I purchased a blood glucose testing machine and experimented with the rigid diabetic diet to find foods that my body digested better than others.

Then I became pregnant. We had moved to a new state and I was determined to have a doctor that would allow me to go into labor and I was determined to manage my diabetes day-to-day myself, and I was determined to be in control of every aspect of the pregnancy and delivery. If there were going to be any late pregnancy consultations or decisions, I was going to be a part of them.

new OB was confident I could manage the diabetes. His greatest concern was that the baby's size would necessitate another cesarean—my daughter weighed 10–5 at birth. But he also assured me that my husband and I would both be involved in any decisions.

. . . At week thirty four, I began weekly sonograms. By week 36, it was clear that the baby was at six pounds and growing at the rate of about a pound a week. I became concerned and asked about induction of labor. At week 38, my doctor agreed if I consented to an amnio to check the maturity of the baby's lungs. They were mature and we proceeded the next morning . . . [During the induction] I monitored my blood sugar level hourly. By early evening I was taken off the pitocin drip and returned to my room. The next morning we followed the same procedure and by mid-afternoon, my body took over and my contractions were steady. On July 30, my eight pound son was born. I had "beaten the odds," and it felt great!

Our third birth was a dream come true. It was two weeks before my due date. I hadn't had any sonograms yet—I was scheduled to have one the next day. I took my children to a lake and I knew I was in labor. I just kept laboring there. I was in a health plan, and one of the doctors was obnoxious. I kept thinking that I had to "beat her out" (with the ultrasound). Well, I did. I got to the hospital later that day and delivered within one and a half hours. It was so fast that the doctor on call (whom I did not know) didn't have time to check my records until after the birth—and then she yelled, "My God, you're a VBAC!" It was an easy birth and the baby was a little over eight pounds.

My fourth birth was a little harder. One week before the due date I had an ultrasound. It said that the baby was over nine pounds. The doctors wanted to schedule me for a cesarean. I said no, I'd have an induction. My contractions started on their own that afternoon, however, and by the time they had hooked me up to the pit, I was in active labor—they didn't turn it on. In two hours, my almost ten pound son was born.

DEB (VBAC—after myomectomy)

I had a uterine scar from a myomectomy, and was told that my future babies would have to be delivered by cesarean. Well, I didn't want to have more surgery. My first baby was born this week. She was ten pounds one oz.—and I'm not a big woman!—and I had a natural birth.

TANIA (VBAC—with herpes)

I had herpes during the last month of my first pregnancy and the doctor told me I had to have a section. He said the baby would die. Then I read a study done at Stanford that said that infants born vaginally to mothers with herpes have only a very small chance of contracting herpes themselves. Even the mothers who had visible lesions in the birth canal at the time of delivery did not contract herpes; all the babies' blood contained antibodies that protected them from the virus. Was I angry! When I had my second child, as luck would have it, I had a lesion on the labia, possibly one inside, too. We took precautions—we put a salve on the lesions and on "suspicious" areas. Mother and baby are fine. One section was enough for me, I'll tell you. I read Lynn Richards book and learned that babies who were born by cesarean to prevent herpes sometimes get the virus anyway—so I really feel as if I made the right choice for me.

MARY (VBAC—with fibroids)

Remember I wrote you looking for information about fibroids. We talked for a while and I said I'd call you back. I kept thinking that if I didn't allow them to do an ultrasound, they wouldn't have noticed the fibroids—after all, I wasn't bleeding or anything, so maybe they had been there a long time and were minding their own business. I had no pain, and the baby was growing fine. I kept visualizing them getting smaller and smaller—and if they couldn't do that, the least they could do was get out of the way for the birth. The doctor said they would interfere and I'd end up with an emergency. They didn't, and he was wrong. Add me to your list of VBACs!

No one can tell what will happen in your particular circumstances, or what decision would be right for you in any situation, but I thought these stories might demonstrate to you the determination, commitment, intelligence, wisdom, strength, and beauty that is out there in the birthing world. I work with so many women who have VBACs in spite of their doctor's concern (or outright disapproval) that I continue to believe in the process of birth and in the possibility of VBAC even when conditions aren't ideal. I have heard from DES daughters who have had VBACs and women with "infections of unknown origin" and women with physical challenges and uterine abnormalities and problems with neighbors and you name it. My belief in birth is almost always affirmed.

I Did My Best

Sometimes things do not go according to plan. Our limits are defined, or something we didn't expect crops up, forcing us to make different decisions, and sometimes literally punching us in the gut.

Some women I have heard from wanted a VBAC but eventually decided on a repeat cesarean for one of a dozen reasons (fetal distress, exhaustion, breech presentation, etc.). Their reactions range from relief to disbelief to tremendous sadness. But as Julia tells Lillian in Hellman's book, *Pentimento*, "Lilly, if you can't, no dishonor. I love you, Julia."[37]

Three women whose circumstances did not permit VBAC should be mentioned here. Two were women who had a bandhl's ring around the uterus in labor. (This is a muscle ring that contracts but does not relax. If it continues to contract, it prevents the descent of the baby, can increase the chances of a uterine rupture, and can compromise the baby's well-being.) I wonder if chiropractic, acupressure, homeopathy, or other forms of healing could assist. I'll let you know when I learn more about this problem. One of the women had an "uneventful" cesarean section, and the other had an extremely difficult cesarean with excessive bleeding and a very long recovery.

The third letter came from a woman who had a hysterectomy at the time of her repeat cesarean. She had labored with the expectations of a VBAC, only to find that something was wrong. She felt no pain, but concurrently with a severe decrease in fetal heart tones, noticed a bulge on the side of her abdomen. An emergency cesarean confirmed that the uterus had opened and that the baby was in the peritoneal cavity. The baby was okay and the mother is, too, but the tragedy of a lost uterus was a big price to pay. This is an extremely rare occurrence.

Worry Ward

In the year 1500 Jacob Nufer's wife had a cesarean section. Jacob Nufer performed it himself. His wife gave birth to six more children, and they were all vaginal births.[38]

So many women who want a VBAC find that their days are filled with concern and anxiety: Will I be able to do this? What if something goes wrong? When is intervention appropriate? How will I feel if it is another cesarean? To these women I suggest that they set aside a certain time each day and just worry. During "Worry Time," you can really get into the worrying! You can obsess and imagine that everything goes wrong. You get to call your midwife, your friends, the hospital, the doctor. However, once that predesignated amount of time is over, you then must begin to train yourself to stop the worrying. Tomorrow, when worry time comes around again, you can worry about all the things you forgot to worry about today, or re-worry over any of the things you didn't worry about enough. If, during "regular hours" you find yourself worrying, you just put that particular worry as a first priority for tomorrow's session. You do not spend any time worrying about it now.

Worry utilizes our body's resources and depletes us. It even does something to the synapses, the junctions between the neurons, where nerve impulses pass. It robs us of our Vitamin C. After a while, it begins to affect our eating, our sleeping, our posture—everything about us. We deserve pregnancies free from the kind of internal posture that worry establishes. One woman realized that she spent the better part of a day thinking about VBAC. It occupied her thoughts day and night. When I asked her how many hours in twenty-four she thought she worried about it, she answered "twenty-three." I asked her whether she was willing to cut her worry time to, let's say, five hours. It took her a few weeks, but she said that over that period of time, she had learned to forget about worrying in the afternoons. (She signed up for a class three days a week and began painting the other two.) By her eighth month of pregnancy, she had cut her worry time to fifteen minutes a day and finally to two minutes.

After worry time, you might want to take a shower or go outside in the fresh air to blow away the negativity and take in a breath of new energy. So many women have said that giving themselves permission so to speak not to deny their fears leaves them so much freer, enabling them just to be pregnant for the rest of the day.

VBAC Lexigram

The letters in VBAC—vaginal birth after cesarean—contain I/he/she can breathe!; I learn and see; This is great! I can have it!I heal a scar; I have a great birth canal!; There is a tale here; I bear/bare it; She is a sage; She is alive—living, breathing, serving, caring. The words star, seer, girl, Christ, grail, grace, create, faith, right, space, breast, sea, tears, bears, heat, hearth, gift, and life are also contained in the letters, as are scar, treason, flag, trial, veil, fight, and fear. (Okay, so there is also rat, larvae, gas, fart, slice, rage, fingers, rant and rave: This could go on forever!) My favorites: I see light! The earth is green. Her face is serene. She leaves a trail. AT LAST, I GIVE LIFE!

Yes!

Because of the women who refuse to be resectioned, VBAC is becoming firmly entrenched. Some doctors are now at the point of "watchful neglect" with VBAC, and a number of smaller hospitals now permit VBAC so that their operating room can be open for "real" emergencies. Judy, a woman from Minnesota who had two cesareans and then her VBAC, says, "I believe these births are correcting many sins." Jana, a first-time mother from Kentucky, said, "I learned more from the cesarean-VBAC moms at my local La Leche League meeting than in my childbirth classes. They really helped me to have a good birth the first time around." Again, the fact that VBAC is so easily attained is not an excuse for doctors to section women quickly the first time around.

Becka writes, "I am so elated to be able to tell you that I brought forth my second son at home in our bed just as the birds started singing at 4:50 A.M. I did it, Nancy! His name is Gabriel and he weighed ten pounds, 2 ounces. It was hard work, but no one can ever take away the grand-ness of this experience! I can't begin to express how satisfied I feel and how full my heart is as a result of this birth." Judy wrote, "And they said I couldn't do it! I wanted to scream, 'Look everyone, look at my healthy new baby!' I wanted the Goodyear blimp to fly over the city." Michelle said, "I thought you VBAC people were all lunatics, right on the fringe. I'm in. I talk to everyone—everyone—about my VBAC!" And Joan wrote, "There was something almost cleansing in the pain, so that after it was all over, I felt euphoric. I also felt the sweet peace of victory. My quest ended. My child's life begun."[39]

15 *Voices Raised!: Starfish*

I recognize the revolutionary power of each woman's telling her own story, taking herself seriously enough, trusting her own experience enough, to detail for the rest of us the consequences of the many large and small moments of connection in her life. I know now that if just one woman were to describe the moments when feeling and thought came together in a new way, and for just a moment we were free, we would begin at last, and not a moment too soon, to "remember" the path. . . . To recover that long-lost, deeply hidden path and to walk it steadfastly together is to grasp our destiny.

—Sonia Johnson[1]

The announcements arrive in the mail daily now. I have "wallpapered" a room with them: "We are proud to announce . . . " "We welcome with love . . . " "A joyful beginning . . . " "We are thrilled to tell you about . . . " "Born at home! . . . " "A VBAC birth!!"

Many of the women who contacted me after *Silent Knife* was written said that they read the birth stories over and over again: they found them to be tremendously inspiring. "More, more!" they cried. With pleasure.

I have received hundreds of letters from women who believed in themselves and in the process of birth—and in so doing, have kept the dream alive for others.

CLAUDIA (Montana)

We did it! A VBAC after two cesareans! Trying to negotiate with eight doctors in the area took too much energy. After lots of discussion, our midwife friend agreed to be at home with us. During labor, I tried to forget everything I knew about birth and follow my instincts. Two days of labor and Logan was born—never once did I lose confidence!

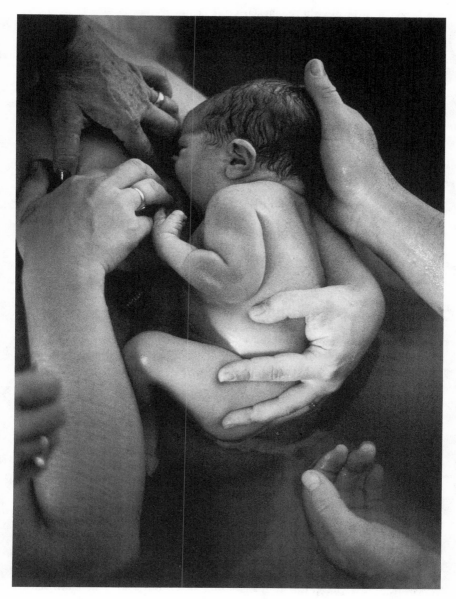

© Suzanne Arms Wimberly.

MARION (Virginia)

I wanted to let you know our success! It was a difficult delivery at the end. Since I hadn't dilated past eight centimeters for several hours, the doctor wanted to do a cesarean. Since the baby was in no distress, I wanted more time, and I would not sign the consent form. The doctor was very upset and threatened to transfer us to another hospital. We requested a second opinion and fortunately got "Dr. Right." He was at the hospital within a half hour. I was still at eight centimeters. He was very patient and calm and suggested if I felt like pushing to go ahead. After two hours we had our baby.

JANINE (Texas)

I was sectioned at age sixteen by an impatient older doctor who admitted me in my "warm up" phase of labor. He sent me for an x-ray and cut me for a "slightly flattened sacrum"—all other measurements normal. The second was a repeat cesarean with a different incision. Now I had a "T."

I had about seven hours of early labor and six hours of active. I pushed for about 90 minutes and the placenta came out an hour later. At one point, my midwife had a "heart to heart" talk with me. She said I had to want it to get stronger. She told me she would hold my hand and lead me to the next phase, not to be afraid. She moaned with me and then asked me to change my moan to a whisper and say "yes." Ten minutes later I said, "I've got to push!"

Incidentally, my mother was at the birth. She was a tower of strength, having undergone an unnecessary section with her third child (same old doctor).

SHEILA (Massachusetts)

I got a message during my pregnancy from the baby. He said, "Birth is not a big issue for me—I know it is for you. I'll be fine and I'll help you be fine, too. He was born twenty minutes after I got to the hospital. (VBAC-T incision)

HELEN (Pennsylvania)

When I had my cesarean, the doctor cut a low vertical incision but couldn't get the baby out and he started snapping at the anesthesiologist for giving me an epidural, not a general. He asked for the knife again and the next thing I knew the baby was born. Four and a half years later I found out what he had cut in his "moment of madness" was a Y incision with one fork extending into the lower fundal part of the uterus, making the cut technically a classical.

It took more than 18 months for me to get my energy back. My son was speech delayed and I'm sure it was because I felt too bad to talk to him. I sought out the most progressive doctor in the state. She said, "Your old doctor really screwed you up. I'd be real bitter, too. But woman to woman, I'd never have this baby vaginally. You have everything to lose: the baby and the chance to have any more." She recommended I have the c-section at 38 weeks. I left her office totally demolished, $100 poorer, with my arms around my belly fearing it would split apart at any minute. I thought about all the rich and glamorous women in the world who had cesareans, like Queen Elizabeth and Jacqueline Onassis and all the movie stars, as if to equate a section with beauty and sophistication. That lasted about two whole minutes until I realized its absurdity.

I realized that I had to try for a VBAC, even if it meant staying in the hospital parking lot. Sometimes I felt like defying the whole system and staying at home.

Other times, I wanted to be in the hospital under close observation, to have that safety net in case the scar did rupture. For as much as I believed it would hold, I had a small but nagging fear that perhaps it wouldn't and I would be solely responsible for that consequence. To me, a trial of labor within the system was the most reasonable course of action. I went to another doctor, expecting him to put another nail in the coffin, closing forever any hope for a VBAC. He was concerned about peer pressure and told me he had never had a patient with my kind of incision. I told him he had the opportunity of a lifetime.

MARY (Michigan)

When I got to the hospital—one that doesn't do VBACs—I didn't actually lie, but everytime they asked me how Kevin was born, I managed to have a contraction. It didn't feel good to have to field their questions, but I got my vaginal birth. My cesarean had been a horror show. With this birth, I expelled a lot of poison along with the baby.

The third doctor I met was wonderful. Everytime I came in he was excited about a VBAC he'd just been to. He told me all the talk about rupture was garbage. He didn't deliver the baby—my husband did. [No, Mary, YOU did!] Pushing was excruciating but it only took a half hour. I gave birth in a full squat, no episiotomy. It was a wonderful experience I will never forget. I can't understand why so many women allow themselves to be sectioned over and over again, without considering VBAC. By the way, I closed up 4 cm. when I got to the hospital. I had to go through transition twice. I was nervous going to the same hospital where I had been sectioned, I just closed up. But we told the nurses I'd just been in labor a few hours—I feared they'd label me failure to progress if they knew it had been over 26 hours.

I was told I'd never have a vaginal birth. My abdominal muscles had been so badly ripped at the section that in my 8th month of this pregnancy you could see the split—6 inches apart—a ridge, the entire length of my abdomen. My VBAC baby was 10 lbs. 2 oz.! They said the baby would look like a banana-head. They said I was so small, he'd be born with a big point like a mountain. There was no molding at all. She was adorable, pink and round.

JEANNE (North Dakota)

I give my thanks for my VBAC to a woman who had to have an emergency cesarean. I was being prepped for a cesarean—my doctor was tired and impatient. But because he had to go and do her, he didn't come back to check me for 2 hours. During that time I dilated fully and began to push and he had no choice but to allow me to deliver vaginally.

PEGGY (Maryland)

I was 40 years old when my VBAC baby was born. Our cesarean baby was born without any labor—my doctor said I'd be too small to birth normally, that I had a severely contracted pelvis and wouldn't be able to birth a 5 lb. baby.

Eleven days after my "due date," on a Wednesday, my labor began. By Saturday things were really moving along. I didn't let on how difficult the contractions were because I was afraid my husband and the doctor would freak and I wanted to remain at home for as long as possible. Sunday at 3:00 a.m. I got into a warm tub and didn't get out til 5:00 a.m. I kept looking at my labor guide and I was still on page one. At 5:30 a.m. I found myself leaning on the hassock with my knees on pillows. The urge to grunt was clearly there and began to get uncontrollable. That worried me. I felt lonely and desperate, I was tired of trying not to grunt and I didn't care about being quiet anymore. I felt something would break loose inside of me. I wished I had a knowledgable support person with me. Was it time to turn myself in or was it still too soon? By 8:00 a.m. I was sure I wouldn't make it, thinking I could hardly endure this stage, how could I endure the worst yet to be? I could hardly cope now even with my freedom at home—I knew I couldn't stand to have all their tubes hanging on/around me and being immobile. The next minute I knew that I wouldn't have to worry about that. I felt the baby move down. I called to my husband and within a few minutes our baby was born—right there.

LINDA (West Virginia)

I was very tired. My blood pressure was rising. I was waiting in my mind for someone to suggest a c-section, and wondering what I would say. And I thought I might say yes! I wonder if this is common to women—to almost want a cesarean even if they know what it means? Maybe a desire to choose the thing rather than be forced to it? Anyhow, with great relief and pride I gave birth vaginally.

GAIL (West Virginia)

I strictly avoided any how-to birth books and classes. Toward the end of my pregnancy several cows in our field were calving and I kept having a mental image of their huge pelvic bones! Our second daughter was born vaginally—she was the exact same weight as our first—9 lbs. 3 oz.—a kind of poetic justice for me as I had heard many times I was too small to have a baby. I thought I would know all about birth if I could go through it, but it remains a mysterious, confusing experience. Still, I am so pleased to have given birth vaginally. Biologically, it is satisfying to complete this process, and socially if feels to me a rite of passage completed. Emotionally it is something of mine—something that I'll always have.

JULIE (Indiana)

Changing doctors at forty-one weeks was traumatic, and probably one of the hardest things I've done. It meant self-preservation for me. I had felt tricked and misled. At the beginning, I felt her criteria for VBAC was acceptable, even up to a few weeks before my due date. One week before the date, she "upped" the criteria. At first I was angry—at the system, at doctors who get cold feet, and at their ignorance. Then I got scared, scared about the defensive medicine our system practices. Being a nurse, I continually see apathy and ignorance within the system. But what scares me the most are the responses I get from other childbearing women; "I wouldn't want anything but a c-section!" It shows the brain-washing our system has accomplished. . . . Although I left the doctor's office crying, it was the best decision I could have made.

ELAINE (Ohio)

I worked at reshaping my attitudes and beliefs about birth. I had always hoped for a healthy baby born vaginally in a hospital. I got that and more. My VBAC homebirth was the most wonderful and meaningful life experience. I can't begin to tell you in words. The joy, pride, and peace will last a lifetime.

GEORGIA (Massachusetts)

My cesarean was done after twenty-two hours of numerous interventions. I had dilated to ten centimeters and was at plus two station. The cesarean was for failure to progress! After five years and one miscarriage, I delivered an eight pound baby girl. My labor was five hours and I had no interventions. This birth was a private miracle for not only did I have a low vertical incision, but the baby was born with a loose knot in her cord. I birthed in a standing position, had no episiotomy, and needed virtually no recovery time. I feel a great sense of accomplishment.

JOY (Colorado)

I read an interview with you, Nancy, and I was really resentful. However, I found myself wondering, and the idea of VBAC stuck in my head. I found myself wondering, "Is it really possible, even for me, with a small pelvis?" My next trip to the library was the clincher: I found your book, went home, and read the whole thing in one night. I was astounded. I read that book three more times cover to cover. I read part of it to my husband. He was astounded. I took it to my doctor and made him listen. He was astounded. "You realize your uterus may rupture and the baby may die?" No, doctor, I doubt that. . . . If I hadn't read that magazine, I'd have had another section. It planted the seed. I have enclosed, for you, as a gift, a year's subscription. God bless you people.

JULIA (California)

My first child was delivered by cesarean in Kabul, Afghanistan after a very long, midwife-assisted home labor. For our second child, we returned from West Africa, where we were living, to Massachusetts. We took VBAC classes and had a natural birth. Without the LSP that we had chosen, the meconium staining I had during labor might well have been justification for a repeat cesarean. Our third child was born in our California home. . . . Oddly enough, it was not the first birth that caused the most upset and turmoil in my life. Rather, it was the last. The delivery was not the problem—I had a short labor and everything was fine. It was the rigidity of the medical establishment that nearly drove me crazy. Our pre-paid health plan, selected for its reputation as having the most liberal birthing practices in the area, immediately classified me as "VBAC," putting me into their "high-risk" category. According to the plan's protocol, that meant I would have to be monitored, have an IV, etc. at all times. Despite the irrefutable fact that I had already delivered a child vaginally without any of these procedures, I was told that "rules are rules." For six months I battled with the plan through review boards and consumer grievance procedures only to be told that the trouble with women like myself was that I didn't appreciate what a great deal they were offering me— a chance at VBAC their way. The decision to have our last baby at home was the result of my fear that control over the birthing process would be wrenched from me the moment I walked in the hospital door. We would have preferred the security of the hospital setting in case of emergency, but that option was closed to us unless we agreed to the procedures that were, by the medical director's own admission, not proven to be necessary or effective. In the end, the vision of an electrode being inserted into my unborn child's head and my older children watching their mom give birth tied to an IV pole and monitor wires was simply too far from what I knew could be the joy of birth. So, when the moment of decision came, we simply stayed at home.

MARIE (Pennsylvania)

The doctor initially said yes to me for a VBAC, "as long as it didn't happen between 11 P.M. and 7 A.M." because of limitations of the facility. Well, I sure didn't know how to guarantee him that that wouldn't happen, so I told him I was leaving his practice. He seemed insulted—he thought he was being supportive.

BARB (California)

The best thing about this birth was that my family was never separated. My seventeen month old slept on the bed next to us while her daddy helped me push her sister into the world! By the way, labor began as Jenn was nursing, progressed faster as she nursed, and when I was "stuck" at nine for what seemed like forever, she latched on and helped me get to ten. A hospital staff would never have allowed it, let alone understood it. I thank God for the marvelous ways our bodies work, for my wonderful midwife, and my dear friends who helped make this birth more beautiful than I ever thought possible.

KATHY (New York)

For Naomi's birth, we decided to "do-it-ourselves." One c-section, one midwife-attended home birth, and one on our own. I'm beginning to teach birth classes!

HADASSAH (Connecticut)

I had four previous cesareans and one of my babies died. . . . For my fifth birth, labor was on-again, off-again for a few days. When it began picking up, I felt a "click"—it felt as if the baby was going between the bones. My LSP came to check me at three in the morning—I was fully dilated and the baby's head was coming through! We went to the hospital and I was beginning to push. We named the baby Raphael which means "Angel of Healing." . . . My sixth baby was two weeks overdue. My midwife came at 9 a.m. By ten, I had to push. At 10:15 the water broke. Seven minutes later, out she came!

LISA (California)

I am a VBAC!!. . . . My baby was posterior and my midwife helped me with various positions. The birth center here has a waterbirth tub, and I stayed in it for a long time: I knelt down on all fours in the water so I had less pain in my back. I pulled up my abdomen and held it often. My husband held me. I had a lot of pain. (My first labor had been easy. My second child was born by cesarean.) I pushed for a long, long time. I finally pushed her out—right in the water, right into my arms! I was so thrilled!. . . . My four year old cut the cord—she is so proud of herself! I delivered the placenta myself and then I walked to the bed from the tub. Two hours later, I was walking around. I felt good and healthy. I am a brave lady and happy. My goal is to teach birth. I am deaf, and there is a great need for education among the hearing impaired. Wish me luck!

BEVERLY (Kentucky)

I did it! I've had a vaginal birth. After two cesareans! The doctor was so supportive—she did not push any interventions on me. She told me she was very nervous, but she went to the trouble of calling doctors in California who had had experience with VBACs and multiple cesareans. Everything went smoothly and afterwards I must say I was somewhat of a celebrity. All the student nurses would come and look at me like they couldn't believe it. Me? I was overwhelmed and overjoyed at the whole experience. I'll never forget it. Three pushes and he was out, all by himself. My family and friends had all worried about this, but I knew it would all be alright.

DONNA (Massachusetts)

I had three sections for "cpd." After I read your book, I knew I could do it. I was going to have another baby—naturally this time. I found a doctor who was willing to try, even though he thought I would be too small. He gave me a thirty percent chance. . . . I arrived at the hospital thinking I was close to delivery. I was only two centimeters! I cried and said, "I can't do it, forget it, all this labor and only two cms." All the fears came back to me. The labor room was so small and cramped. Now I was bleeding from the examination. I couldn't breathe from the heat. My midwife spoke some sense into my head. "You are going to do it. You must take one contraction at a time." I set my mind for a long hard labor and I determined to relax. It was hard to do that in the hospital. At about nine p.m. I felt like I had to go to the bathroom, real, real bad, but I couldn't. The nurse examined me and said I was nine cms. I was yelling with excitement—9 CEN-TIMETERS!!! "I am really going to have this baby. There is no turning back now. He's coming, he's right there. He has to come out!" I couldn't stop laughing, talking, yelling, crying. The excitement was indescribable. I delivered Nathan who was a whopping TEN POUNDS 5 OUNCES!! My others had been 8–3, 7–14, and 7 even, respectively. My recovery was the best. I got up immediately and took a shower. I left the hospital the next morning. Praise God! It was wonderful!!!

SANDY (New York)

Seems my pattern is to take a few days to get to 2 centimeters. Then another chunk of time to get to 3–4, and then it is only a couple of hours to delivery. This time we didn't check at all for dilation. So Amy's labor was 44 hours and the most painful experience I've had in my life. The first thirty hours I was handling it with a good mental attitude and focusing on "baby" and "open" and "let it hurt." The next ten hours, I was tired and wondering if "this baby would ever come out" and "how can anything hurt this much" and "keep letting it hurt." The next four hours I was wondering if I was going to live through the pain. My back hurt and there was even a bulge where the head was pushing against it. My hips hurt and of course the stretching cervix. We took several walks. My seven and a half year old and I finally went for a walk together and that is when the baby turned. Twenty minutes of pushing and making "moose" noises and her head was born. Push more. No body. Amy stretching her head. No body. Midwife trying to get her armpit and corkscrew. No body. Shoulder dystocia. Midwife says to flip me to hands and knees (from sitting). Out! Pinking up. Crying. Pink. Bright-eyed. Apgars 8 and 10. Beautiful baby. Super nurser. Much celebration. Placenta born fifty minutes later. Five year old brother cut the cord. More celebration! No lacerations. I felt like I had been in a war and took a week of resting to feel like I had any energy again. . . . We are all fascinated with her. She is constantly in someone's arms and sleeps in our "mega-bed." Birthing her was hard and I have compassion for others who have had difficult births. I am grateful for the support that was given to me, and I have grown and passed the love along whenever possible.

HANNAH (Rhode Island)

I had four cesareans. My fifth was a VBAC in the hospital, and my sixth was a homebirth. I feel "grown-up" now.

ROCHELLE (Illinois)

The baby broke his clavicle on the way out of birth—I have terrible hemorrhoids—but this birth was tremendous! He's fine and healthy—I am fine and healthy and we went home the day after the birth.

PEGGY (Ohio)

My husband and my sister were with me throughout the labor. My midwife arrived about two hours before the birth. At 6:30 or so I stood up and started pushing. Then I sat in my comfortable rocker and pushed. At 6:55 I just slid off the rocker (my bottom) and pushed my baby right into my husband's hands. It was exhilarating, wonderful, exciting. I'm sure you know the rest! You may be interested to know that my doctor was there for the birth—she took the pictures and only wanted to come because she had never seen a homebirth. She did not have any part in the birth except as an observer.

DIANE (British Columbia)

After two cesareans, the second after an attempt at VBAC, my Inner Spirit kept urging me on to completion. My doctor said, "Look, lady, with your track record, forget it." His associate said, "What is it about you women that you must have your babies naturally." He reluctantly agreed to a trial of labor as long as I had a short labor and agreed to forceps. . . . I just knew I was not going to have one of those short, text-book labors. The thought of forceps haunted me. After much prayerful deliberation, my husband and I agreed on a homebirth. We felt it was the safest place to ensure that we would receive the best possible experience and the quality care we wanted. My doctors did not know my change of plans. . . . My agreement with my midwife was not to have her rescue me from pain. But when I had been in labor for many hours, I was possessed with how I could annul that agreement. Overwhelmed, I expressed myself freely and without reserve. My midwife calmly let my words trickle by her like water off a duck. It was that calm that let me know I was acting normally and I got on with accepting my labor. I started pushing at about 1:00 a.m. I was squatting, supported by my human goal posts, pushing like I never pushed before (literally!) My midwife encouraged me to stop and touch my baby's crowning head. She held a mirror so that I could see. At last! One more push . . . gently . . . and Ta-da!—a beautiful ten pound baby boy. . . . As I listened to the "Hallelujah" tape my friend was playing, it was as if all the universe was rejoicing with me and indeed I am sure it was. I felt a sense of completion and wholeness and perfection. My husband cut the cord and my children delighted in seeing their brother born. After thirty hours, we were all exhausted but exhilarated. . . . I will never be the same. I am a changed woman.

CHRIS (Ohio)

I took the heart tones on my own. When I was completely dilated, my water broke. There was a moderate amount of meconium. After a number of hours, I said to myself, "No one else can do this for me. I might as well get to it." And so I did.

MARY (Minnesota)

When you said that each of us knew deep inside in our womanplace where we wanted to give birth, I knew immediately that I should be at home. It was something I had totally rejected intellectually before—being a nurse, "I knew better." But there it was, clear as a bell. . . . Due to a difficult political situation in town regarding midwives, I decided to go to the hospital and not get involved in a legal battle. I went through three days of labor at home, and I wonder if it would have been different if I knew I was staying at home. Also, I never did go into labor with my first, so I guess I was making up for that. I was disappointed not to have a homebirth, but I will next time. The birth, other than that, was wonderful, just what I wanted. I am one happy woman.

CATHY (Nevada)

What a gift, this birth. When I got to the birthing room, the nurse said, "It's your day. You call the shots." After two sections, I couldn't believe my ears. Naturally I ended up with the doctor who didn't like our VBAC plans. But things went so fast that I only saw him once. He never even had time to put on his gloves and do an episiotomy. So much for being too small. I had my eyes closed during contractions—I opened them just in time to see the baby's face.

LISSA (South Dakota)

I did it! It's a boy! Two years of hard work paid off in a wonderful birth experience for us. I can hardly believe it! I have healed my cesarean scar. I am woman! . . . Things slowed down a few times but no one got concerned. I just got in the shower and stayed there until I felt a strong desire to push. It took me a little while how to best direct my energy toward effective pushing. . . . His head circumference was nearly an inch bigger than his brother's who was born by section for cpd. Ha! I had no episiotomy and no tearing, thanks to perineal massage during late pregnancy, kegel exercises, more massage during crowning, and a slow easy delivery assisted by my midwife. . . . There was some fetal distress just before the birth, but a change in position helped that. The cord was looped around his head twice, but Shelly slipped it over his head and left it unclamped.

GAYLE (Washington)

A lot of feeling is going into a few words. Something has grabbed hold of my heart and won't let go. I got butterflies in my pregnant tummy just knowing I was going to make it this time! My daughter was born, not without effort, but naturally and drug-free—the most memorable and important event in my life. I feel so peaceful and now I want to help others.

SUNNY (Alabama)

Yes! We have a beautiful, gorgeous, rosy baby girl. A short 5 hour vaginal birth— all natural with daddy and firstborn attending. Wow. . . .

OLIVIA (North Carolina)

Looks like another OB put his foot in his mouth—said it couldn't be done. Well, now the joke's on him. Our almost nine-pound son was born at home! He weighed nine ounces more than our first, who was born by cesarean. We found a midwife who flew across country to attend our birth—angels really do fly. . . . After the section I wasn't allowed to hold my baby and my arms ached for him. Having David in my arms this time has meant the world to me. The pushing was hard, but it felt good emotionally. The midwife thinks my labor was long because I was "working through" some things "upstairs." Her attention to my emotions was a big help—she feels a VBAC is no different physically from any other laboring woman, but there may be some other things that have to be addressed. I think my anger helped me birth this time. It motivated me to keep on going. I thought that after the birth my anger would subside—not so. The birth center here, unfortunately the most progressive birth option around, still will not accept VBACs. I went to talk to the CNM there and she was icy cold. Aren't happy births resulting in beautiful children more important than adhering to the "SYSTEM"? I am amazed at how many people are offended by a homebirth when they ought to be rejoicing over a VBAC and a healthy baby.

TINA (Oregon)

The doctor who did my section said that my pelvis could only accommodate a six pound baby. Well, he was off by at least two pounds! This doctor said I had plenty of room! My husband held me throughout the labor, and I kept talking to the baby, "Baby, come." I sang songs and hymns to myself. Oh, on the way to the hospital, we stopped at the Pancake House! Then we walked around a shopping plaza. While we were in a hardware store, the contractions were coming about every 5 minutes. . . . Later, I got really scared. I wanted the contractions to get weaker. Things slowed down. I finally told all the people in the room that I had to be left alone. I told them that I had been depending on them too much and I really needed to go it on my own. Within an hour, the contractions started back up again really strong. . . . I had no tearing and no episiotomy. There was a gush of blood as the baby was born, something like a blood vessel that was protruding. I had three stitches and everything was fine. To top it all off, we had our first girl after three precious little boys.

CINDY (Florida)

Nancy and Lois, words cannot express how grateful I am for your wonderful book *Silent Knife*. After years of depression and no true understanding, it has come as an answer to prayers. The whole issue is so complicated, yet you make it suddenly seem so simple. A woman is either in control or she isn't. There is and can be no compromise. . . . Everyone was screaming at me at my first birth that I wasn't doing it right—and they made me feel responsible for all the intervention. After the birth, I had years of questioning and deep sorrow and regret. With my second child, I did not have a cesarean—I had a VBAF—vaginal birth after forceps, which is just as painful, I think, and just as humiliating. With my third, I had a completely pure birth. . . . Thank you for validating my feelings and really looking at the whole thing logically.

DAN (Mississippi)

We were so stunned when the doctor said about a week before the birth that he might have to do a cesarean because the baby was breech. Sure enough, he did. "We don't like to deliver the first one vaginally if it's breech." Poor Daniel! He didn't know he was the first one! . . . Well, after this disappointment, we decided to do some research on all this. Somehow we felt we had been duped. . . . With our second, we went in with our eyes wide open. The first doctor we talked to seemed positive on a VBAC, but with restrictions—monitors, etc. When he found out about the low vertical incision, he said that with a VBAC, the best we could hope for would be a hysterectomy, the worst death to all. . . . Thank God for Dr. B! We found him a month before the birth. We had planned a homebirth—staring hysterectomy and death right in the face—but our midwife was not experienced in breech birth. So, in active labor, 6 cms. dilated, we drove seventy-five miles so this doctor could assist with our little bottom-first baby. What a joy! With no medication from start to finish, no intervention, no restrictions on walking, squatting, or anything else—and best of all, with no knives, my wife delivered a beautiful girl. It was such a joy, we named her Rebekah Joy. . . . Thank you God, and thank you [VBAC people] for helping us get back to His original plan for childbirth.

KAREN (Germany)
Three and a half years ago, my heart was broken when the homebirth we had planned for years ended in a cesarean of questionable necessity. Due to problems I had had with early miscarriages and my advancing age, it did not seem likely that I would ever be pregnant again, much less have a homebirth. Nevertheless, before my incision was barely healed, I heard about a woman who knew about VBACs. Today we have a beautiful new baby daughter, born at home, a dream come true. You may remember that I flew to the States from Germany and met all of you wonderful people at a Cesarean Prevention Movement conference. It was one of the most moving events I have ever experienced, and I will always cherish the memory of those two days. Just think, without my cesarean, I never would have met so many wonderful people, or had the courage to leave my family when I was six months pregnant. Now that's an unexpected fringe benefit! Life takes such curious turns sometimes. We will be moving back to the States soon, and I plan to become a birth activist, too!

CATHY (California)
For three years I maintained my cesarean was unnecessary and six months ago I proved it! My cesarean was for cpd-ftp—a 6–15 baby with a 13 and a half inch head. My son was nine and a half pounds with a 15" head. . . . I left the group of doctors I had because they refused to allow me to labor, although they did promise me a meaningful cesarean. I switched to a doctor who said he supports VBACs. When I was nine months pregnant, he changed his mind. I changed again. The hospital where I work as an aide won't tell you the truth, but they do almost 70% cesareans, they really do.

LEAH (Idaho)
I've been meaning to write and let you know our most wonderful news. Nine years of grief and pain because of my c-section is over. I have learned about faith, courage, and trust in oneself. This was a pregnancy of many changes, new things to discover, battles to fight within, and fears to overcome. . . . As it turned out, there was some fetal distress as my little girl came through my bones. I heard the urgency in my midwife's voice and then all the strength of an Amazon woman poured through me and I pushed her out. I am so happy, I walk around smiling all the time.

ARDEAN (New York)
When I was pregnant with our fourth, having had three previous cesareans, I met a local midwife casually downtown. She told me there was no reason why I couldn't deliver vaginally. What a wonderful pregnancy it became—looking forward to a

natural birth instead of a surgical nightmare. I had many periods of fear and doubt, but underneath I had a continuing confidence: "I can do it." . . . I have four days of contractions. My midwives come and go. "It must get closer and more intense," they tell me. They ARE closer and more intense. Augh! Another day of contractions. When? When? I hit a period of depression and near exhaustion. I rest a bit, as much as I can. I get up and walk. Suddenly it is like cannonballs, escalating intensity, four in a row—I barely get up the stairs and in three and a half hours I am pushing out our 9 lb. 5 oz son (so much for CPD!). I am exultant, triumphant, ecstatic, speechless, amazed, astounded, and thankful. I am SCREECHING with JOY!

JUDY (Minnesota)

I had our baby, born VBAC, after a gradually progressive, almost enjoyable ten hour labor. I thought I was destined for a third cesarean, but saw a poster advertising a Cesarean Prevention Movement workshop. I had written down the particulars on a piece of cardboard with lipstick because I was without paper and pen at the time. The number was smudged and I had to call eleven different people before I heard the blessed words, "Hi. This is CPM. May I help you?"

NANCY (Florida)

During this pregnancy, I was diagnosed as a gestational diabetic. I ate well and walked over a mile every day. My doctor wanted me in the hospital on insulin for the last twelve weeks of my pregnancy and on a diet of 1800 calories. He said they'd "take" the baby at 38 weeks. I left that doctor. . . . Labor began within a few days of my due date. We stayed at home with a midwife for 28 hours and then presented ourselves at a hospital. The first doctors were rude and bullies. The shift changed and we got a better crew. . . . We lied like crazy. We made no mention of my previous cesarean or the diabetes. We told them I had only been in labor for 2 hours. We told them I had taken a Lamaze course. (We had taken a homebirth course which the hospital wouldn't accept.) Our doctor made the comment we had really practiced our Lamaze breathing. They don't let husbands in for delivery if he hasn't had Lamaze. I let him in nine months earlier even though he hadn't had Lamaze. . . . I was in labor a total of 39 hours. I pushed out a ten pound baby, beautiful, healthy, and alert.

JACKIE (Minnesota)

I have four children. Each birth was totally different ranging from a c-section to a beautiful "pure" birth for the last. Twice I used doctors. They both worried. They felt like they must be in control, even if they had to use coercion to keep it. They performed unnecessary routine vaginal exams because they can't tell what's going on without them. Everything was done for their comfort and convenience. Twice I used midwives. They were gentle and understood my fears. They listened quietly and watched to sense where the labor was. Everything was done for my comfort and my convenience.

MARY (Minnesota)

My first child was born six years ago. I had a normal, uncomplicated pregnancy. I was ten days "overdue" when my water broke. I went to the hospital and went through the whole routine. You know the story—cpd and ftp. Two years later I had a repeat cesarean. . . . I was five days past my due date this time. My contractions began, but never having had a "normal" labor, I couldn't judge how far things were progressed. I had prepared myself as best I could for a real marathon. Alone at home, I concentrated on relaxing. I rocked during the contractions, and was determined to stay with it. . . . Shortly after my husband got home, we left to go to the hospital. As we got closer to the city, the traffic got heavier. When we got to the hospital, I couldn't get out of the car—I was pushing! Within twenty minutes, I pushed my son out. I knew I could have a VBAC, but I never dreamed it could be so fast and that easy. Oh to have known with my first and my second what I know now.

SHEILA

I knew I couldn't trust most doctors—after all, they didn't trust ME in my ability to give birth—but I found one who was trained in Holland who attends homebirths. I found a labor assistant which made my husband feel like he'd been replaced, but actually put him much more at ease when I was actually in labor. And finally, I forgot about learning HOW to breathe. I talked for hours to a friend who was also having a VBAC—about our fears, our anger, our disappointment over the first birth, our excitement, our beliefs, our feelings, getting in touch. . . . I listened to my body. It wouldn't let me sit still. I paced the floor all night, leaned against the wall during contractions. I didn't go to the hospital until I felt ready, which my LSP said was about seven centimeters. The best part was, I YELLED a lot in the hospital! The first time I had taken classes that told me how to keep quiet and be good so you could control your birth. This time I enjoyed letting it be in control. I WALKED to the delivery room, and I would not get on the table there: I squatted, which helped turn the baby from a posterior position. How nice to have a woman support person and be able to say, "DAMN, THIS HURTS!" and she says, "I know, I know." It helped my husband feel better, knowing it's okay to hurt for a while. If I didn't have her there, I might have told the staff, and they'd have given me drugs. I had no idea it would be so hard to push. I had no idea it would hurt so much. And I've never been so happy. I'll gladly go through with it again in two or three years! I'm having so much fun BRAGGING now! I didn't tell people I was planning a VBAC, just let them assume what they wanted. Now I'm telling EVERYONE, strangers, bank tellers, the mailman that I had a 10 lb. 1–1/2 oz. boy NATURALLY, didn't even get stitches, went home from the hospital that day. I thank the many, many people who were behind me on this one—I love you all.

LORETTA

My doctor remarked that waiting for our baby was like having three coronaries. He stayed at the hospital all night—he slept in the doctor's lounge. He'd never attended a woman with one cesarean before, let alone me—with two. . . . The nurse told me to be a "good girl" and leave the fetal monitor belts on. I informed her that "good little girls" end up with c-sections, that women get pregnant and have babies, not girls. . . . I will definitely enjoy "tooling" around the city in my car with the C.P.M. bumper sticker on the back!

PAULA

After 24 hours, I got hung up at 7 cms. for two hours at which point the doctor suggested the possibility of resorting to a c-section. A nurse suggested that I try pushing since I had been fighting it anyway. What a God-send she was. It worked! One and a half hours later my healthy baby boy was born.

ROSIE

I was able to achieve my fantasy about childbirth—at home with a midwife. Amazingly, I labored for only two hours—it began when I put my first two down for a nap and Sophie was born when they woke up! It was a real family event. The boys made a birthday cake and we had balloons and flowers delivered to the house. An hour after she was born, we celebrated her "Very First Birthday." What I liked best was nothing in our normal daily routine was changed. The boys went to bed their usual time that night. As a result, the boys accepted her arrival very matter-of-factly, naturally, and without jealousy. What a difference from my cesareans.

JOHN

Here is a humble letter of our experience from a VBAC woman's husband. Our first baby was born in a hospital—a healthy boy. I felt so unworthy of being a Daddy, our whole lives would be changed now, it was a change we looked forward to, so when I stood there looking at him, secret tears of joy stole to my eyes. Two years later, on Friday the 13th which turned out to be unlucky for us, our doctor was on vacation and the other one said they had to do a c-section because one hand wanted to come out first. I had to wait in the waiting room until they were ready for me. My wife hated the spinal. One and a half years later we were disappointed when the doctor said we'd have to have a repeat cesarean because my wife's incision was made the wrong way, up and down, so we went and accepted another c-section. We had a little girl, she wasn't really "born" to us, or was she? I think she was stolen out through that ugly cut. My wife thought the spinal was worse than any labor could be. One year later my wife started labor so we rushed to the hospital as the doctor had been warning us that it was very dangerous to be in labor after a cesarean. But at the hospital nobody seemed to be in a hurry, and we were put in a room and had to wait for hours, the labor getting stronger, if only we had a way of making this baby hurry and pop out, but a nurse warned me that it could never be done. Finally, after six hours of labor our surgeon was ready to perform our fourth c-section. In the meantime, some of our friends were having VBACs after [cesareans] and two without the doctor's consent. So we decided then and there that labor wasn't as serious as the doctors like to say it is. A year later, my wife had a miscarriage without a cesarean; was the road really opening up for a VBAC for us? The following summer my wife again became pregnant, she was determined not to see her doctor, try a VBAC, she so dreaded those spinals. We found a wonderful, experienced, encouraging midwife, but such dreadful thoughts would run through my mind as the time was coming nearer and nearer. Would I be wifeless and the children motherless in the twinkle of an eye? But no, I could not have such thoughts, but would look to a higher hand for courage and comfort.

We were both hoping it would be early, so it would be over with sooner but that was not to be. When labor began, it was 2:30 a.m. My wife didn't make fast progress although the midwife said she was opening up, so time went on all day long. At 7 p.m. things started to get more exciting, won't be long now, and lo and behold at 7:45 out popped a bounding baby girl. We did it, it can be done. Where are all those doctors out there that say it can't?

MINDY

This time I went with midwives at a birthing center. What a difference! Nobody even mentioned my scar—and with a "T" on my uterus yet! After a long beginning, I arrived at the center at 8 cm. and fifteen minutes later the baby was born! It all seemed so right, so logical. It amazes me how birthing in this country has gotten so far away from the natural process.

LIZ

I did not want a VBAC. I was fully prepared for another cesarean. My doctor said I should go into labor and then have the section. It took extra time in traffic to get to the hospital, and the hospital wasn't ready when I arrived. I was checked and found to be at 8 centimeters. I would have had a section even then, although I know you people would think that was ridiculous. One nurse there had had a VBAC and she told me the recovery was so much easier. I have to admit, it was.

GEORGEANNE

For so long, I felt as if there was something missing. Now I feel different. My husband, too, says he can see something different.

DEBORAH

I live in a remote little village in Mexico, eight hours by highway and an additional three hours by exit road to San Diego. I was willing to go anywhere to avoid another section. My husband and I sold our fishing boat in order to have enough cash to pay for the birth. We stayed in California for two weeks prior to the birth; I cooked for the family that housed us. As with my first labor, this one set no speed records—but my daughter entered the world peacefully at the home of my friends.

PAM

And then your book came out! It took a long, long time, but I threw away my x-rays. I went to the most "supportive" doctors around—prepared to discuss the non-relevance of the term "CPD"—lots of ammo—but they stopped when they heard I had had two sections and wouldn't go on. I finally found a group to "give me a trial" after two sections—so I decided to change my medical records so CPD would not be an issue. I picked up all my previous records, copied them on the copy machine, cut-paste and retype—and then recopy the paste up. It looked as good as the original and the doctor looked it over, said it was in order, and filed it. During this time, I was trying to find an attendant for a homebirth—and my husband and I prepared to stay home with or without an attendant. We did find someone near the end. After three days of very active labor, I was zero (!) percent dilated and my baby still not engaged. We figured my pelvis was really blocked and went to the hospital. The doctor thought labor had just begun and didn't rush for the section. I was willing to try anything, so I agreed to a shot of morphine to "rest" and hope labor would resume and work. In 1/2 hour my water broke and Danny was born in less than two hours. With baby #4 I NEVER saw a doctor— I had a beautiful LONG labor. All three children cut their brother's cord. He was born on the day I had my "Blessingway."

LESLIE

I studied everything I could about it. My husband was so sick of hearing me talk about birth but subconsciously must have realized that this was needed by me, and was my best listener and supporter. I don't think he was convinced about a normal birth until my eighth month when he decided he'd better take me seriously. The following month, we had our baby at home. Little did I know that I was on my way to becoming a childbirth activist! I found myself speaking about VBAC to my friends and then in front of groups. When I became pregnant with my fourth, there was no doubt about having another homebirth. This pregnancy was so relaxed—it was wonderful. I will never say never again—I was never going to have a vaginal birth, never a homebirth, never breastfeed a baby past six months, never let my babies sleep in my bed, never homeschool, etc. And this all started because a few of the women out there cared about me having an unnecessary cesarean section.

SUE

A new nurse came on shift. She began to set up an IV bottle and tore the tape to attach it! I stared at the bottle and thought, "please no." Another battle. I asked, "What's that?" in a superstitious tone. The nurse responded, "You have to have an IV." Dave told her I wasn't going to have one. She said, "ALL laboring women have IVs." He said, "No they don't." She looked really shook. She then said, "But your wife might rupture." "I doubt that," Dave said. "The doctor okayed no IV." Then she really got upset: "Well, your doctor is not here and your wife needs it!" My husband said that the doctor was well aware of the consequences. The nurse said, "Well, he didn't tell me and I am in charge at this point." The doctor, by the way, was in the Caribbean. We stood our ground, and she left, never to be seen again. . . . When I was fully dilated and pushing, the nurse instructed me to lie on my back and grab my knees. (Where were my knees?) This is 1989, I thought—women don't lie on their backs in labor anymore. I told her I wanted to squat. She mumbled something about "this is the way it is done" and then left the room. Didn't see her again either. . . . I remembered you saying the pelvis opens up more in a squat. I sat upright and announced "I WILL NOW SQUAT!" Everyone was very surprised. I felt the baby's head move on the first push. I told the nurse and she checked me and was amazed at how far the baby had come down. I hope she won't argue with the next woman who wants to squat. [I hope she will suggest it.] The somewhat skeptical doctor came in. The doctor used a scare tactic—he said that the baby was going "back up" between contractions. I said to him, "It's supposed to, you dummy." He was very anxious, this being a VBAC (probably his first though he wouldn't admit to it) and all. He started tugging on the baby and told the nurse to push on my tummy [Note: this is a very dangerous thing to do.]—I thought this to be a rather strange practice. Nevertheless, my baby was born in one piece. She was covered from head to toe in meconium. [This may very well have happened because of what the doctor and nurse were doing.] The doctor tugged and pulled my placenta out [another absolute no-no] and then actually scraped the inside of my womb with his hand. I shouted, "WHAT ARE YOU DOING?" He said he had to "get it all." I didn't think that was necessary and it sure did hurt. I was given my baby and I said to her, "We are going to spoil you rotten." She started to cry but I explained to her that the term spoiled rotten wasn't bad. She continued to cry and I told her we would have plenty of time to talk this out, but that right now she should nurse. She did, pulling off every now and then to make a comment. Who knows exactly why she was upset? . . . But even now, at seventeen months, she has a lot to say about the world in general. She weighed 9 lbs. 9 oz. and I signed myself out of the hospital 12 hours later.

JON

I called you a few months ago. My wife has a classical scar from a cesarean section. Although we have never met, I knew you would be happy to know the result—a beautiful homebirth with a midwife. Her labor was 57 hours and she pushed for an additional three. The baby was 9–4.

JEAN

It only took four hours from start to finish, and five minutes later I felt marvelous! That's how birth should be, isn't it? A 10 lb. VBAC son!

JODI

Joseph is here. Born on February 25. He weighed 10 pounds! A full two pounds larger than my cpd cesarean baby. My water broke and within twenty minutes I felt like pushing. I realized my midwife wasn't going to make it. I knelt down in my living room and draped myself over the couch and basically never moved from the spot. I called a friend who called a local midwife who sensed the urgency of the event and she flew over here. It was good she was here as Joseph had "tight" shoulders—not true dystocia but nonetheless a tight squeeze. It was all so intense . . . so powerful, very little relief between contractions, mostly non-stop. It was over—start to finish—in two hours. It really took my breath away. I realized the fine line between birth and death. It was good for the midwife who helped—it was her first VBAC. She's not allowed to do them. She never worried about uterine rupture or even thought of it while she was here. She saw that VBAC babies come out.

CONNIE

I never had a section, but my pelvis was partly crushed in a car accident two months before my baby was born. The doctors all told me I'd have to be sectioned, and of course, I was very worried about the baby. But my sister is a very strong natural childbirth advocate. I'd absorbed, by osmosis, all that "stuff." I decided to try to have the baby naturally. Everything went fine!

RUTH

When my cesarean born twins were six months old, I realized I was pregnant again. I had a wonderful home VBAC.

MARILYN

No doctor was going to calm his fears by putting a knife in my belly! My VBAC was great.

LAURIE

It took me two years to recover enough from the trauma of Kate's birth to even want to be pregnant again. I find now, after Joey's birth, that a part of me will always hurt for her and me and what we lost, but I can begin to let go. Yes, my labor was long, and yes it hurt, but none of that is important anymore. In fact, after three weeks I was sure I had the greatest birth experience imaginable. I know with Kate that I did what I had to do, but we are not programmed to forget that land of birth trauma.

MARY

My cesarean was done because the baby's arm was trying to come out next to her head. They said it was bad enough, a head coming out alone, but two things at once? This time, it was "just" the head, and I had a vaginal birth.

LYNNE

My cesarean was done for cpd. What a laugh. This baby, born at home, was what they called a compound presentation. His hand was up next to the side of his head and just as the head was showing we saw a hand—the arm—up there, too. My son still sleeps with his arm near his head!

ELLEN

There were so many things working against me that it is nothing short of a miracle that our daughter was born healthy and happy. You know of my precious cesareans, one a classical, and then I developed gestational diabetes, a rare anti-body was detected during pregnancy, causing doctors to recommend weekly aminos in the last two months to ensure the baby's health which we of course refused. The doctor we had found ended up losing his privileges in our last two months of pregnancy and we were forced to start the search all over again. We were unsuccessful at that and ended up having to acquaint ourselves with a homebirth and all that one goes through to come to accept that route against all advice of doctors and family. When it became evident that I had to transfer to the hospital, our midwives were concerned I would end up with a section since they felt the staff would be so angry with me that they would simply sit back and let me suffer a few more hours until I begged for a section. Luck came my way, though, when the doctor on call refused to treat me and a more sympathetic doctor who had just come off his holiday came into the hospital. Against all odds, she is here—she is beautiful—and we will never forget all the support you VBAC people gave.

NANCY

It snowed today, and I am remembering last year at this time—I think wistfully of myself with my big belly, my parka not snapping at the bottom, our baby's birth imminent, and all the hopes and dreams and fears. And this year, she is here, a dream come true, spreading joy as she crawls through the house, babbles and waves at us. She is a complete delight, in a way our cesarean born never was. I am sure some of it is because she is our second, but I can't help but believe that being born instead of being yanked out, and emerging into loving arms instead of into those cold strangers and sterile isolettes must have something to do with it, too. I am at peace with myself for the first time in my life, not only because of the birth, but because of the issues I had to resolve first, in order to find the strength and confidence that enabled the birth to happen. She was born at home, but I was undecided at the beginning of labor. We remained flexible and decided we would wait and see how we felt as things progressed without a head trip or failure thing.

ROSALYN

Unfortunately our planned homebirth ended in a hospital delivery room. Because of meconium and low heart tones during pushing, we went to the hospital. I am glad to say, however, that the actual birth went much better than I would have expected being in the hospital. The doctor was supportive—he even went out on several "limbs" for us which he has taken some criticism for. Most of the hassles actually occurred after the baby was born. He was fine, but they wanted to do all kinds of tests on him. We got out as soon as we could but not soon enough for our new little son who was subjected to numerous blood work-ups because of incompetence on the part of the technicians and deprived of his mother's arms until I finally got my hands on him and left. While I am disappointed that I had to go to the hospital to "finish" the birth, I am so glad I had the strength and courage to ask for and demand the things I wanted and needed. I am also excited that I really proved I don't have cpd! This baby was 9 lbs 7 oz! By the way, my due date, according to my last period, was Oct. 18. He was born December 10. The doctor was insisting on induction in November. I said no. Although it was hard to follow my heart, I am glad I waited.

ADREAN
An update! We just had our second home VBAC after four days with broken membranes. Midwives are so patient! "Automatic" labor didn't click in until the fourth day, lasted for about 45 minutes—and then, seven minutes of hard, over-whelming pushing and it was all over! In a way, I feel as if I "missed" it, since it was all so fast. She arrived with her little arm right alongside her head. The birth ended up quite a party—the midwives who were taking turns here all stayed, all four of our other kids were there, and my dear friend was camerawoman! This birth confirmed how different each labor/delivery is even in the same woman and to keep it in the confines of a chart or graph is so ludicrous! A lovely woman in the community has asked me to be at her birth. "All I have to do is look at you and I know I can do it, too!" she says.

VICKIE
This was my eighth baby, numbers four and five being c-sections, the rest vaginal deliveries, number 7 being at home. Dr. #1 said it would be impossible to "birth from below." Dr. #2 said we could give it a try as long as there is nothing that concerns him. Dr. #3 said she would transfer me to the high-risk clinic for "close observation." Dr. #4 said it can't be done—why would any sane mother risk her life and the life of her baby simply to forego a little discomfort. . . . I asked him why in the world should I let anyone cut me again, when I already had vaginal births after my cesarean. He said this might be the one that "broke the camel's back." I went to the hospital to ask questions. After a runaround, the woman I was finally referred to was the head nurse on the maternity floor. She came to the U.S. many years ago, delivered five babies the American way, and then stayed at home to have her sixth! She has been making changes in that ward, having the hospital revise their protocols. When I told her what the 1st doctor had said, she said, "There is no room for a doctor like that on my team." Well, there was no room on my "team" either—I stayed home.

MARIE
My first was a c-section after being fully dilated for seven hours. The baby remained in a persistent posterior position. I suffered from a severe uterine infection and

ultimately a pulmonary embolism—and three months later, severe depression over the whole thing. His birth certificate said CPD, though a pelvimetry (they'll never do that again) showed I had plenty of room. This baby was born after a 12 hour labor—my husband saved the day—he refused to give up when after pushing for two hours, squatting, the doctor determined that she was a transverse head (my pelvis may not be conducive to anterior positions?)—he put me on my hands and knees. Six contractions later, she was born on the labor bed, coming so fast that they (thankfully) didn't have time to do anything except catch her! My 11 lb. 3 oz "little" girl knew what to do once her daddy corrected the problem. I had a couple of superficial tears—within a week I felt WONDERFUL. She's five weeks old and already 14 lbs and gorgeous. One of my nurse friends in OB tells me they're still talking about us. I hope our experience helps to calm the fears of many people.

JOANNE

I was twenty-three years old and pregnant with my third child when I discovered a varicose vein in the birth canal. Horrified, I immediately phoned the doctor and rushed to see him. He examined me and told me that when the time came, I'd have to have a cesarean. I agreed, but then, I might have agreed to a lobotomy. How stupid I was! My 6 lb. 2 oz. baby (my two others were 8 lbs.) entered the world via IVs, monitors and drapes. I cried throughout the ordeal and my husband was not allowed in because of the "emergency" nature of "this particular birth." I was convinced that three children was enough, and agreed to a tubal ligation right then and there. Over the next eight months I was haunted—did I really need a c-section? Was my baby smaller than he should have been (he was taken early). I sought out another doctor—the most beautiful woman from India, I think. When she was taking my history she asked the reason for my section. When I told her, she hesitated, and then she said that in her opinion, a varicosity never constituted a section—but it was done and over with. I couldn't get her words out of my head. I was also feeling bitter about the tubal ligation. Not for long though—I questioned the doctor about the percentage of them that were successfully reversed, and she referred me to a doctor who had a very high rate of tubal reinastimosis. I scheduled my surgery with caution—again I would be cut! But this time I was making the decisions. I had selected this surgery and my head was really psyched for it. I had it done, and went home and waited to get pregnant. It took eight months, but I did become pregnant! I went back to my wonderful new OB and she encouraged me to have a VBAC the whole way. I ate so well and I went swimming almost every day. The one haunting thought—I still had that varicose vein. Would it rupture during birth? Would I hemorrhage? . . . When I got to the hospital, my doctor was waiting. I asked her about a fetal monitor and IV and she said that she would hate to interfere with the natural process that I was doing myself. The entire time she boosted me up, gave me support, and encouraged me. She did not do one vaginal exam. After several hours, I felt like pushing. I asked about the vein. The doctor said she could see it and everything was fine. She told me that everything in the vaginal area has the capability to stretch, so get to work and start pushing! I did and my 7 lb 5 oz daughter came into the world honestly. I nursed her and my husband and I cried together. I felt like Wonder Woman! That I could move a mountain! I thank the doctor and I thank you for your powerful book—it stayed by my side the entire time. I am even considering a 5th child. I love children and I would love to relive the beautifulness of it all. I'd love to go on Phil or Oprah and tell my story!

JAN

An interesting thing happened. Four months after my homebirth, all the depression of my cesarean came out. I felt my incision "coming apart." This may seem silly, but I had been made to feel (by the doctors who told me I would die if I stayed at home) that my body would not hold together. Now I know my incision was healed—you cannot imagine the relief that one feels when they are healed of this wound.

CLAIRE

My pushing phase was eight hours. I had read about a VBAC woman who pushed for twelve. I was hoping not to win the record, but knowing that there is wide variation to all phases of labor helped me. I am so proud.

LISA

I was told that I was too small to have a baby vaginally. When I was pregnant with my second child, I went to a fair. There was a drawing to win a teddy bear. There were hundreds of people at that fair, and only one teddy bear. I paid the fifty cents for the raffle ticket, and as I dropped it in the box, I said to my friend, "I have about as much chance of winning the bear as I do of having a VBAC. If I win that bear, I'm going to try for a vaginal birth." I left the fair, and that night, I got a call to come and pick up the bear—my ticket had won. Six months later, teddy bear under one arm, VBAC baby in the other, I came out of the hospital humming, "And this is the day the teddy bears have their picnic!"

PAM

I came into the hospital much further along than I realized. I said to the nurses, I am in labor, but I have time. I want to go to the bathroom before you check me. I felt as if I needed to have a bowel movement. In the bathroom, I sat and grunted for a few minutes. Then all of a sudden, I realized—THIS IS THE BABY! I felt the baby's head come out—it was soft, smooth, velvety, rippled and warm. I shouted for the nurses. They came in immediately, and hoisted me up. They wanted me to move to the bed, but we only got a few feet. I yelled as I pushed, Oh God! and I pushed her all the way out—what a fantastic relief! I did it! I yelled as Jim walked in—he had been out parking the car. The doctor walked in and said, "Well, you don't have to worry about that IV and monitor we have been fighting about all these months."

SARAH

It seems important to relate that my maternal great grandmother gave birth to her 12th child on their dining room table. Her youngest, my grandmother, had her first two in the hospital, but the next two at home because they didn't have the money for the hospital. She stated she didn't like being at home because her husband didn't like handing the instruments to the doctor, so by the time the fifth was born they had enough money and she went to the hospital again. She had an emergency cesarean and my grandfather was asked to choose if his wife or the baby should be saved. Both were saved and fifteen months later my grandmother had her last child—a VBAC!!! in the 1940's! My mother had her first 5 babies after unmedicated labors but with spinals at the last minute—(except for one surprise breech that just "flew out" while she was alone in the labor room). She says that looking back, spinals were ludicrous because all the work was over with by then. Her last child was taken by cesarean at eight months due to an RH problem. He was tiny and required two complete exchange transfusions to save his life. After this experience, my parents betrayed their religious beliefs and began using artificial birth control. Neither my mother nor my grandmother ever said anything positive about birth. I never saw their cesarean scars, but heard them described as ugly and hideous. . . . When I went into labor, there was a little bit of meconium. I remembered the horror stories I had been told in nursing school and I was terrified. I called my mother who said, "I wish I could do this for you." Nothing I had learned in childbirth classes helped. . . . The suave and debonair partner came in— he had done two sections in the ninety minutes I had been at the hospital. . . . I refused to get out of the Lazy-Boy chair in the labor room—I was the first woman to be monitored and pitted in the chair. There was a medical student on my case— I secretly began calling her Frank. I wished she wasn't there but I didn't know how to ask her to leave. . . . The doctor came back and said I looked "too comfortable." I was tired and HUNGRY! A few hours later, not enough progress made, I was presented a consent form to sign for a c-section like I had a choice, but I didn't feel like I did. . . . My baby was taken to the nursery. My husband went to see her, and said that she looked like she was searching for me, but she did seem to recognize him as someone important to her. When I first saw her, she had a scabby mark on her scalp from the internal lead. She had poppy eyes—she looked like E.T. I felt ashamed and was glad when they took her back to the nursery. A bossy nurse gave me a bath—I couldn't bathe myself!—and instructed me in "peri-care" for my intact perineum. I am glad my pride was dulled by demerol and phenergan. I had two days of grease on my hair. I made Vic put balloons in the room to make things seem more festive. What a joke. I nursed the baby out of a sense of duty, not longing (although now I am proud—she never had formula or a pacifier or sugar water). Since I had no "bowel sounds" I was unable to eat. It had been days. . . . I hadn't planned on purchasing the newborn pictures, but she really was beautiful after all, so we bought the whole set. The night before we went home, we went to the physicians' fancy-schmancy dinner where we had a nice meal and our babies got "babysat" for the whole evening. A little American enculturation early on. My doctor avoided me for the whole hospital stay. When I finally saw him, he said that it was too bad things didn't work out—it always seemed like the couples who wanted a natural birth ended up with c-sections. Then he said I could have intercourse in two weeks. Yea, I can hardly wait. Get out of town. It took more than six weeks for me to start connecting with my daughter. She was a "gaze-averter" for a long time and not very affectionate. My incision healed, although I hated it and tried to hide it from my husband. It was tender for several years afterwards. . . . So, now perhaps you can understand why I had this baby at home.

ANNE

I did it! What an experience! As I was getting dressed to go to the hospital, suddenly, after nine months of optimism, I was frightened. I said, "Mom, I'm scared," relieved at having said it. We talked about how I felt and I said I'd never forgive myself for not trying. Then I laughed and said that since we had moved overseas to Holland I didn't have a choice—they don't do repeat c-sections here! My husband took pictures of me standing next to the monitor instead of hooked up to it, like I was in America. . . . When the baby was "stuck" the doctor was called in . . . to adjust the position slightly. He used forceps, but inserted them so slowly and gently—he did not want to injure my perineum. Then he took them out and told me to continue pushing—gently. He said he didn't want to do an episiotomy— that it would make things easier today if we did, but it would be harder on me in the days to follow. I found out that the section rate here is 4% and that midwives attend the vast majority of all births.

KIM

After 45 hours, my first labor concluded at the end of a physician's blade. None of the nightmarish contraptions avoided. I dealt with insensitive nurses and bullish doctors. Then came the grand finale: an infection on my incision and a very high fever that brought me close to death. There was the added bonus of not being able to hold my baby once for one long agonizing week after the operation. My body and psyche were both nearly killed in that operating room. Many will argue that those machines and procedures were there for the safety of myself and the baby— I am certain that they inhibited me and made it impossible for my body to carry on with the natural function of birth. When I became pregnant again, panic set in. Not because I didn't want the baby, but because I thought the only way that it could be born was another gash into my belly. All the doctors I talked to said that with my previous complications after surgery, another cesarean was the safest route. I thought the operation caused the complications? . . . As I pondered my situation, I realized that I could die in the hospital as well as at home. At least I would die free of interference. My husband would not hear of it . . . But then we met our midwife, who gave me the courage to look into myself and fulfill my ultimate dream. She knew VBAC was safe—she had been attending them for twenty years! Blessed midwife, who taught me that fear was in my head, that it was all up to me. . . . I brought only the highest thoughts into my head and my heart. The negative was there only as an opponent to overcome. My will became that of a sorceress! I was an eagle flying high above all evil. . . . Labor was okay, but transition was difficult. I was ten centimeters with no desire to push. I kept having delirious, exhausted fear that my cesarean scar would burst. Three hours passed. I tried different positions. Four hours. Finally, summoning my last ounce of personal power, I remembered the pugilist in me again. My screams were those of a warrior doing combat on the battlefield of life. If I lost, it would be death with dignity rather than life with only half my soul. . . . My four year old stroked the baby's head as it came through the opening. My husband held my legs as they surrendered this new being to the light. As it turned out, the cord was wrapped around her leg. But it all ended well with my little flower opening her eyes to find me, instead of the blare of hospital lights.

VAL

My first husband and I separated and later divorced. He never understood my grief over the section, and that was a big contributing factor, although of course there had been some problems before that. Four years later, I married my present husband. On our first serious date, I asked him if he would read your book. He didn't know it then, but a lot was riding on his response to that request. He read it, and got as angry as I was about the injustices at birth. I knew I had found a soul mate. Two years later, we had a baby—at home. I had twelve minutes of pushing! I used to read your book and wonder if a story of mine would ever go into a birth book like that. Well, here it is!

JANET

I wrote a letter to our local paper to tell them about VBAC and to warn people about unnecessary cesareans. The doctor who delivered my first baby (with no labor) wrote back, explaining why cesareans are done. It was rather insulting—he said, "I hope this increases your medical knowledge." It just proves the point that OBs feel they must "save" women from their own stupidity. It was my superior education coupled with my intelligent brain that led me to do the research that proved that his medical knowledge is a lot of you-know-what.

DIANE

As you know, I dragged my husband to your seminar—kicking and screaming all four hundred miles of the way. What a "conversion"! He told everyone at work about our home VBAC—one of the women there said, "ICK! You must have been lying in a real mess—it must have taken forever to clean it up." He said that it was the most wonderful warm mess he's ever been in—something he'll never forget. The woman thinks we are from Mars. . . . I don't think I told you that I had infertility problems after our first child. My doctor told me—after many tests— that we had only a 5% chance of ever getting pregnant again. I went home and cried. I just gave up. I didn't want sex anymore. It was too painful if it wasn't leading to a baby. A few months later, when signs of ovulation came, I just couldn't let the month pass. Somehow, I knew within days that I was pregnant. I didn't rush out and get a blood test or anything. I decided that I had to start then and there trusting my body. One of my friends says when in doubt she uses the Caroline Ingalls—of "Little House on the Prairie"—theory: What would Caroline have done? In this case, she would have waited. . . . At ten weeks, the doctors could hear no heart tones. They told me to come back in a week. Still nothing. They said a sonogram was necessary. The day before my appointment I saw Dr. Robert Mendelsohn on TV talking about the danger of ultrasound. I called the doctors and they said ultrasound was perfectly safe. I went in and of course the baby was fine. Another lesson: TRUST. . . . The doctors said they were concerned about my emotional health. They questioned my stability if a cesarean "became necessary." I began to feel like an animal searching for a place to give birth—nothing felt right. We had little money and insurance didn't cover midwives at home. We considered birthing at a midwife's house about three hours away, one who was very comfortable with VBAC. . . . My dreams were very vivid during the pregnancy and often violent. I dreamed of people chasing me up mountains and of people forcing me to do things I didn't want to do—I physically fought them off: my fears reflected. . . . I started labor when my husband and son had the flu. I think I stopped it with my thoughts—I just kept saying, "this isn't the right time." Two days later—a full moon—I knew this was really it. I asked everyone to be quiet during each contraction—the people with me understood. When I was close to full dilation, I became ravenously hungry—I had never heard of that! I had eaten lightly, lots of fruit juices and tea to this point. I ate a big chicken sandwich, carrots, and more juice!! I squatted with contractions between bites. After this feast I took what I knew would be my last walk before the birth. Tom and I walked around our hilly backyard with him helping me over the "mountains." I felt as if there was a bowling ball between my legs. The sun was setting and it was cool and beautiful. I loved being outside! I came in and took a shower. I knew it would be soon. . . . As her head came out, I felt as if my whole body was being ripped apart—but actually, I didn't even have a tear! What a relief as she slithered out of me! She didn't look all that big to me—what a surprise to find out her head was 16". CPD? Not on your life. I didn't know she was a she for a long time after the birth. All I cared about was that I was holding my baby. As I write this, two years have passed, and the glow still comes over me. It is something that nobody can ever take away from me. I want to do it again. I want to feel the strength and power of those contractions. I want the peace, the intensity, the bursting forth of life. Even if I never have a baby, again, I will always have this with me. [Note: Just three months ago, Diane had her third child—another wonderful home birth.]

KAYLA
Hold on to your hat! A home VBAC with TRIPLETS! The midwives knew that there were two babies, but didn't know about the third until the delivery. The sad part for all of us is that because of the status of homebirth and midwifery in this state, we have to keep it quiet.

CASSIE
My first was a section for a breech—the doctor was honest enough to say that she didn't know how to deliver a breech vaginally. The cesarean didn't bother me all that much. My second pregnancy was a cesarean—the doctor said that this was the safest route to take—and I really didn't mind. I believed that cesarean babies were prettier! But on the table the second time, I felt pain. My doctor said that was impossible—I was anesthetized and I really couldn't be feeling anything, which caused me to apologize and quiet down—you see, I had to be the perfect patient. My feelings were different after this one. I knew I would never have another cesarean or any more children. I had heard about VBAC before, but until then, it was of no interest to me.

CLARE
Mine was a hospital birth—22 hours during which I empathized with the girl in your book who was secretly wishing for a section to stop the pain—anything! They gave me something so I could relax between contractions. During that time, I dilated like crazy (fear of rupture, fear of pain, fear of fear may have prevented my cervix from opening up before. It took 1 1/2 hours of pushing to get her out. The delivery was performed under bright lights with stirrups but I didn't care! The episiotomy was nothing compared to the belly rip. My husband was always there— we were both as high as kites. I kept up a stream of nonsense in my joy and relief that my prayers were answered: I had a vaginal delivery! It may not have been natural, but I did not have pain medication as such (novocaine for the epis.) or an IFM. Bonding was straightforward—I got her for about an hour in the recovery room. It was love at first sight. . . . I do think that women who go for purebirth are very brave. I'm not sure it's for me. A homebirth presupposes one has help

with the other children—although I actually couldn't rest well in the hospital. What I really mean is that for me a hospital situation where you are not regarded as ill is perhaps more restful. My attitude to the baby was quite different this time. Previously I had felt 'dumped on' and inadequate to care for him, as I was recovering from the operation. The nursing staff was largely impatient with this. This time, I had mobility so soon after the birth and that has been marvelous—I don't feel so desperately exhausted or depressed. It will be VBACs always for me!

FRAN

After a cesarean, probably the two most important ingredients for me with my VBACs were: not to have expectations—that means positive or negative, to let my body do whatever it needed to do and accept it, to keep an open mind to the many possible challenges (such as a long labor for me, different presentation, whatever); and to surround myself with positive people who agreed with VBAC and keep telling me how great I was doing. . . . Chuck and I both got concerned when I got to 8 cms.—the place I never got beyond in my first pregnancy. We were both struggling to pass that point. The midwife helped us, though, she kept pointing out how well things were going, and never showed any doubt at that time or any other. . . . There was a slight "lip" over the baby's head, and with my permission, the midwife slipped it back and I was really ready to push. I wanted to be on my hands and knees. My sister was massaging my back with a wonderful herbaloil and Chuck was holding warm washcloths on my lower back. It all felt wonderful in spite of the tremendous contractions. It all worked together—the position, the contractions, the compresses, the tea, the massage, the support. When Tyler's head crowned, the tremendous love I felt as my sister's eyes met mine and I saw the sparkle and the ear to ear smile—it was an intense moment. We had always been close—sharing a room for fifteen years—but this was different, it was so special. Indeed, the whole birth was special. My 3 and 1/2 year old daughter was with us the whole time. She had been putting cool compresses on my forehead. She fell asleep minutes before the delivery—she has maintained a very loving warm relationship with her brother—she has never shown a shred of jealousy. It is perhaps only conjecture, but I have to believe that this special bond between them is due to the fact that they (we) were not separated at all. . . . Enough—I could go on and on! Edit whatever you want. We love you. [I love you, too.]

KRIS

I started writing you a letter about my births and now, twenty pages later my husband thinks I am the one writing a book. I just couldn't stop—once the words started coming it was like the pen was just jumping out of my hand! Three days in the hospital isn't all that much for a c-section, I was told—but for me, every minute was torture. Once home, I became a "leaky faucet" at the mere mention of a c-section. You put me in touch with a woman nearby who had a VBAC—I called her and cried and talked for three hours on the phone to her—she didn't even mind! . . . When I got pregnant again, I cried. I was so scared. The doctor said my babies would keep getting bigger but my small pelvis would never change size. Every doctor I saw said I had an unusually small pelvis and so it would be a no-go. One said he wasn't about to "quake in his boots" while I was trying to get this baby out. Finally I located a supportive doctor—his wife was 4' 11" and had delivered three good sized babies. I went to a medical library and heard the words "Index Medicus" for the first time in my life. I read everything. My mother was screaming at me that I should listen to the first doctors. She thought this new one must be a quack if he didn't agree with everyone else. . . . Well, after all, the VBAC did happen. My dreams came true.

IRIS

My first was a vaginal birth. The second time, I had a prolapsed cord and had a section. The next three were all sections. When I got pregnant with my sixth, I was sure I'd have another operation. My sister-in-law is a doctor and she said I'd die if I attempted a VBAC. I was so tired of surgery! A friend lent me a book called Silent Knife. I decided I would have a VBAC. My husband had a big problem with this. We had a lot of fights. I told him to read the book, he said he would but he was really busy at work. One evening the kids were in bed and I gave it to him and said one chapter—that's all. Well, he read three. He apologized and said he was sorry for all the c-sections I had been through. We had to travel pretty far, but we had our VBAC. Even my sister-in-law now thinks I made the best choice. I got a call from a local newspaper. They may do an article on this!

ANDREA

I didn't know about VBAC or the CPM until recently, but I groped my way through my vaginal delivery on my own. I felt so strongly that even when the midwife and doctor said they could no longer take responsibility for me as their patient, my husband, friend, and I simply closed the hospital door and labored on our own. Once we did that, I began, finally, to have intense contractions and to "make progress." Thank you so much for your delight in my birth.

JOAN

I am a La Leche League Leader and have been meaning to write to you for years. I am a VBAC—but ours was one before it was given a name. My section was in 1967. I was devastated. I read, I researched, I cried and cried, I swore at God. My husband was totally bewildered. My doctor was my salvation. Through unsurpassed understanding, obstetric expertise, and a tough skin to weather the professional criticism, he guided me through my vaginal delivery just one year after my section—a first for both of us. Afterwards he said, "God was I nervous." I have had two more vaginal deliveries. I am immensely proud of my obstetric history and don't for a minute forget the nightmare of emotions following my section. I help as many women as I can to avoid cesareans—I am a pioneer of sorts, I guess, too!

TERRI

I couldn't enter an operating room for a fourth time. So, after three sections, I said it's a birthing room for me from now on. My previous doctors just got word of my VBAC—they were flabbergasted.

LINDA

CPD? Please. My son was 9 lbs. 1 oz. with his fist up under his chin—chest plus arm 16″ in diameter. My cpd baby was 8 lbs. 1 oz. If there is anybody in my state who needs help—for the rest of my life they can call me.

ALICIA

After three sections I thought I was doomed for another. I had called you before the birth of my third child but ended up with a section—after he was crowning. I was so discouraged! This time, I laboured at home five days (five!) and after I got to the hospital a very supportive doctor helped me. I got just a drop of pitocin and the doctor massaged the cervix. After four hours in the hospital and only twenty minutes of pushing, my daughter was born. Only a few people truly believed in us.

REBECCA
My family is now complete. But a VBAC doesn't happen just once in a woman's life; I know I relive it over and over and over again.

PEGGY
The labor was awful. I was miserable the whole time. I felt lonely and desperate for relief. I lost all confidence in myself and went to the hospital to be checked. One centimeter. ONE CENTIMETER? That's all my body can do in three days of labor? What have I gotten myself into? Me and my big ideas! God is punishing me for rebelling. . . . The nurse checked me two hours later and I was still at one centimeter. We were told we would have to go to another hospital where a cesarean could be performed. Forty five minutes later, in the car, I felt a burning, stinging sensation. I thought, this is the biggest stool I have ever passed—or could it be the baby? No, it's probably something else. But could this grunting be the "pushing" I have heard about? If it would just come out, this thing, I would feel better and could handle the contractions better. We arrived at the hospital—too late to do a section—this was the baby coming! . . . The episiotomy that they did, the stitching of it, was worse than anything else. The first nurse misjudged my dilation—if she hadn't, I would not have been so discouraged. (She had also said to me that a few days earlier a VBAC woman had said that the exploration of the uterine scar after the surgery had been so painful that she didn't know how she endured the pain. That was all I needed to hear at the time. But it did serve its purpose—I said no to that.) After my cesarean, Jim and I cried like babies. We didn't cry this time—maybe all the built up emotions came out with the afterbirth. I am mostly thrilled about this birth.

HELENE
The main reason for my first three pregnancies ending in cesareans was that I was suffering from undiagnosed chemical sensitivities which caused me to be schizophrenic. By the time I was expecting my fourth I knew about the allergies and was in the process of recovering, so I knew that I could birth normally. However, quite a few people in my area, still seeing me as neurotic, did not think I would succeed with a normal birth. I think anyone who wants to have a VBAC should try, even if counselled not to. . . . For the first birth, my husband remained outside of the room for the most part, praying. This was more comfortable for me than if he had been in the room with me. The placenta came quickly. I only wanted to sleep after the birth—my husband took the baby. My midwife said that she had seen this lack of interest in the baby in another woman who had had a VBAC after three cesareans. After being kept away from our babies three times in the hospital by force the mothering instinct is affected perhaps? . . . With my fifth child, second VBAC, my midwives felt the baby was small—it was one week before my due date—and they thought a homebirth might be dangerous. I made an appointment

with the doctor and he wanted to do an internal. I felt this would be dangerous, so I went home and began eating more—more protein and more in general—hoping the baby would be late. Two weeks later, I started labor. It was on again, off again . . . for three days. There was a lot of pain. Things picked up and for the next two days, I had contractions. I felt really discouraged. I started thinking about going to the hospital to be sectioned and just get it over with. I decided to sit in the tub and think. In the water, I realized that the contractions had become regular. My husband arrived home and said that I had a blessing from a holy person we knew, and as soon as he repeated the blessing, the labor became painless. I called my midwife and then my LSP. She arrived with a friend I had never met. I got nervous since this is usually considered wrong at a homebirth, but we talked in the kitchen, and I felt fine. My midwife checked me—9 cm—a painless transition. I stood up and as soon as I did, I felt strong pushes from inside. I said the baby is coming but no one really believed me, and the baby pushed herself out while I was standing up at 9 cm. This time I was much more interested in bonding with the baby and much less exhausted. After an hour, I squatted and the placenta came out. I had much less blood loss this time, I think because my prenatal care from the midwives was so good, and they told me to eat things like liver and alfalfa sprouts. I tore a little but was actually less sore afterwards than when I didn't! My first three births probably would have been vaginal if I had had a midwife at home, and the last two would have been cesarean if I had been in the hospital, the first for 96 hours ruptured membranes and the second for getting discouraged and being impatient, both things a midwife can handle and most doctors can't.

GRETTA

I called you when I was four weeks overdue. I went into labor four days later, and had a perfect baby and a great birth. Quick, relatively easy. Home in eight hours.

KAREN

I spent the better part of this pregnancy working to get into the birthing room. VBAC is still considered high-risk, and since I had two sections and had a T-incision (inverted), I gave up the fight. They hooked me up to a mal-functioning fetal monitor and told me they couldn't get the baby's heartbeat. My LSP had brought her trusty fetoscope—and the heartbeat was strong and steady throughout. (The hospital said they couldn't find their fetoscope!) A friend came to be with us in labor—they said she couldn't stay. My husband told them that he was a lawyer (he's not) and they didn't say anything else about that. I have an enlightened doctor and once he got there, things went well.

MICHALENE (Ohio)

Rachel Catherine is one blessed week old today. I want to tell you: "I AM HEALED!" All the hurts and guilt and upset over the cesarean I had are gone. I can hardly believe the healing power of this experience. I feel whole and normal and finally at peace . . .   My water broke and my first reaction was panic. The baby wasn't due for four and a half or five weeks—I was positive when I had conceived. Our house was torn apart. My husband was painting the baby's room and our bedroom. Nothing was ready . . . Our midwife arrived and her gentle attitude helped me immediately. She told us to get a good night's sleep. I was worried! What if the baby is too premature? What if I can't open up? What if I can't do it? I was impatient, but she reminded us that maybe our early baby needed a little more time, a little more gentle labor stimulation. . . .

The day passes. I take shower after shower to stay relaxed. I cry out—not in pain—but in sheer frustration. I pace the house. I eat a little. My midwife straightened up the house!! Bless her heart! My hips begin to hurt a bit. . . .

Labor picked up and I was feeling a lot of pain. I labored and labored and labored and stayed at eight centimeters for twenty-four hours! I no longer believed anyone when they told me that it was all happening. I am MAD. My husband— never a discouraging word. I complain. I'm terrible. My midwife tells me my body is wise, to trust this all. As each hour passes, I think, "If it doesn't happen in an hour, we'll go to the hospital." At the end of the hour, I think, one more hour, and so on throughout the most frustrating day of my life. All this time, one of our cats is in heat. She walks around the house yowling and screaming. Hi cat. I know how you feel. . . .

Near evening, in this day three, I've lost track. I decide to have a little castor oil. Within an hour, I feel terrible. Sick, like the flu. Clutch. Maybe infection is setting in. We've been so careful—taking my temperature, clean sanitary pads, clean everything, only two vaginal exams. My face is burning hot. Alas! This is only a reaction to the labor, and the contractions getting stronger and closer. We order pizza.

Someone says I look beautiful. It feels so good to hear that. It's getting so difficult to stay relaxed. "My God, how long?" Our friends are here, watching MASH reruns.

I ask if we should go to the hospital. I want to hear everyone say the word "No." Do I want to go to the hospital? I say it: No. I feel like a crazy person.

I cry. I sob. Everyone seems discouraged. I lose track of time. I tell God I hate Him (forgive me, Lord!) I can't stand the pains. They aren't doing anything. I fall apart. I tell Don I can't do this anymore. I have reached my limit. No more. To the hospital. He says no! I almost beg. I am digging my nails into his arms and beginning to scream. He wraps his arms tight around me and tells me it will take one hour to get to the hospital and another hour to get ready for a cesarean.—He says he KNOWS I can have this baby then. I say no, no, I'm really going to die. Don't hate me for giving up. He holds me tighter and tighter. He tells me to go ahead and scream. So I do. And I start to moo! Just like a cow. Louder and louder. Mary's 18 month old daughter is sleeping and I know I am going to wake her but I can't stop now. I was afraid to start making noise. I grunt. Don starts yelling, "You're pushing, you're pushing!" "I AM NOT!" I yell back. He half carries me out of the bathroom, yelling "It's baby time! It's baby time!" I am astounded at the pain and I never dreamed I could make so much noise. Never, never again, I think. Next time, a scheduled cesarean. I couldn't believe how hard I was working. I needed cheerleading. Don was so excited, so happy, he was uplifting me, he was magnificent. He understood.

My midwife offered me a mirror. Till now, it was important for me to see it. Now, I just wanted to do it. Finally, finally I could feel the baby in the birth canal. I felt it slip under the pubic bone and then move down more. Then the head crowned!! I could FEEL it! Then it turned and the midwife told me to reach down and feel the baby's head. I felt this wrinkled mass and cried, "My baby!" I pushed again and again. And then THERE WAS OUR BABY BETWEEN MY

LEGS!! Don and I reached for "it." Pink, clean, creamy, wonderful. We can't see if it's a boy or a girl. A blanket covers "it." The baby is perfect. I am awe struck. No cesarean, no cesarean. Not even any tears on my perineum. We did it.

After a while, Don cuts the cord and clamps it. Our daughter is on her own. My heart clutches. I love her so. I try to thank Don, our midwife, and my friends for believing, for helping my two and a half year dream come true. I can't get the words out. Everybody is crying.

I smelled awful after the cesarean. My baby was taken away. I couldn't move. This time I take a shower and fall asleep fresh and clean and clear-headed, with my baby in my bed.

The magic of this experience will last forever. I realize that I set myself up to win. It has changed me/us. I have given birth. I am humbled. Not just by the birth but by the overwhelming support everyone has given me. With no strings, and with complete total devotion. This is the most exciting, exhilarating, strongest experience of my life. We are all winners.

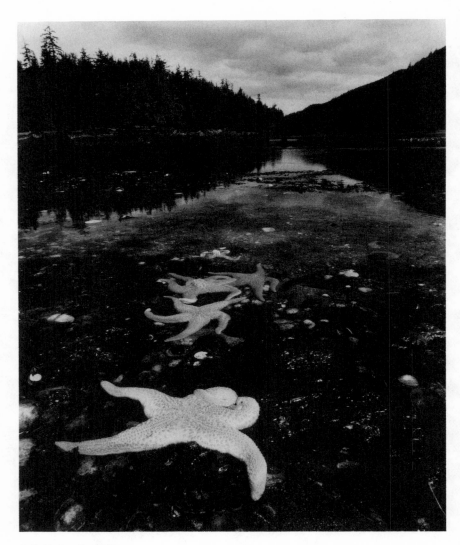

© Keith Lazelle 1991.

16   *Open Season!*

Open Season

"For what do I go to this far land which no one has ever reached? Oh, I am alone! I am utterly alone!"

And Reason, that old man, said to her, "Silence! What do you hear?"

And she listened intently, and she said, "I hear a sound of feet, a thousand times then thousand and thousand of thousands, and they beat this way!"

He said, "They are the feet of those that shall follow you. Lead on! Make a track to the water's edge! Where you stand now, the ground will be beaten flat by ten thousand times ten thousand feet." And he said, "Have you seen the locusts how they cross a stream? First one comes down to the water-edge, and it is swept away, and then another comes and then another, and at last with their bodies piled up a bridge is built and the rest pass over."

She said, "And of those that come first, some are swept away and are heard of no more; their bodies do not even build the bridge?"

"And are swept away, and are heard of no more—and what of that?" he said.

"And what of that—" she said.

"They make a track to the water's edge."

"They make a track to the water's edge!" And she said, "Over that bridge which shall be built with our bodies, who will pass?"

He said, "The entire human race."

And the woman grasped her staff,

And I saw her turn down that dark path to the river.[1]

Although the original title of the above passage is "Track to the Water's Edge," Shirley Luthman, in whose book I first read it, calls it "The Soliloquy of the Pioneer." I invite you to read it one more time. The first was for your head; the second time is for your heart.

Each of you reading this book is a pioneer. You have helped to make and to keep a path to the water's edge. I bow to you all.

Shortly after I had chosen the title for this book, I was writing the abbreviation for it on a computer disk. I realized that it spelled the word "os." An os is a mouth or an opening into the interior of an organ. It is time that we open our mouths and our hearts. We do not need to have our bellies or our bottoms cut open in order to see inside.

"Namaste" is an Indian word. The term means: "I honor the place inside of you where the entire universe dwells. It is a place of love and of truth and of light and of peace. When you are in that place within you, and I am in that place within me, we are one." In a very real sense, the entire universe dwells within each pregnant woman. To cut her body unnecessarily is to destroy a world.

In many cultures, pregnancy and birth are not times of stress or abrupt change in people's lives. Women birth wherever they happen to be, pick up their babies, and get on with their lives. While I prefer a little more ceremony, or perhaps even a celebration of sorts to welcome a new being into the world, I always believed that continuing to work in one's rice paddy, or finishing the chicken plucking within minutes after birth, seemed a bit far-fetched. I was certain that this information was a plot perpetrated on the American woman for the purpose of inducing guilt. Most women in this culture are so physically exhausted and emotionally debilitated after birth that they are barely able to eat the rice or the chicken, let alone prepare them. Indeed, they themselves have often been picked over and plucked apart. (I happily made pancakes hours after my last birth!)

I once saw a statue of a woman holding her newborn baby up to the Gods. I wondered how many women in our country would have the strength to stand up moments after birthing, lift their babies to the sky, and say "Look here, Dear Universe! Look Stars! Look Sun! She's here! She's wonderful, isn't she! And I am, too." No, for the most part, women in these parts are too weak, too worn out, too sad and too stunned.

We have a stake in each other's births. One woman birthing in a way that feels powerful and free can influence so many others around her. I remember attending a gathering just before I became pregnant with my third child. I talked with a woman there whom I had met several times before. She had recently had a homebirth, and there was something about her that was different. I couldn't put my finger on what the difference was, but in her presence I felt magic. She emanated joy. Months later, when I went into labor, I consciously placed an image of her face in my mind's eye. I heard her voice and I made it my own. I gave birth.

Childbirth educator Jody McLaughlin reminds us that the women's birth movement is not a pressure group unified for conquest; however, we do have an intangible unity which has carried us through centuries of persecution and domination.

The miracle is that no one has to do it singlehandedly. Everyone who is willing to do his or her own part completely is joined by many others who are inspired to do their part completely. When we were born on earth, each of us was given a certain sphere of activity to influence—some larger, some smaller—eventually touching all. Throughout our whole life our job is simply to exert the best possible influence on the part of the world we touch. The flowers we cultivate in our own garden will drop their seeds in the patch next door. This is how in our own gentle way we transform the world.[2]

In "Images of a Planetary Family" we are told that Light is an image for evolutionary convergence of consciousness. Wherever there are people with an understanding of the unity of all life, "whether they are relatively isolated individuals, in the midst of industrial civilization, or members of a new age community, there stands a point of light. Ultimately . . . there will be . . . just . . . Light."[3]

Sonia Johnson reminds us that we can bestow grace and power mightily on one another. "I've been one of the very lucky ones," she says. "When I stand before a group of women to speak, I am almost lifted off my feet by the flood of passionate energy and invincible spirit that pours forth from them. Though this can also be felt to some degree in the audience, I always wish every woman there could stand where I'm standing and get the full impact of it. None of them would ever lose heart again."[4]

I am one of the very lucky ones, too. From Maine and New Hampshire, where I have met so many beautiful "Northern Lights," to Florida and Louisiana, my life has been enriched; and I have also felt the energy, commitment, and spirit which Sonia speaks of. It gives me hope. In Colorado I have met women who have moved mountains; every woman I have met in Canada is royalty. No, I will never lose heart again: They all have left "heartprints."

We do not have decades to make changes, nor can we afford any more self-delusion. As women, we long for a new world "where human hearts can rest and love." To have that world, Sonia says, we must be at rest now; we must love now. "There is no future apart from this moment. So there is no need to feel frantic about time, terrified that we haven't enough of it in which to change things. Panic about the shortness of time . . . paralyzes us as does all fear. If we can feel hopeful and confident and full of life and vigor right now, we have made the future one of hope and power and life."[5]

We must be cautious, lest we become the hunters, and those who have been interfering in our births, the hunted. There is no more hunting season. We are all free to roam.

I wonder if you ever change human beings with arguments alone; either by peppering them with little sharp facts or by blowing them up with great guns of truth. You scare them, but do you change them? I wonder if you ever make any real difference in human beings without understanding them and loving them. For when you argue with a man, you are somehow trying to pull him down and make him less; but when you try to understand him, when you like him, how eager he is to know the truth you have; and you add to him in some strange way, you make him more than he was before; and, at the same time, you become more.[6]

Florence Luscumb, a suffragist born in the late 1800s, was considered a radical and spent her life working for change. She wrote: "There is nothing in the world that is so transitory and fragile as a snowflake, and nothing so irresistible as an avalanche, which is simply millions of snowflakes. So that if each one of us, little snowflakes, just does our part, we will be an irresistible force."[7]

Better get out your mittens. Elaine tells me that there are now flurries in north Alabama, and Cathy and Michelle have been shoveling in New Jersey for a long time. Vickie tells me that even some of the Texans are getting out their boots—their snow boots this time. Flurries have begun in Wisconsin and Illinois. Luce's taken out her sled in Missouri. In Connecticut, there's enough to build a whole family of snowpeople. There's a blizzard in New York, of course, and even California's blanketed. This is some storm, believe me! Not ominous, magnificent! I have word from Deborah in Pennsylvania and from Patti in Indiana: they're covered. It always snows in Minnesota, right, Bev? Laurie's skiing in Nevada and there are reports of squalls in Arizona. And in Ohio Kim and Mary are making snow angels. No, I will never lose heart again.

To all of you who have read this letter, I thank you once again. Together we will all make a difference. As for me, I have been sitting at this typewriter for so long, I don't even know what season it is. I thought it might be summer, but I just looked outside and it is snowing here, too. Actually, I am about to take a walk. I'm on my way to the beach. There's a starfish in my hand.

Postnote

On the very day that I delivered the final manuscript of *Open Season* to my publishers, Amy Clarke went into labor. I had the distinct privilege of being the LSP for Amy and her husband, Wally Spear. When the labor was over, I called Greenwood Publishing Group and yelled, "Stop the presses!" I knew that Amy and Wally's story needed to be included in the book.

Amy had had two previous cesarean sections, both for "cpd" and failure to progress. She is a small woman, under 5'2". When she was forty-two years old, she became pregnant: she wanted a home birth. Several months into the pregnancy, she found out that she was carrying twins. As the pregnancy progressed, she learned that baby "A" was breech.

Amy and I had numerous phone conversations. She and Wally live more than a two hour drive from my house, but they came to see me several times. We found it somewhat interesting that each time they came to see me, there was an unpredicted torrential rainstorm.

Amy spent almost every waking hour of her pregnancy looking for a midwife who would attend her at home. She located several who said that they wished they could help her out, but that her situation was just too much of a political risk. After meeting with Amy and Wally, several other midwives called me and told me they felt that the couple was a poor psychological risk. They were extremely concerned that the couple would manifest serious complications during delivery.

I disagreed. The more I got to know Amy and Wally, the more convinced I was that everything was going to be fine. Many women are "working things through" in their post-cesarean pregnancies. Amy reminded me of myself "back when": thank goodness there had been someone who had enough faith in me to attend my birth. I believed with all my heart that this birth would not be a disaster, but a healing, and I told Amy and Wally that I would help them find skillful, willing care if we had to search the four corners of the earth.

We didn't even have to get to the corners. We found her in the middle of the United States, that is—a midwife who not only has attended more than two thousand births, but teaches other midwives as well. She believed that Amy was one of many "heavy birth casualties" in this culture and that she deserved to try. At the end of Amy's ninth month of pregnancy, despite pressure from other midwives, she flew to their state and awaited the onset of labor. I had called my dear friend who is a midwife and she agreed from the start to assist a primary midwife, so together we drove to the birth.

There is so much story to tell! Suffice to say that after three (fun, exhausting, connecting, difficult, wonderful, Soul-Searching, etc. etc.) full days and nights of active labor, Amy pushed Rachel (surprise! The doctor who insisted upon an ultrasound reported that both babies were definitely boys) into the world even as she held "breech baby A," Benjamin, in her arms. That beautiful picture is imprinted on my heart and soul; none of us who were there would have missed it for the world.

Wally and Amy worked very hard for this birth. Each difficult step along the way, each "rejection" was an opportunity for them to question, to reevaluate, to refocus, and to gain strength. I once heard it said that when the rug is pulled out from underneath us, we can learn to dance on a shifting carpet. This birth was an incredible experience and I mean INCREDIBLE. We are all grateful, awestruck, and delighted. In addition, we felt angry at an obstetrical system that would cut Amy open yet a third time, and frustrated that the fear that that system induces limits and influences so many midwives. By most standards, Amy was at least a "seven-point c-section"! Instead, she had two big, beautiful babies (almost fifteen pounds total!) a whole new view of herself and the world at large. ("Why not go out on a limb? That's where the fruit is." —Will Rogers.)

To Valerie El Halta, all I can say is WOW! To the other member of our "Dream Team," Heather Laier, what more can I say? As Khalil Gibran says, "Believing is one thing, doing is another." To Steffie Goodman, Emily Osgood, and Annie, my deepest respect and gratitude. To Nicholas and Damaris: you were super! To Leo: thanks for your graciousness. Lucian de Crescenzo once said, "We are each of us angels with only one wing. And we can fly only by embracing each other."

And to Amy and Wally: you taught us all, we taught each other. "The eyes that have tears belong to souls that have rainbows." Did you hear the rain that third night? There was a torrential downpour. And all was well.

(Moving) Forward

Now that you have read *Open Season* you may look at life a bit differently. In fact, watch out, giving birth and claiming all the insight into how powerful and capable and valuable a human being you are because you are a woman (emphasis on wom(b)) is extremely threatening to the balance of power in this world. Suddenly, or in some cases slowly, women are beginning to reach out of their drugged (by television, by public education, by over-the-counter drugs, by their births, and so on) comfort zones and are starting to grasp their full potential. They are making bold decisions that they never before would have dared to make. Like the woman many years ago, who returned recently purchased plums to the store: The plums were rotten. She had had a VBAC after two cesareans. She knew now she had a right and responsibility to speak up. She amazed herself with her new-found courage. She said, "I would never have dared to do such a thing before I birthed my third child. My life has been truly changed."

Awakened women choose the uncertainties of divorce over suffocating, denigrating marriages. They quit meaningless jobs. They explore their spirituality and some of the feminine roots of that spirituality that were pulled up long ago. They ask questions and require intelligent answers. They hold meetings where women can have a safe place to cry, laugh, scream, and share. They pursue life paths of healing—midwifery (underpaid, underappreciated, and often illegal), homeopathy, herbalism, and activism. They care and they act on it.

You know who you are and as I often say to women across this country, this earth, "I'm so glad you're there. Keep the presence. There are more of you coming. Keep the lights on."

Open Season, like *Silent Knife*, once read, will reap new energies from people. Many more "starfish" will be gently and lovingly rescued. I knew what *Open Season* said before I read it, because Nancy and I hear the "same" stories, read the "same" articles, shed the "same" tears, and hold the "same" women close to our hearts. We are truly kindred spirits. With six children, two husbands, and many miles between us, and oh so much work to do, Nancy and I have often both kidded, "Wouldn't it be nice if I had a clone?" Ah, Nancy, we fooled them again. We don't need their reproductive technology, we are the closest thing to clones that you can get and we did it naturally!

Yes, so much work to do! Haven't we tried to quit so many times? Why us? We are not alone. The number of people who care about this issue are growing and they come from many walks of life. But you're right, Nancy—it isn't happening fast enough. There seems to be a rapidly growing number of young women, ages twenty to thirty—about the age we were when we were knifed— who don't see it coming. Worse yet, they vehemently ask for it, whether it be the whole course—a cesarean, or just an appetizer—some demerol, forceps, an epidural, and so on. Well, because of this disturbing scenario something more has to happen. What is it going to take, a fifty-percent cesarean rate? I hope not.

Ten years ago, the concept of the Cesarean Prevention Movement, Inc. (CPM) was born at our first nationwide workshop on VBAC. It took a full year before I somewhat reluctantly took the reigns in hand and launched CPM with the publication of the first CLARION. By 1983 *Silent Knife* was out. And the old OB cesarean boat started rocking. We got the medical profession's attention. And the women, brought together and encouraged by *Silent Knife* and the CPM, began the work of changing the cesarean consciousness to a cesarean prevention consciousness. We need more of us. We are up against ignorance, apathy, and one of the biggest, wealthiest lobby groups in the United States.

Yes, something has to be done. So it seems quite fitting, although it wasn't planned, at least by us, just as *Open Season* goes to press that the CPM is about to go through a change, a change of image but not of philosophy or content. Thus the women of CPM are at this moment getting used to the feel and sound of the new name, the International Cesarean Awareness Network (ICAN). Why the change? Because of what I said before. We need more of us. No coopting is taking place. Just some smart marketing. The name CPM shocked people. It led them to ask questions like "Why would you want to prevent a cesarean? I thought they were done only if necessary." CPM brought together the dedicated, courageous few who were willing to do the work, often under less than desirable circumstances—seemingly not enough money, not enough time, not enough people, not enough support. But there was enough of all of that and more. And now my pioneer sisters, it's time to welcome our more timid, our more wary sisters into the fold. Perhaps our new name won't scare them off quite so often as our old one did. They will, however, most definitely get more than they bargained for. And let's give it to them with love in our hearts first and foremost. Many of them are freshly wounded, as we were. They are confused and scared. Some are very angry. Most are emotionally numb. As we continue to put holes in the OB cesarean boat, let us help our sisters ride the waves of labor with inner knowledge, faith, and courage.

Nancy, I think we are going to make it. We have to believe that, because if we didn't, we would quit. We are going to see that day when the circle of women is complete and strong again. We will be older and grayer than we are today, but we will see it. Because the women—the healers, the activists, the path finders are not giving up. As givers of life we hold a power and understanding that we have no intention of relinquishing without a fight. Compassion and love conquers all.

Esther B. Zorn
President, CPM/ICAN

Appendix 1: Values Clarification

(Please number each according to importance.)

Birth Experience

To have my partner present during the labor and birth

To have a medical doctor present

To be able to welcome the baby gently (dim light, warm room, etc.)

To labor and give birth in the same place

To feel at one with the energy, my partner, the attendants throughout the birth

To be in my own home

To be able to do what I choose

To be totally accepting of whatever may happen during labor and birth

To have minimum interference

To have the baby with me after the birth (no separation)

To be in quiet, peaceful surroundings

To have the ultimate in safety equipment

To feel at one with the energy, my partner, the attendants throughout the birth

To avoid pain

Wild card (write your own):

To maintain a spiritual perspective throughout the birth

To be in a birthing room in a hospital

To have an obstetrician present
To have a lay midwife present
To have other children present
To avoid pain
To have other supportive people present
To be in a birthing center
To have a nurse midwife present
Wild card (write your own):

Attendants

They will be available throughout the experience, but not interfere with us unless we ask them
They have a high regard for me and my partner's intuition and knowledge
They have much knowledge of complications and how to handle them
They maintain a spiritual perspective throughout the birth
They and we feel like friends rather than having a professional-patient relationship
They have much knowledge and experience with normal birth
They encourage our responsibility and will consult with us before doing anything
They charge a low fee
They can use drugs, do suturing, and have hospital privileges when needed
Wild card (write your own):

They will participate totally, tuned in to our feelings
They can be depended upon to do the right things, make decisions, and take over in an emergency
They will be with me during labor, birth, and if there are complications
Wild card (write your own):

We will repeat this exercise in a few weeks.

Adapted by Anne Frye from an exercise by Penny Camp. © Informed Homebirth.

Appendix 2: Addresses

National Cesarean Prevention Movement (and affiliates)
P.O. Box 152
Syracuse, NY 13210
315–424–1942

American Academy of Husband Coached Childbirth
P.O. Box 5224
Sherman Oaks, CA 91413
800–423–2397

American Foundation of Maternal and Child Health
30 Beekman Place
New York, NY 10022

American Society for Psychoprophylaxis in Obstetrics (ASPO)
1141 K St. N.W.
Washington, D.C. 20005

Compleat Mother magazine
P.O. Box 209
Minot, ND 58702
In Canada:
P.O. Box 399
Mildmay, Ontario N0G 2J0

C/SEC, Inc. (Cesarean/Support, Education and Concern)
22 Forest Rd.
Framingham, MA 01701
508–877–8266

Friends of Midwives (Massachusetts; write for affiliates)
P.O. Box 3188
Boston, MA 02130

Garden of Life Birth Center
(Specializing in natural birth and VBAC)
5460 Schaefer
Dearborn, MI 48126

Informed Homebirth
P.O. Box 3675
Ann Arbor, MI 48106

International Childbirth Education Association (ICEA)
P.O. Box 20048
Minneapolis, MN 55420

La Leche League International
9616 Minneapolis Ave.
Franklin Park, IL 60631

Midwifery Today
P.O. Box 2672–MP
Eugene, OR 97402

Midwives Alliance of North America
P.O. Box 1121
Bristol, VA 24203

Mothering Magazine
P.O. Box 8410
Santa Fe, NM 87504

NAPSAC
P.O. Box 267
Marble Hill, MO 63764

Nutrition Action Group (NAG)
Thomas Brewer, M.D.
66 High St.
Exeter, NH 03833
603–778–1476

Positive Pregnancy and Parenting Fitness
51 Saltrock Rd.

Baltic, CT 06330
203–822–8573

Stopping Hospital and Medical Errors (SHAME)
3701 Staunton Ave.
Charleston, WV 25304

VBAC Canada
8 Gilgorm Rd.
Toronto, Ontario M5N 2M5

Notes

Introduction

1. Linda Goodman, *Star Signs* (A *Practical Guide for the New Age*) (New York: St. Martin's Press, 1987), p. xxv.
2. Quote by Hugh Prather.
3. Poem by e.e. cummings.

Chapter 1

1. Story sent to me by Barbara Keeler, founder and director of Eagle Star, P.O. Box 62127, Colorado Springs, Colorado 80962. It was included in an article by Bob Welch. The source is unknown. Barbara says she has heard variations of it many times.
2. Grace Akinyi Ogot, "Educate a Woman and You Educate a Nation," *Boston Globe Magazine*, January 26, 1986, p. 54.
3. Alice Walker, *The Color Purple* (New York: Washington Square Press, 1982), p. 178.
4. Suzanne Arms, "Push, A Woman's Western" Impact Productions, 1725 B Seabright Avenue, Santa Cruz, California 95062.
5. Lewis Carroll, *Alice's Adventures in Wonderland and Through the Looking-Glass* (New York: Bantam Classic Edition, 1981), p. 156.
6. Kenneth Keyes, *The Hundredth Monkey* (Coos Bay, Oreg.: Vision Books, 1981), p. 18.
7. This is a line from a movie entitled *Marathon*. No other information is available.
8. Judith Herzfeld, *Sense and Sensibility in Childbirth* (New York: W. W. Norton, 1985), Dedication.

Chapter 2

1. Sue Roberts, "You Wonder Why Sometimes," *MAMA* (Mid-Hudson Area Maternity Alternatives), Vol. 2, No. 7 (Summer 1980): 4.
2. Kathleen Stocking, "The Rebirth of Home Birth," *Michigan: The Magazine of the Detroit News*, February 12, 1984, p. 18.
3. Quote by Harry S Truman.
4. Ginny Cassidy-Brinn et al., *Woman-Centered Pregnancy and Birth* (Pittsburgh: Cleis Press, 1984), p. 10.
5. Cesarean Prevention Movement of Southeast Florida, Coral Springs, Florida. From a conference brochure, February 22, 1990.
6. Nina McCain, "More Childbirth Control for Women Urged," *Boston Sunday Globe*, November 17, 1985, p. 46.
7. From a lecture on "The Art of Labor Support" given by midwife Janet Leigh in Boston, 1988.
8. Cassidy-Brinn, *Woman-Centered Pregnancy and Birth*, p. 9.

Chapter 3

1. Poem by Grantly Dick-Read in *Childbirth Wisdom*, (Goldsmith), p. 206.
2. "Scientific Theories Suggest a Light at the End of the Tunnel," *The Tarrytown Letter*, March 1982, p. 2.
3. From a lecture given by Sheila Kitzinger in Toronto in November 1984.
4. Gayle Peterson and Lewis Mehl, *Pregnancy as Healing*. Vol. 1 (Tucson, Arizona: MindBody Press, 1984), p. 28.
5. Beverly Beech, "The Politics of Maternity: Childbirth Freedom Vs. Obstetric Control" in Susan Edwards, ed., *Gender, Sex, and the Law* (London: Croom Helm Ltd., 1985), pp. 50–76.
6. Roy Masters, "What Is the Cause of Homosexuality?" *New Dimensions*, Grants Pass, Oregon, Special Issue, 1989, p. 55.
7. Fredelle Maynard, "The Emotional Highs of Successful Childbirth," *Woman's Day*, September 1, 1978, p. 70.
8. "Hunting Rare Animals Morally Wrong Act," *Needham Chronicle* (May 1988): 4.
9. The discussion on wildlife laws come from two pamphlets: "Abstracts of the Fish and Wildlife Laws" from the state of Massachusetts, Division of Fisheries and Wildlife, Saltonstall Building, Government Center, Boston 02202, 1985; and "Waterfowl Hunting Regulations," from the state of Minnesota, Department of Natural Resources, St. Paul, Minnesota 55146, 1986.
10. "Doctors of Deceit" *First Woman*, Vol. 1, No. 4 (April 1989): 1.
11. Ivan Illich. *Medical Nemesis*, p. 245.
12. Ibid.
13. "Doctors on the Defensive: A Nationwide Crisis," *Ladies' Home Journal*, April, 1986, p. 88.
14. James W. Prescott, "Body Pleasure and the Origins of Violence," *Bulletin of Atomic Scientists* (November 1975): 10–20.

15. From a seminar entitled The Awakening Heart, Insight Transformational Seminars, 2101 Wilshire Boulevard, Santa Monica, California 90403.

16. Tim Lowenstein, "Gentle Places and Quiet Spaces," Conscious Living Foundation, Vol. 2, No. 2 (Spring 1986): 2.

Chapter 4

1. Steven Wright, "I Have a Pony," Warner Brothers Records, Inc., Burbank, California 91510, 1985.

2. Merle Shaine, *Hearts That We Broke Long Ago* (New York: Bantam, 1983), p. 6.

3. Allan Parachini, "Cesarean Sections: Are There Too Many?" *Los Angeles Times*, November 19, 1987.

4. Carol Gentry, "Cesarean Births Rise, Especially in Florida," *St. Petersburg Times*, September 21, 1986, p. 6B.

5. Public Citizen Health Research Group, "Unnecessary Cesarean Sections: How to Cure a National Epidemic." Available for $15.00 from PCHRG, Dept. PR, 2000 P.St., NW, Rm. 700, Washington, DC 20036. See CISEC Newsletter, First Quarter, 1988 and CPM/VBAC Newsletter of Dallas, Texas. Winter/Spring 1988.

6. Available through the National Cesarean Prevention Movement, P.O. Box 152, Syracuse, New York 13210, August 1987.

7. Jack Pearson, "Cesarean Section and Perinatal Mortality," *American Journal of Obstetrics and Gynecology* Vol. 1, No. 48 (1984): 155.

8. Allan Parachini, "U.S. Maternal Death Rate May Be Wrong," *Boston Globe*, August 19, 1984.

9. Erik Eckholm, "Curbs Sought in Cesarean Deliveries," *New York Times*, August 11, 1986.

10. Colman McCarthy, "The Rise in Cesarean Childbirth," *Morning Call (PA)*, January 9, 1985.

11. Robert Schneider, *When to Say No to Surgery* (Englewood Cliffs, N.J.: Prentice-Hall, 1982), p. 42.

12. Report on the Consensus Development Conference on Cesarean Childbirth, U.S. Department of Health and Human Services, National Institutes of Health, Bethesda, Maryland, October 1981. Publication #82–2067.

13. Final Statement of the Panel from the National Consensus Conference on Aspects of Cesarean Birth, Department of Clinical Epidemiology and Biostatistics, Health Sciences Centre, Rm. 2C12A, McMaster University, 1200 Main St. W, Hamilton, Ontario, Canada L8N 3Z5, February 1986. Also see *Canadian Medical Journal*, Vol. 134, No. 12 (1986): 1348–1352.

14. Alan Otten, "Physicians Group Seeks to Lower High Rate of Cesarean Deliveries," *Wall Street Journal*, October 27, 1988.

15. Sonia Johnson, *Going Out of Our Minds: The Metaphysics of Liberation* (Freedom, Calif., Crossing Press, 1987), p. 125.

16. "M.D.'s Question Rising Cesarean Rate," *American Medical News*, January 18, 1985.

17. Alicia Blaisdell-Bannon. "Expectant Mom Gives C-Notes," *Cape Cod Times*, January 12, 1986.

18. "Going with the Odds" (Letter to the Editor) *Allentown (Pa.) Morning Call*, March 6, 1985.

19. Angela Barron McBride, "The American Way of Birth," in Margaret Kay, ed., *An Anthropology of Human Birth* (Philadelphia: F. A. Davis Co., 1982), p. 415.

20. Shirley Luthman, *Energy and Personal Power* (San Raphael, Calif.: Mehetabel & Co., 1982), p. 38.

21. From a number of letters I have received.

22. Barbara Katz Rothman, "The Meaning of Choice in Reproductive Technology," in *Test-Tube Women*, p. 25.

23. Richard Knox, "Surgery or Not? Study Finds Divergence in Massachusetts," *Boston Globe*, August 15, 1984, p. 1.

24. Ron Wilson, "Affluent Women More Likely to Have Cesareans Than Poor," *Wall Street Journal*, July 27, 1989, p. B4.

25. Ibid.

26. Ibid.

27. Gina Corea, "Childbirth 2000," *Omal*, V, no. 7 (April 1979): 107.

28. Constance Garcia-Barrio, "High-Tech Help for High-Risk Mothers," *American Baby*, September 1988, p. 45.

29. Chase Collins, "Random Voo Doo," *Ms. Magazine*, August 1977, pp. 59–65.

30. Lewis Wall, "Historical Note: Cesarean Section in Traditional Africa," *Resident and Staff Physician* (July 1984): 55–59.

31. Ibid.

32. Carolyn Kleefeld, *Climates of the Mind* (Los Angeles: Horse and Bird Press, 1979), p. 222.

33. Jane Butterfield English, *Different Doorway: Adventures of a Cesarean Born* (Point Reyes Station, Calif.: Earth Heart, 1985), p. 1.

34. Judith Goldsmith, p. 155.

35. English, *Different Doorway*, p. 3.

36. Ibid., p. 78.

37. Ibid., p. 139.

38. Ibid., p. 63.

39. Lynn Richards, From a Conscious Childbearing letter sent to me October 28, 1988, p. 3.

40. Ibid.

41. Carl Jones, Personal Communication, 1989. Also see *Birth Without Surgery: A Guide to Preventing Unnecessary Cesareans* (New York: Dodd, Mead, 1987).

42. Richards, p. 37.

43. Kimberly Wulfert, "The Psychophysiological Nature of Birth," *Positive Pregnancy Fitness Newsletter*, Vol. 1 (Winter 1988): 1.

44. Mecca, Cranley, et al., "Women's Perceptions of Vaginal and Cesarean Deliveries" *Nursing Research* 32 (No. 1 January/February 1983): 10–14.

45. Marilyn Moran, "Medically Unattended Home Birth Viewed As Positive Alternative" (Letter to the Editor), *NAPSAC News* (Fall 1977): 19.

46. Russ Rymer, "What You Hear Under the Knife," *Hippocrates* (May/June 1987): 100–102.

47. From a weekend seminar I attended presented by Bernie Siegel, M.D., in Boston, 1985.

48. Ibid.

49. Eleanor Trawick, "Teenage Oppression and Reproductive Rights," in *Test-Tube Women*, p. 131.

50. Poem by Patricia Newell, printed in the *Cesarean Prevention Clarion* 3, No. 2 (1985): 1.

51. Patricia Newell, "Secondary Infertility After Cesarean," *Cesarean Prevention Clarion*, 3, No. 2 (1985): 1.

52. Frank Kendig, "Keeping Them in Stitches," *Technology Illustrated* (July 1983): 55.

53. Laurie Colwin, *Another Marvelous Thing* (New York: Penguin Books, 1987), p. 101.

54. Mark Gerzon, *A Choice of Heroes: The Changing Face of American Manhood* (Boston: Houghton Mifflin, 1982), p. 208.

55. Colwin, *Another Wonderful Thing*, p. 115.

56. Barbara Katz Rothman, *Recreating Motherhood: Ideology and Technology in a Patriarchal Society* (New York: W. W. Norton, 1989).

57. Gerzon, *A Choice of Heroes*, p. 208.

58. Richards, p. 35.

59. Norma Benny in *Reclaim the Earth*, p. 141.

60. Michel Odent, *Birth Reborn* (New York: Pantheon Books, 1984), p. 102.

61. Leo Sorger, "The Art of Breech Delivery," *C/SEC Newsletter* 10, No. 1 (January 1984): 1.

62. Luthman. *Energy and Personal Power*, p. 30.

63. Cathy Romeo, "Visualization of Breech Reversal," *Positive Pregnancy Fitness Newsletter* 5, no. 2 (Fall/Winter 1989): 4.

64. Gloria Eng-Enorvac, "Baby Came Breech," *Compleat Mother* (Summer 1988): 18.

65. Richards, p. 89.

66. Margaret Catanese, "Vaginal Birth After Cesarean: Recommendations, Risks, Realities, and the Client's Right to Know," *Holistic Nursing Practitioner* (November 1987): 35–41.

67. Community Blue Ribbon Commission, Blackstone Valley, Rhode Island, April 29, 1985.

68. From a lecture given by Attorney Mark Mandell in Providence, Rhode Island in 1987.

69. "A Successful Program to Lower Cesarean Section Rates" *New England Journal of Medicine* 319 (December 8, 1988): 1511–1516.

70. Erik Erikson, *Ghandi's Truth: On the Origins of Military Non-Violence* (New York: W. W. Norton, 1969), p. 425.

71. Clark Norton, "Absolutely Not Confidential," *Hippocrates* 3, No. 2 (March/April 1989): 52.

72. Anne Finger, "Claiming All of Our Bodies: Reproductive Rights and Disabilities," in *Test-Tube Women*, p. 281.

73. Marsha Saxton, "Born and Unborn: The Implications of Reproductive Technologies for People with Disabilities," in *Test-Tube Women*, p. 298.

74. Ibid., p. 307.

75. Goldstein, p. 110.

76. Boston Women's Health Book Collective, *The New Our Bodies, Our Selves* (New York: Simon & Schuster, 1984), p. 7.

77. Trudy Keller, "Teaching Cesarean Birth in Standard Childbirth Classes," *C/SEC Newsletter* 15, No. 1 (1989): 1.

78. Richard Graham, *American Journal of Obstetrics and Gynecology*, May 1, 1984.

79. Paul Starr, *The Social Transformation of American Medicine: The Rise of a Sovereign Profession and the Making of a Vast Industry* (New York: Basic Books, 1982), p. 9.

80. Jay Katz, *The Silent World of Doctor and Patient* (New York: Free Press, 1984), p. 41.

81. Starr, *The Social Transformation of American Medicine*, p. 28.

82. Stanley Gross, "The Myth of Professional Licensing," *American Psychologist* 33, No. 11 (1978).

83. Virginia Lubell, "Is There a Better Way?" Unpublished Manuscript sent to me in March 1990.

84. Katz, *The Silent World of Doctor and Patient* (New York: Free Press, 1984), p. 83.

85. Robert Howard, in *Genesis* (Newsletter for the American Society for Psychoprophylaxis in Obstetrics), 1411 K. Street N.W., Suite 200, Washington, D.C. 20005, April/ May 1983, p. 15.

86. Katz, *The Silent World*, p. 51.

87. Goldstein, p. xi.

88. Thanks to Alison Rausch for providing these anecdotes.

89. Margery Eagan, "Midwifery Bears Fruits of Labor," *Boston Herald*, February 2, 1989.

90. Richard Moskowitz, "The Great Malpractice Scandal," *The Santa Fe Reporter*, April 16, 1981, p. 15. Also see Moskowitz, Dick "Healing the Malpractice Crisis," *Mothering Magazine*, Winter, 1989, p. 27.

91. Ibid., p. 16.

92. Ibid.

93. From personal correspondence, 1989.

94. Ibid.

95. Ibid.

96. Esther Rome, "How to Prevent Unnecessary Cesarean," *Middlesex News*, November 23, 1987.

97. Leslie Belay, personal communication, May 1990. Co-editor of *Midwifery Advocate*, P.O. Box 237, Newtonville, Mass. 02160.

98. Doris Haire, "A Forum on Malpractice Issues in Childbirth Proceedings," in Diony Young, ed., International Childbirth Education Association, Minneapolis, Minnesota, 1985. pp. 14, 15.

99. "Doctor Proposes No Fault Insurance to Help Reduce Medical Malpractice Suits," *Boston Globe*, February 20, 1986, p. 76.

100. David Stewart, and Lee Stewart, "A Forum on Malpractice Issues in Childbirth Proceedings," in Diony Young, ed. International Childbirth Education Association, Minneapolis, Minnesota, 1985, 35, 36.

101. Ibid.

102. Steven Goode, "Cesarean Sanction." *Insight*, June 22, 1987, p. 58.

103. George Annas, "Forced Cesarean: The Most Unkindest Cut of All." *The Hastings Center Report*, June 1982, p. 16.

104. Goode, "Cesarean Sanction."

105. Annas, "Forced Cesarean."

106. Ibid.

107. Ibid.

108. Ibid.

109. Ibid.

110. Ibid.

111. Alan Dershowitz, "Mothers Vs. Babies' Rights," *Boston Herald*, May 10, 1988.

112. Brenda Coleman, "Doctors Warned on Courts," *Sun Sentinel* (Fla.), March 6, 1988.

113. Bridgett Jordan, "Court Ordered Cesareans: An Ethical Dilemma," *National Cesarean Prevention Movement Newsletter, The Clarion* 5, No. 3, (1987): 1.

114. This case was discussed at a lecture entitled "Politics of Childbirth Series: Court-Ordered Cesarean Sections," Boston, March 8, 1989. Sponsored by the Massachusetts Friends of Midwives.

115. Robbie Davis-Floyd, "Birth as an American Rite of Passage," in Karen Michaelson, ed., *Childbirth in America: Anthropological Perspectives* (South Hadley, Mass.: Bergin & Garvey, 1988), p. 153.

116. Ibid.

117. This quote appeared in midwife Nan Ullricke Koehler's *Artemis College Newsletter*, 131 Frati Lane, Sebastopol, California 95472, April 1990.

Chapter 6

1. Heather's letter appeared in the *VBAC of Toronto Newsletter* (Fall 1987).

2. Thomas Kuhn, "Scientific Theories Suggest a Light at the End of the Tunnel," *The Tarrytown Letter*, March 1982, p. 16.

3. Ibid.

4. Ibid.

5. Ibid.

6. Letty Cottin Pogrebin, *Growing Up Free* (New York: Bantam, 1981), p. 542.

7. Lynn Richards, *The Vaginal Birth After Cesarean Experience* (South Hadley, Mass.: Bergin & Garvey, 1988), p. 25.

8. Judy Herzfeld, *Sense and Sensibility in Childbirth: A Guide to Supportive Obstetrical Care* (New York: W. W. Norton, 1985), p. 129.

9. Carolyn Kleefeld. See chapter 4, note 32.

10. Samuel Thomson in Katz, p. 37.

11. Perri Klaus, "Bearing a Child in Medical School," *New York Times Magazine*, November 11, 1984.

12. Antoine de St. Exupery, *The Little Prince* (New York: Harcourt, Brace & World, 1943), p. 17.

13. Ann Frye, *Understanding Lab Work in the Childbearing Years*, Informed Homebirth, (New Haven, Conn.) 1985 (1990 edition will be available through CPM). Robin Blatt, *Prenatal Testing* (New York: Vintage Books, 1988).

14. Judith Goldsmith, *Childbirth Wisdom from the World's Oldest Societies* (New York: Cogdon Weed, 1984), p. 7.

15. Sharon Stephenson, and David Weaver, "Prenatal Diagnosis—A Compilation

of Diagnosed Conditions," *American Journal of Obstetrics and Gynecology* 141 (1981): 319.

16. Barry Seigel, "The Promise and Problems of Prenatal Testing," *American Baby*, November 1987, pp. 95–101.

17. Gina Corea, "Childbirth 2000," *Omni* 7, No. 1 (April 1979): 50.

18. Constance Barrio-Garcia, "PUBS—A New Prenatal Test," *American Baby*. July 1987, pp. 49–51.

19. Gina Kolata, "First Trimester Prenatal Diagnosis," *Science* 221 (September 9, 1983): 1031.

20. Barrio-Garcia, "PUBS."

21. Ibid.

22. "New Test May Rival Amniocentesis," *Ladies' Home Journal*, 1985, p. 56.

23. Barry Seigel, pp. 95–101.

24. Gina Kolata, "Ethical Issues in Prenatal Diagnosis: Mass Screening for Neural Tube Defects," Hastings Center Report, December 1980, p. 8.

25. Marjorie Sun, "FDA Draws Criticism on Prenatal Test," *Science* 221 (July 1983): 440–442.

26. "Unnecessary Hospital Testing: A New Study," *McCall's*, March 1986, p. 73.

27. Matt Clarke, et al., "Questions About the Pap Test," *Newsweek on Health*, Spring 1988, p. 8.

28. Mary Spletter, "Just Testing: Common Medical Tests Yield Mixed Results," *Hippocrates*, (May/June 1987): 86–90.

29. Moira Longo, "All Those Lab Tests," *Great Expectations*, (Spring 1985): 2

30. Barrio-Garcia, "PUBS."

31. Peter T. Rowley, "Genetic Screening: Marvel or Menace?," *Science* 225 (July 13, 1984): 138.

32. "Prefers Nipple Stimulation for Antepartum Testing," *Obstetrics/Gynecology News*, August 25, 1985.

33. R. Lenke and J. Nemes "Use of Nipple Stimulation for Contraction Stress Test," *Obstetrics/Gynecology* 63 (1984): 345.

34. Margery Eagan, "A Test About Just Who We Are," *Boston Herald*, March 3, 1988, p. 10.

35. Barbara Katz Rothman, *The Tentative Pregnancy: Prenatal Diagnosis and the Future of Motherhood* (New York: Viking Penguin, 1987).

36. M. Eagan, "A Test About Just Who We Are."

37. Barbara Katz Rothman, *The Tentative Pregnancy.*

38. "Are We Hooked on Tests?" *Health and Nutrition: News & World Report*, Washington, D.C., 1988.

39. John Robbins, *Diet for a New America* (Walpole, N.H.: Stillpoint Publishing, 1987.).

40. From personal correspondences, 1985–1988.

41. Ibid.

42. Goldsmith, p. 141.

43. Nancy Hatch Woodward, "Obstetricians and Nutrition," *Tampa Tribune*, February 2, 1986.

44. Personal Correspondence.

45. Ibid.

46. Ibid.

47. From the *Nutrition Action Group Newsletter*, March 6, 1987.

48. Eugenia Allen, "Medical Update: Even Moderate Amounts of Alcohol Cause Smaller Babies," *American Baby*, April 3, 1989, p. 123. Barry Zuckerman, "Alcohol Use During Pregnancy," *Boston Parents' Paper*, September 1986, p. 3.

49. Sent to me in a letter from 1989. No source available.

50. Nan Ullricke Koehler, *Artemis Speaks*, 13140 Frati Lane, Sebastopol, California 95472.

51. Ivan Illich. *Medical Nemesis*, p. 155.

52. Ibid., p. 106.

53. Suzanne Arms, *Immaculate Deception: A New Look at Childbirth* (South Hadley, Mass.: Bergin & Garvey, 1984).

54. Goldsmith, p. 194.

55. Ibid., p. 46.

56. Ruth Hubbard, "Personal Courage Is not Enough: Some Hazards of Childbearing in the 1980s," in Rita Arditti, Renatti Klein, and Shelly Minden, eds. *Test-Tube Women* (Boston: Pandora Press, 1984), p. 338.

57. Rita Baron Faust, "Why Doctors Mistreat Women," *Redbook*, May 1989, p. 193.

58. Ruth Holland, and Jill McKenna, "Regaining Trust" in Arditti et al., eds., *Test-Tube Women*, p. 414.

59. Jay Katz, *The Silent World of Doctor and Patient*, (New York: Free Press, 1984), p. 97.

60. Maureen Ritchie, "Taking the Initiative: Information Vs. Technology in Pregnancy," in Arditti, et al., eds., *Test-Tube Women*, p. 402.

61. Janice Raymond, "Feminist Ethics, Ecology, and Vision," in Arditti et al., eds., *Test-Tube Women*, p. 435.

62. Corea. "Childbirth 2000," p. 104.

63. Joseph Bruchac, "Long Memory," The Dance Free Press, P.O. Box 225, North Billerica, Massachusetts 01862, Vol. 3, No. 2, Summer 1987.

64. Diana Tonnessen, "Epidurals," *American Baby*, March 1990, p. 5.

65. Christine McCarthy Smith, "Epidural Anesthesia in Labor," *Journal of Gynecological Nursing* (January/February 1984): 17–21.

66. Tonnessen, "Epidurals."

67. "FDA Cites Danger in Childbirth Anesthetic," *Boston Globe*, August 24, 1983, p. 17.

68. Ann Murray, "Effects of Epidural Anesthesia on Newborns and Their Mothers," *Childbirth Development*, Society for Research in Child Development, Inc., Foundation 41, The Woman's Hospital, Sydney, Australia, Vol. 52, pp. 71–82.

69. Ibid., p. 78.

70. Murray, Ann, et al., p. 81.

71. Michele Odent, *Birth Reborn* (New York: Pantheon Books, 1984), p. 17.

72. Illich, *Medical Nemesis*, p. 144.

73. Judith Nolte, "The Boomerang Effect," *American Baby*, March 1990, p. 4.

74. Illich, *Medical Nemesis*, p. 145.

75. "Now That You're in Labor," *American Baby*, April 1987, p. 12.

76. Laurie Nadel, "The Touch That Heals," *American Baby*, April 1987.

77. Doris Haire, "Drugs in Labor and Birth," *Childbirth Educator*, Spring 1987.

78. Illich, p. 44.

79. From a conference entitled "Birth as Perinatal Continuum," Escalen (California),

1980. See also "Being Born," 1983—CBC Transcripts, P.O. Box 500, Station "A," Toronto, Ontario, Canada M5W 1E6.

80. Arms, *Immaculate Deception*.

81. "Do-It-Yourself Anesthetic," *Cosmopolitan*, November 1989.

82. "Manufacturer Pulls Bendectin Off Market," National Women's Health Network, P.O. Box 5055, FDR Station, New York, New York, 10105. July/August 1983, p. 8.

83. Ibid.

84. Peter Gosselin, "FDA Admits Delay in Seizing Devices," *Boston Globe*, February 26, 1990.

85. Herzfeld, *Sense and Sensibility*, p. 49.

86. Ritchie, "Taking the Initiative," p. 409.

87. Scarlett Pollack, "Refusing to Take Women Seriously," in Arditti et al., eds., *Test-Tube Women*, p. 145.

88. From a telephone conversation in 1988. Also see Jones *Birth Without Surgery: A Guide to Preventing Unnecessary Cesareans* (New York: Dodd Mead, 1987).

89. Corea, "Childbirth 2000," p. 106.

90. Ibid.

91. E. A. Friedman, "The Obstetrician's Dilemma: How Much Fetal Monitoring and Cesarean Section Is Enough?," *New England Journal of Medicine*, 315, No. 10 (1986): 641–643.

92. Kenneth Leveno, et al. "Fetal Monitoring," *New England Journal of Medicine* 315, No. 10 (1986): 615–619.

93. Dolores Kong, "Doubts Raised Over Fetal Monitor," *Boston Globe*, March 1, 1990, p. 1.

94. Myra Gerzon Gilfix, "EFM, Informed Consent, and Malpractice," *ICEA News* 24, No. 3 (August 1985).

95. "Fetal Heart Monitors," *SMAPSAC Newsletter*, No. 7, January 1986.

96. G. S. Sykes, "Fetal Distress and the Condition of Newborn Infants," *British Medical Journal* 287, No. 6397 (October 1, 1983): 941.

97. "ACOG: EFM Equal to Auscultation," *C/SEC Newsletter* Vol. 15 # 1, 1st Quarter 1989.

98. "Items in the News," *Transitions* (Newsletter of the CPM of S.E. Minnesota) Vol. 7 #1, April 1990.

99. "Monitors: More Harm Than Help." *American Baby* (November 1986) p. 32.

100. Jurgen Morgenstern, "A Device for Continuously Measuring the Rotation of the Fetal Head," *American Journal of Obstetrics and Gynecology* (November 15, 1984): 798.

101. Lauren Wolf, "Tens—A New Alternative," *Cesarean Birth Update* 9, No. 5, (November 1985): 9.

102. *V.D.T. News* (Microwave News), Box 1799, Grand Central Station, New York, 10163. Elaine Clift, "VDT's Can Bring on Medical Problems," *New Directions for Women* 18, No.4 (July/August 1989).

103. "Childbirth Hype: Don't Be a Victim," *Woman's Day*, April 1988.

104. "Everything You Always Wanted to know About Pregnancy," *Cosmopolitan*, February, 1986.

105. "Positive Episiotomy" (Letter to the Editor), *American Baby*, February 1987, p. 12.

106. Diana Korte "What Doctors Don't Tell You," *Parade Magazine*, July 7, 1985, p. 13.

107. "Episiotomy," *Childbirth Educator,* Spring 1989, p. 46.

108. Nancy Perry, "How Safe Is Episiotomy and Second Stage Forced Pushing?," *CENMASAC Newsletter* 1, No. 3 (March 1985).

109. *Compleat Mother,* Spring 1986, p. 7.

110. R. F. Harrison, et al., "Is Routine Episiotomy Necessary?," *British Medical Journal* 288, No. 6435 June 30, 1984: 1971.

111. Sandra Dowie, "Birth Without Episiotomy: Cutting Out the Unkindest Cut of All," *Medical Self Care,* p. 56.

112. "Milestones," *Childbirth Educator* (Spring 1982): 54.

113. Tom Verny, in "Being Born," CBC Transcripts, P.O. Box 500, Station "A," Toronto, Ontario, Canada M5W 1E6. See also Verny's book *Secret Life of the Unborn Child* (New York: Summit Books, 1981).

114. Diane Mason, "The Facts About Forceps," *American Baby,* March 1985 p. 77.

115. Odent, *Birth Reborn,* p. 98.

116. P. E. Treffers, University of Amsterdam, February 22, 1984. Personal correspondence.

117. "New Hep-Lock PF," ESI Elkins-Sinn Inc., Cherry Hill, New Jersey. Readers' Service Card no. 8.

118. Laurie Colwin, *Another Marvelous Thing* (New York: Penguin Books, 1987), p. 104.

119. Goldsmith, p. 143.

120. J. P. Lenihan, Jr., "Relationship of Antepartum Pelvic Examinations to Premature Rupture of the Membrane," *Obstetrics/Gynecology* 83 (1984): 33–36.

121. Dave Barry, "A Long Over-due Look at Natural Childbirth," In Nan Koehler, ed. *Artemis Speaks* (1985), p. 424.

122. Goldsmith, p. 60.

123. Ibid.

124. Goldsmith, p. 77.

125. Shay Huffman, "Ancient-New Method of Cord Care," *CENMASAC Newsletter* 3, No. 3 (March 1987): 1–4.

126. Ibid.

127. Goldsmith, p. 77.

128. *Compleat Mother* (Summer 1988): 33.

129. Alice Martin, "Can Ultrasound Cause Genetic Damage?" *Journal of Clinical Ultrasound* 12 (January 1984): 11–20.

130. Robin Mole, "Possible Hazards of Imaging and Doppler Ultrasound in Obstetrics," Royal Society of Medicine: Forum on Maternity and the Newborn: Ultrasonography in Obstetrics, Birth, Special Supplement, Vol. 13,(December 1986): pp. 23–33.

131. Doris Haire, "Fetal Effects of Ultrasound: A Growing Controversy," *Journal of Nurse-Midwifery* 29, No. 4 (July/August 1984): 241–246.

132. I. Peterson, "Ultrasound Safety and Collapsing Bubbles," *Science News* 130 (December 13, 1986): 372.

133. "Fetal Effects of Ultrasound," Cable News Network, April, 1982.

134. "Sesame Street Baby," *American Baby,* May 1989, p. 12.

135. "Vacuum Extraction," *Childbirth Educator* (Spring 1984): 13.

136. A. Vacca and A. Grant, "A Randomized Controlled Study to Compare Vacuum Extraction with Forceps Delivery," VIIIth European Congress of Perinatal Medicine 15, No. 4–6, August 1983.

137. *News West* (Massachusetts) 3, No. 50 (May 11, 1988).

138. Goldsmith, p. 48

139. Pamela Summey, and Marsha Hurst, "The Making of an Obstetrician," *Childbirth Educator* (Spring 1984): 14.

140. "Questions an Obstetrician Is Most Asked," *Cosmopolitan*, February 1986, p. 178.

141. Hugo Lagercrantz and Theodore Slotkin "The 'Stress' of Being Born." *Scientific American* (April 1976): 100–107.

142. Ibid.

143. Ibid.

144. Goldsmith, p. 162.

145. Ibid., p. 67.

146. Ibid., p. 121.

147. Barbara Williams, "PKU: Do You Have a Choice?," *Mothering*, 34 (Winter 1985): 59.

148. Jonathan Coe, "The Crime of Circumcision," Center for Orgonomic Education, P.O. Box 383, Careywood, Idaho 83809. For information on this reprint, write Newborn Rights Society, Box 0048, St. Peters, Pennsylvania 19470.

149. *Compleat Mother* (1986): 7.

150. Ann Briggs, *Circumcision: What Every Parent Should Know* (Earlysville, Va.: Birth & Parenting Publishers, 1985).

151. Rosemary Romberg, *Circumcision: The Painful Dilemma* (South Hadley, Mass.: Bergin & Garvey, 1985). Wallerstein, ed. *Circumcision: An American Health Fallacy* Springer Series: Focus on Men Vol. 1, James Hennessey, ed. (New York: Springer Publishing Co. 1980).

152. Michel Odent, in "Being Born," CBC Transcripts, P.O. Box 500, Station "A," Toronto, Ontario M5W1E6.

153. Daniel Grossman, "Neo-Luddites: Don't Just Say Yes to Technology," *Utne Reader* (March/April 1990): 44.

154. Langdon Winner, "Missionaries in Lab Coats—Technology as the Modern Religion," *Utne Reader* (March/April 1990): 48.

155. Shirley Luthman, *Energy and Personal Power* (San Raphael, Calif.: Mehetabel & Co., 1982).

156. Sonia Johnson, *Going Out of Our Minds: The Metaphysics of Liberation* (Freedom, Calif.: Crossing Press, 1987), p. 9.

157. Rita Arditti, Renate Duelli Klein, and Shelley Minden, eds., *Test-Tube Women: What Future for Motherhood?* (Boston: Pandora Press, 1984).

158. Goldsmith, p. 192.

159. Sara Sloan, "Seven Steps to Stagnation," *Nutritional Parenting*. New Canaan, Conn.: Keats Publishing Co., 1982, p. 21.

160. Mary Sharpe, "Being Born," CBC Transcripts, P.O. Box 500, Station "A," Toronto, Ontario, Canada M5W 1E6.

161. Harriet Lerner, *The Dance of Anger* (New York: Harper & Row, 1985), p. 125.

162. Boston Women's Health Book Collective *The New Our Bodies Our Selves* (New York: Simon & Schuster, 1984), p. 99.

163. Herzfeld, *Sense and Sensibility*, p. 66.

164. Luthman, *Energy and Personal Power*, p. 146.

165. Bob Mandel, *Open Heart Therapy* (Berkeley, Calif.: Celestial Arts, 1984).

166. Goldsmith, p. 115

167. Matt Clark, "The Cultures of Medicine: Why Doctors and Treatments Differ the World Over."

168. "Childbirth in New Zealand," (a three-part report on childbirth in New Zealand), *Listen and TV Times* March 12–26, 1990.

169. Goldsmith, p. 201.

170. Ibid., p. 72.

171. Ibid., p. 133.

Chapter 7

1. Andrea Szmyt and Herb Pearce, Workshops and Support Groups, P.O. Box 134, Cambridge, Massachusetts 02140.

2. Linda Leonard, *The Wounded Woman* (Boulder, Colo.: Shambala, 1983) p. 3.

3. Thomas Kuhn, "Scientific Theories Suggest a Light at the End of the Tunnel," *The Tarrytown Letter,* March 1982, p. 18.

4. Robert Johnson, *She: Understanding Feminine Psychology* (King of Prussia, Pa.: Religious Publishing Co., 1976).

5. Ibid.

6. James Prescott, "Body Pleasures and the Origins of Violence," *Bulletin of the Atomic Scientist* (November 1975): 10–20.

7. Ibid., p. 18.

8. Ibid., p. 17.

9. Boston Women's Health Book Collective, *The New Our Bodies, Our Selves* (New York: Simon & Schuster, 1984), p. 103.

10. Ibid., pp. 27–28.

11. Phyllis Chesler, *Mothers on Trial* (New York: McGraw-Hill, 1986), p. 404.

12. Phil Donahue, *The Human Animal* (New York: Woodward/White (Simon & Schuster), 1985), p. 297.

13. Ibid., p. 226.

14. Audrey Allen Tracey, "Childbirth and Ethical Issues Raised," Boston, August 5, 1987, p. 5.

15. Chesler, *Mothers on Trial*, p. 232.

16. Kate Millet, *Sexual Politics* (New York: Doubleday & Co., 1970), pp. 31, 45.

17. Mark Gerzon, *A Choice of Heroes: The Changing Face of American Manhood* (Boston: Houghton Mifflin, 1982), p. 21.

18. Ibid., p. 31.

19. Gwynne Dyer, *War* (New York: Crown Publishers, 1985).

20. Gerzon, *A Choice of Heroes*, p. 55.

21. Ibid., p. 63.

22. Ibid., p. 69.

23. Ibid., p. 205.

24. Ibid., p. 71.

25. Ibid., p. 236.

26. Ibid., p. 83.

27. Ibid.

28. Letty Cottin Pogrebin, *Growing Up Free* (New York: Bantam, 1981) p. 543.

29. Rita Baron-Faust, "Why Doctors Mistreat Women," *Redbook*, May 1989, p. 195.

30. Gerzon, *A Choice of Heroes*, p. 144.

31. Ibid., p. 149.

32. Ibid., p. 235.

33. Ibid., p. 203.

34. Ibid., p. 143.

35. Cathy Perlmutter, "Women Doctors Speak Out," September 1983, pp. 27-32.

36. Anne Schaef *Woman's Reality* (Minneapolis: Winston Press, 1981), Chapter 1: "Fitting In: The WMS and the Other Systems in Our Culture," pp. 1–20.

37. Ibid.

38. Ibid., p. ii.

39. Ibid., p. iv.

40. Ibid., Chapter 2: "The Original Sin of Being Born Female," pp. 23–50.

41. Ibid.

42. Harriet Lerner, *The Dance of Anger* (New York: Harper & Row, 1985), pp. 1–3.

43. Phyllis Chesler, *Mothers on Trial* (New York: McGraw Hill, 1986) p. 233.

44. Ibid., pp. 113–118.

45. Ibid., p. 128.

46. Schaef, *Woman's Reality*, p. 100.

47. From a talk by Sheila Kitzinger called "The Sexuality of Birth" given at Mercy College in Detroit, May 2, 1986. Reported by *Compleat Mother*, Fall 1986.

48. Schaef, *Woman's Reality*, from Chapter 5: "The FS and the WMS: New Ways of Looking at Our Culture," pp. 100–145.

49. Ibid., p. 132.

50. Ibid., pp. 100–145.

51. Ibid., p. 142.

52. Howard S. Levy, *Chinese Footbinding: The History of a Curious Erotic Custom* (New York: Bell Publishing Co. 1967), p. 16.

53. Ibid., p. 23.

54. Ibid., p. 34.

55. Ibid., p. 71.

56. Ibid., p. 83.

57. Sonia Johnson, *Going Out of Our Minds: The Metaphysics of Liberation* (Freedom, Calif.: Crossing Press, 1987), pp. i–iii.

58. Ibid.

59. Ibid.

60. Ibid.

61. Ibid.

62. Ibid., p. 25.

63. Ibid.

64. Ibid., p. 28.

65. Ibid., p. 44.

66. Ibid.

67. Linda Leonard, *The Wounded Woman* (Boulder, Colo.: Shambala, 1983), p. 11.

68. Ibid., p. 164.

69. Thomas Kuhn, "Scientific Theories Suggest a Light at the End of the Tunnel," *The Tarrytown Letter*, March 1982.

70. Gerzon, *A Choice of Heroes*, p. 238.

71. Betty Friedan, "How To Get the Woman's Movement Moving Again," *New York Times*, November 3, 1985, sec. 4, p. 25.

72. Leonie Caldecott and Stephanie Leland, eds., *Reclaim the Earth: Women Speak Out for Life on Earth* (London: Women's Press, 1983), p. 17.

73. Source unknown.

74. Donahue, *The Human Animal*, p. 224.

75. Ibid., p. 231.

76. Gerzon, *A Choice of Heroes*, p. 163 (quote by John Irving).

77. Ibid., p. 119.

78. Norma Benney, "All of One Flesh," Caldecott and Leland, eds., in *Reclaim the Earth*.

79. Donahue, *The Human Animal*, p. 329.

80. Caldecott and Leland, *Reclaim the Earth*, p. 7.

81. Chris Thomas, "Alternative Technology: A Feminist Technology?" in Caldecott and Leland, eds., *Reclaim the Earth*.

82. Ibid., p. 165.

83. Robert Johnson, *She: Understanding Feminine Psychology* (King of Prussia, Pa.: Religious Publishing Co., 1976), p. 75.

Chapter 8

1. Ivan Illich, *Medical Nemesis*, p. 254.

2. Claudia Wallis, "Re-examining the 36-Hour Day," *Time* August 31, 1987, pp. 54–55.

3. Ibid.

4. Stephen Hall, "The Initiation," *Hippocrates* (July/August 1987): 52–61.

5. Wallis, "Re-examining the 36-Hour Day," p. 54.

6. Elwyn Chamberlain, *Gates of Fire* (New York: Random House, 1978), p. 41.

7. Hall, "The Initiation," p. 53.

8. Jay Katz, *The Silent World of Doctor and Patient* (New York: Free Press, 1984), p. 88.

9. Paul Starr, *The Social Transformation of American Medicine: The Rise of a Sovereign Profession and the Making of a Vast Industry* (New York: Basic Books, 1982).

10. Illich, *Medical Nemesis*, p. 29.

11. Ibid., p. 29.

12. Ibid., p. 32.

13. Ibid., p. 99.

14. Ibid., p. 39.

15. Ibid., p. 80.

16. Ibid., p. 80.

17. Ibid., p. 79.

18. Nancy Gibbs, "Sick and Tired," *Time*, July 31, 1989, pp. 48–53.

19. Wallis, "Re-Examining the 36-hour Day," p. 54.

20. Ann Landers, *Boston Globe*, February 20, 1986, p. 71.

21. Wallis, "Re-Examining the 36-Hour Day," p. 54.

22. "Radical Surgery: The Day the MD's Went on Strike," (Philadelphia: Koren Publications, 1987).

23. *Compleat Mother*, (Fall 1986); *Journal of the American Medical Association* 255, No. 6 (February 14, 1986): 806; and *CENMASAC News* 2, No. 3 (March 1968).

24. Illich, *Medical Nemesis*, p. 146.

25. Ibid., p. 275.

26. Ibid., p. 112.

27. Katz, *The Silent World*, p. 37.

28. Martha Weinman Lear, "Down with High-Handed Health Care!," *Woman's Day*, February 7, 1984, "Back Page."

29. Ibid.

30. Doris Haire, "Improving the Outcome of Pregnancy Through Increased Utilization of Midwives," *Journal of Nurse Midwifery*, 26, No. 1 (February 1981).

31. Katz, *The Silent World*, p. xiv.

32. Ibid.

33. Ibid., p. xvii.

34. Ibid., p. 46.

35. Ibid., p. 51.

36. Ibid., p. 83.

37. Ibid., p. 98.

38. Ibid.

39. Ibid., p. 99.

40. Ibid., p. 101.

41. Ibid., p. 126.

42. Perri Klass, "What Should a Doctor Tell a Patient?," *Discover* (October 1985): 20–21.

43. Katz, *The Silent World*, p. 96.

44. Ibid., p. 101.

45. From a lecture given by midwife Janet Leigh in Boston in 1986.

46. Rita Baron-Faust, "Why Doctors Mistreat Women," *Redbook*, May 1989, p. 114.

47. Ibid., p. 115.

48. Ibid.

49. From a lecture by Bernie Siegel given in Boston in 1984.

50. Gerald Bullock, *Apologies of a Reformed Obstetrician*. Unpublished manuscript.

51. David Hilfiker, "Facing Our Mistakes," *New England Journal of Medicine* (January 12, 1984), p. 10.

52. Ibid., p. 11.

53. Carol Cassell, *Swept Away* (New York: Fireside [Simon & Schuster], 1984), p. 25.

54. Cathy Perlmutter, "Women Doctors Speak Out," *Spring* (September 1983): 27–32.

55. Ibid.

56. Ibid.

57. Ibid.

58. Perri Klass, *A Not Entirely Benign Procedure: Four Years as a Medical Student*, G. P. Putnam's Sons, New York, New York, 1987, pp. 48–49.

59. Diane White, "Tootsie Awards," *Boston Globe*, January 22, 1983, p. 7.

60. Kenneth Keyes, *The Hundredth Monkey* (Coos Bay, Ore.: Vision Books, 1981), p. 126.

61. From Santi Bhakti, *Love, Peace*. Edited by Jacob Trapp. UU, 1971.

Chapter 9

1. Cris Williamson, "The Changer and the Changed," Olivia Records, Inc., Oakland, California, 1975.

2. "Midwife Profile: Fran Ventre," *The Midwife Advocate: Massachusetts Friends of Midwives* 2, No. 3 (Autumn 1985): 5.

3. "An Interview with Raven Lang," *The Doula: A Magazine for Mothers* 1, N. 4 (Spring/Summer 1986): 2–12.

4. Ibid.

5. Ruth Watson Lubic, "Insights from Life in the Trenches," *Nursing Outlook* (March/April 1988): 64.

6. Janet Jennings, "Who Controls Childbirth?" *Radical Science Journal* (London, 1982): 2–16.

7. From *Excerpta Medica* International Congress Series No. 412. International definition of "midwife" as accepted by the World Health Organization. Proceedings of the VIII World Congress of Ob/Gyn, Mexico City, October 1976.

8. Judith Goldsmith, *Childhood Wisdom from the World's Oldest Societies* (New York: Congden & Weed, 1984), p. 48.

9. Endesha Holland, "Granny Midwives," *Ms.* (June 1987): 51.

10. Bev Eaton, "Midwives Make a Comeback: The Search for the Personal Touch," *Hartford Courant*, Section E, March 1988, p. 1.

11. Jutta Mason, "Reflections on the Alternative Birth Culture: Does Professional Midwifery Pose a Problem?" Also, "The Dangers of Professional Midwifery." For reprints, send $3.00 to 242 Havelock St., Toronto M6H 3139

12. Sally Inch, *Birth Rights: What Every Parent Should Know About Childbirth in Hospitals* (New York: Pantheon, 1984), p. 178.

13. Laurie Friedman, "Why I Left BCH," *The Midwife Advocate* 5, no. 1 (Spring 1988): 1.

14. Judith Hoch Smith, and Anita Spring, eds., *Women in Ritual and Symbolic Roles* (New York: Plenum Publishers, 1978), p. 130.

15. Ibid., p. 6.

16. Robert Johnson, *He: Understanding Masculine Psychology* (King of Prussia, Pa.: Religious Publishing Co), p. 31.

17. Margery Eagan, "Midwifery," *Boston Herald*, February 1, 1989.

18. Neil S. Rosenfeld, "Midwife vs. Doctor," *Newsday*, September 26, 1982.

19. Ibid.

20. Sloane Crawford, unpublished manuscript on midwifery, 1983.

21. Ibid.

22. Sonia Johnson, *Going Out of Our Minds*, p. 61.

23. "An Interview with Raven Lang."

24. Rosenfeld, "Midwife vs. Doctor."

25. The Midwife Collective of Toronto, "VBAC Politics and Informed Choice," Midwifery Task Force of Ontario No. 12, Summer 1986.

26. From a lecture by Michel Odent in 1987 in Boston.

27. Peg Spindel, "Midwives, VBACs and Politics," letter, January 1986.

28. Massachusetts Friends of Midwives, P.O. Box 3188, Boston, Massachusetts 02130

29. Phyllis Chesler, *Mothers on Trial* (New York: McGraw-Hill, 1986), p. 331.

30. Mark Gerzon, A *Choice of Heroes: The Changing Face of American Manhood* (Boston: Houghton Mifflin, 1982), p. 71.

31. Jack Sweeny, "All in the Family," *The Southern Feminist* (Fall 1987).

32. Gina Corea, "Childbirth 2000," *Omni* 1, No. 7 (April 1979): 106.

33. Gerald Perry, " 'Handmaid's Tale' Depicts Futuristic Puritans in Harvard Square," *Boston Globe*, March 4, 1990, p. B39.

34. Archie Brodsky, "It Isn't About One Person Anymore," *The Midwife Advocate*, (Winter 1986): 5.

35. "MANA Conference '89," *The Midwife Advocate* 7, No. 1 (Winter/Spring 1990).

36. Raymond De Vries, "Regulating Birth: Midwives, Medicine and the Law (Philadelphia: Temple University Press, 1985).

37. Margot Edwards, and Mary Waldorf, *Reclaiming Birth: Heroes & Heroines of American Childbirth Reform* (Freedom, Calif.: Crossing Press, 1984).

38. Corea, "Childbirth 2000," p. 107.

39. Arthur Rivan, "The Health Care System: Public Protection and Personal Freedom," *Western Journal of Medicine* 136 (March 1982): 3.

40. "MANA Conference '89."

41. Archie Brodsky, President of Massachusetts Friends of Midwives, personal communication, May 1990.

42. Jenny Stearns, "In Support of Midwifery—An English Perspective," *The Midwife Advocate* 5, No. 1 (Spring 1988): 4.

43. Chesler, *Mothers on Trial*, p. 405.

44. "Commentary," *The Midwife Advocate* 5, No. 2 (Summer 1988).

45. Chesler, *Mothers on Trial*, p. 405.

46. From Patricia Barki, International Women's Council on Obstetrical Practices, personal communication.

47. Anonymous in *Elisabeth Kübler-Ross Newsletter*, No. 25, Winter 1985–1986, p. 5.

48. Barbara MacFarlane, "Saving the Midwives in New Zealand," *ICEA News* 24, No. 2 (May 1985): 5.

Chapter 10

1. Ellen Switzer, "The Failure of American Hospitals," *Ladies Home Journal*, June 1985, p. 45.

2. "China Reports Panda's Birth in Hollow Tree," *Boston Globe*, December 29, 1982, p. 11.

3. Martha Freeman, "First Class Delivery," *American Baby* (March 1990): 45.

4. Ibid.

5. Martha Weinman Lear, "Down with High-Handed Health Care!," *Woman's Day*, February 7, 1984, "Back Page."

6. Montgomery Brower, "Every Mother's Nightmare," *People*, No. 43, October 24, 1989, p. 123.

7. "Study: Hospital Negligence Kills Thousands," *Burlington* (Vt.) *Free Press*, March 1, 1990, p. 2A.

8. Charles Inlander and Ed Weiner. "You Can Say 'No' to a Hospital Stay," *Whole Life Times* (September 1985): 16.

9. "Answers You Need Before You Say 'Yes' to Surgery," *Family Circle*, October 15, 1988, p. 92.

10. Charles Inlander and Ed Weiner. *Take This Book to the Hospital with You*. (Emmaus, Pa.: Rodale Press, 1985).

11. Laurence Cherry, "A Hospital Is No Place for a Sick Person to Be," *Discover*, October, 1985, p. 96.

12. Inlander and Weiner: "You Can Say 'No' to a Hospital Stay," *Whole Life Times*, September, 1985, p. 16.

13. Ibid.

14. Ibid.

15. Judith Herzfeld, *Sense and Sensibility in Childbirth: A Guide to Supportive Obstetrical Care* (New York: W. W. Norton, 1985), p. 3.

16. Herzfeld. Personal correspondence, 1984.

17. Freeman, "First Class Delivery."

18. Robert Mendelsohn, in a radio interview in Boston in 1987. Please see all his books—they're wonderful!

19. "Perinatal AIDS: Infection Control for Hospital Personnel," Polymorph Films, Inc., 118 South Street, Boston, Massachusetts 02111, 1988.

20. Lois Morris, "The War Between Doctors and Nurses," *Good Housekeeping*, July 1983, p. 93.

21. Ibid.

22. Ibid.

23. Ibid.

24. Ibid.

25. Ibid.

26. Switzer, "The Failure of American Hospitals."

27. Ibid.

28. Ibid.

29. Morris, "The War Between Doctors and Nurses."

30. Switzer, "The Failure of American Hospitals."

31. Sidney Mitchell, "Making Sense of the Hospital Setting," *The Circle News*, 4, No. 2 (Spring 1985).

32. Switzer, "The Failure of American Hospitals."

33. The Newsletter of the Midwifery Task Force of Ontario, P.O. Box 489, Station "T," Toronto, Canada, M6B 4C2.

34. Ibid.

35. Lynn Richards, *The Vaginal Birth After Cesarean Experience* (South Hadley, Mass.: Bergin & Garvey, 1988), p. 185.

36. Informed Homebirth, Box 3675, Ann Arbor, Michigan 48106.

37. Caroline McEwan, *Great Expectations* (Spring 1985): 52.

38. Corea, "Childbirth 2000," 106.

39. Diane Mason, "Giving Birth at Home," *American Baby* (December 1984): 20.

40. "Merryn's Birth," VBAC of Ontario Newsletter, Fall 1987.

41. Deborah Duda, *Coming Home: A Guide to Home Care for the Terminally Ill* (New York: W. W. Norton, 1984), p. 15.

42. Judith Goldsmith, *Childbirth Wisdom* (New York: Congdon & Weed, 1984).

43. Melissa Everett, "Homebirth on Trial: Fighting for the Right to Choose," *Whole Life Times* (April/May 1984): 18–21.

44. Corea, "Childbirth 2000."

45. Ibid.

46. Personal correspondence, 1987. See also Marilyn Moran, "Philosophy of Childbirth," *New Nativity News* 1, No. 2 (Summer 1977): 7.

47. Robbie Gass, with "On Wings of Song." Tape available through Interface, 552 Main Street, Watertown, Massachusetts 02172; or Spring Hill, 675 Mass. Ave., Cambridge, Massachusetts 02139.

Chapter 11

1. "The Tears Are the Healing" is a song by Karen Riem. It is on a wonderful tape entitled "Hello Forever" (a song I often play at seminars and workshops). For information on this and other tapes by Karen Riem, send a SASE to Karen Dreams, P.O. Box 7–611. West Hartford, Connecticut 06107.

2. Dane Rudhyar, *The Astrology of Personality* (New York: Doubleday, 1970).

3. Susan MacKay, "Worse Case Labor Rehearsal: A Response." *ICEA Sharing* 11, No. 3 (1984).

4. Deborah Duda, *Coming Home: A Guide to Home Care for the Terminally Ill* (New York: W. W. Norton, 1984), p. 14.

5. Ivan Illich, *Medical Nemesis*, p. 99.

6. Ibid., p. 102.

7. Doris Wong, "Christian Scientists Indicted in Death of Son," *Boston Globe*, April 27, 1988, p. 1.

8. Ibid.

9. Personal correspondence from Steven Schatz, September 27, 1986.

10. Illich, *Medical Nemesis*, p. 195.

11. Ibid., p. 205.

12. Duda, *Coming Home*, p. 187.

13. Boston Women's Health Book Collective, *The New Our Bodies, Our Selves* (New York: Simon & Schuster, 1984), p. 56.

14. Pablo Casals, from his book *Joys and Sorrows*, reprinted in: "Learning and Teaching Peace: The Best Gift of All," by Mary Whitten, *Needham Chronicle* (Massachusetts), February 24, 1988.

15. Geneen Roth, *Breaking Free from Compulsive Eating* (New York: Signet, 1984), p. 75.

16. From an unpublished paper by Jeannie Parvoti Baker, "Healing Cesarean Section Trauma: A Transformational Ritual," Utah, January, 1990.

17. Quote by Rilke.

Chapter 12

1. Judith Goldsmith. *Childbirth Wisdom from the World's Oldest Societies* (New York: Congdon and Weed, 1984), p. 134.

2. Sheila Kitzinger, from "Being Born." CBC Transcripts. P.O. Box 500, Station "A", Toronto, Ontario M5W1E6.

3. Ann Cowlin, *Dancing Through Pregnancy/Afterbirth*, Box 3038, Stony Creek, Branford, Connecticut 06405.

Chapter 13

1. Linda Goodman. *Star Signs (A Practical Guide for the New Age)* (New York: St. Martin's Press, 1985), p. 32.

2. Alan Watts, *The Wisdom of Insecurity* (New York: Vintage, 1951), p. 24.

3. Shirley Luthman, *Energy and Personal Power* (San Raphael, Calif.: Mehetabel and Co., 1982), p. 130.

4. David Cayley, in Sheila Kitzinger, "Being Born".

5. Goodman, *Star Signs*, p. 262.

6. Ibid., p. 263.

7. These quotes come from a variety of posters, letters, postcards, etc. and the like, which I have found or have been sent to me.

8. From her brochure "Creating The One", 5526 Oyer St. Suite 1138. Dallas, Texas 75206–5024.

9. Kimberly Wulfurt, *Positive Pregnancy Fitness Newsletter*, 4 no. 1 (Winter 1988): p. 2.

10. Luthman, *Energy and Personal Power*, p. 75.

11. Ibid., p. 95.

12. Ibid., p. 96.

13. Ibid., p. 29–36.

14. Ibid., p. 14.

15. Ibid., p. 63.

16. Ibid., p. 50.

17. Ibid., p. 28.

18. Shirley Luthman, *Collection of Intimacy* (Tiburon, Calif.; Mehetabel Co., 1980), p. 34.

19. Ibid., p. 144.

20. Lewis Mehl and Gayle Peterson, *Pregnancy As Healing: A Holistic Philosophy for Prenatal Care* Vol. I (Tucson: MindBody Press, 1984), Chapter 1.

21. Luthman, *Collection of Intimacy*, p. 59.

22. Michel Odent, *Birth Reborn* (New York: Pantheon Books, 1984), p. 110.

23. David Chamberlain from Sheila Kitzinger "Being Born."

24. Ibid.

25. Goodman, *Star Signs*, p. 424.

26. Stephanie Dematrakopoulos, *Listening to Our Bodies: The Rebirth of Feminine Wisdom* (Boston: Beacon Press, 1983), pp. 25, 283.

27. Ibid., p. 29.

28. Phyllis Chesler, *Mothers on Trial* (New York: McGraw-Hill, 1986), p. 3.

29. Linda Leonard, *The Wounded Woman* (Boulder, Colo.: Shambala, 1983), p. 131.

30. Elisabeth Dodson Gray, ed., "Giving Birth" in *Sacred Dimensions of Women's Experience*. (Wellesley, Roundtable Mass. Press, 1988), p. 50.

31. Anne Schaef, *Woman's Reality: An Emerging Female System in a White Male Society* (Minneapolis, Minn.: Winston Press, 1981), p. 80.

32. Jeanne Ball, "A Journey into Other Lives," *Boston Globe Magazine*, January 26, 1986, p. 15.

33. Schaef, *Woman's Reality*, p. 80.

34. Luthman, *Energy and Personal Power*, p. 96.

35. Virginia Sandlin, Box 1983, Cathedral Station, New York 10025. From a brochure explaining her workshops.

36. *Elisabeth Kübler-Ross Newsletter*, no. 33, Winter 1988.

37. Ange Stephens, "The Spirit of Healing," Mothers Southern Alliance of Midwives, P.O. Box 29507, Atlanta, Georgia 30329.

38. Luthman, *Energy and Personal Power*, p. 67.

39. Goodman, *Star Signs*, p. 113.

40. Judy Lockwood, *Rim of Fire: Meditations for the Modern Madonna*, April 1988.

41. Nancy Caldwell Sorel, *Ever Since Eve: Personal Reflections on Childbirth* (New York: Oxford University Press, 1984). From *Ms. Magazine* September, 1984, p. 56.

42. Ivan Illich, *Medical Nemesis*, p. 134.

43. Ibid., p. 136.

44. Ibid., p. 137.

45. Lynn Baptiste Richards, "Home VBAC: A Midwife's Perspective," *Mothering* (Winter 1987).

46. Fredelle Maynard, "The Emotional Highs of Successful Childbirth," *Woman's Day*, September 1, 1978, p. 140.

47. Judy Chicago, "The Birth Project," March 11-April 3, 1988, Northeastern University. From the brochure.

48. Luthman, *Energy and Personal Power*, p. 86.

49. Ibid., p. 87.

50. Ibid., p. 86.

51. Network Chiropractic, Network Lifeline, Inc., Vol. 1, Issue 1, 336 Chestnut Street, Needham, 02192, 1988.

52. Christine Brown, "Therapeutic Effects of Bathing in Labor," *Journal of Nurse Midwifery* 27, no.1 (January/February 1982): 13–16.

53. Network Chiropractic.

54. P. Klass, "Birth, Interaction, and Attachment," Pediatric Round Table no. 6. Johnson and Johnson, 1982, p. 85.

55. Sally Kirwin, "Labor Support," Transitions, *CPM Newsletter* SE Minnesota, Vol. 6 no. 3 (December 1989–March 1990).

56. Archie Brodsky, *The Midwife Advocate* 5, no. 3 (Summer 1988): 3.

57. Carl Jones, Henci Goer, and Penny Simkin. "Labor Support Guide—For Fathers, Family, and Friends" (Seattle, Wash., Pennypress) ($1.00).

58. From Marilyn Moran's Philosophies of childbirth, personal communication and Birth at Home League, Box 6223, Leawood, Kansas 66206.

59. Marilyn Moran, *New Nativity Newsletter* no. 2 (Summer 1977): 7.

60. Ann Cowlin, *Dancing Through Pregnancy/Afterbirth*, Box 3083, Stony Creek, Branford, Connecticut 06405.

61. Jasmine Miller, "Easing Pregnancy and Birth Through Massage," 288 Old Oak Trail, Coventry, Connecticut 06238.

62. "Colors—Their Impact on Our Well-Being," The Natural Choice, Livos Plantchemistry, Sante Fe, New Mexico 87501, Spring/Summer 1989.

63. Goodman, *Star Signs*, p. 266.

64. Ibid., p. 260.

65. Goldsmith, *Childbirth Wisdom*, p. 174.

66. Ibid.

67. Tim Lowenstein, "Gentle Places and Quiet Spaces," Conscious Living Foundation, Vol. 2. no.2 (Spring 1986).

68. Goodman, *Star Signs*, p. 262.

69. "River" by Linda Arnold, available through Ariel Records, Box 2229, Santa Cruz, California 95062.

70. Goldsmith, *Childbirth Wisdom*, p. 13.

71. Michel Odent *Birth Reborn* (New York: Pantheon Books, 1984), p. xvii.

72. Sheila Kitzinger, "Being Born," CBC Transcripts, P.O. Box 500, Station "A" Toronto, Ontario M5W 1E6.

73. Odent, *Birth Reborn*, p. 73.

74. Sylvia Klein Olkin, *Positive Pregnancy Fitness* (Garden City NY: Avery, 1980). See Chapter on "Inner Bonding."

75. Unpublished manuscript sent to me by Virginial Lubell in 1987, p. 57.

76. William Poole, "The First Nine Months of School," *Hipppocrates* (July/Agust 1987): 70.

77. Laurie Colwin, *Another Marvelous Thing* (New York: Penguin Book, 1987), p. 94.

78. Colleen Stanton, in Kitzinger, "Being Born."

79. David Cayley, in Kitzinger, "Being Born."

80. Odent, *Birth Reborn*, p. xi.

81. Tina Raymond, "Participatory Conception Class, A.D. 2089," *Childbirth Educator* (Winter 1988–1989): 48.

82. Scarlett Pollack, "Refusing to Take Women Seriously," in Rita Arditti et al. eds, *Test-Tube Women: What Future for Motherhood?* (Boston: Pandora Press, 1984), p. 146.

83. Robert Wechsler, "Hostile Womb," *Discover* (May 1988): 83.

84. Alan Watts, *This Is It* (New York: Random House, 19), p. 66.

85. Odent, *Birth Reborn*, p. 10.

86. Richard Knox, "Risk of Late Pregnancy Downplayed," *Boston Globe*, March 8, 1990, p. 1.

87. Elizabeth Noble, in Kitzinger, "Being Born."

88. Adrienne Lieberman. "Is Natural Childbirth Dead?" *American Baby* (April 1990): 55.

89. Lynn Richards, *The Vaginal Birth After Cesarean Experience* (South Hadley, Mass: Bergin and Garvey, 1988), p. 50.

90. Elizabeth Davis, "Passing Judgement," *Mothering* no. 50 (Winter 1989): 68. Also see Marlena Ekstein, "Commentary: Global Agenda, Personal Choices," Massachusetts Friends of Midwives 6, no.1 *Midwife Advocate*, (Spring 1989): 1.

91. From a series on PBS, Moyers: *Joseph Campbell and the Power of Myth* (interviewed by Bill Moyers), 1988.

92. Joseph Campbell, *The Power of the Myth*, (New York: Doubleday, 1988), p. 148.

93. Harriet Lerner, *The Dance of Anger* (New York: Harper and Row, 1985) p. 27.

94. Dave Barry, "Deliver Us from the Delivery." *Boston Globe*, May 12, 1985. See Also *Artemis Speaks*.

95. Alan Watts, *The Wisdom of Insecurity* (New York: Vintage, 1951), p. 9.

96. Lisa Alther, *Other Women* (New York: Alfred A. Knopf, 1984).

97. Luthman, *Energy and Personal Power*, p. 86.

98. Goodman, *Star Signs*, p. xxi.

99. Read *Star Signs* by Linda Goodman. See also, Robert Brody, "Music for Labor," *American Baby* (February 1990): 40.

100. Suzanne Arms, "Five Women, Five Births" Suzanne Arms Productions. 1977, Available Through CPM P.O. Box 152, Syracuse, New York. 13210.

101. Betty Friedan, "How to Get the Women's Movement Moving Again," *New York Times*, Section VI, November 3, 1985, p. 26.

102. Sondra Ray, *Ideal Birth* (Berkeley, Calif.: Celestial Arts, 1985), p. 58.

103. Odent, *Birth Reborn*, p. 54.

104. From personal correspondence, 1989.

105. From a letter from John Davis, 1987. Research by Steve Maier, University of Colorado, Boulder, and Mark Lodenslayer, University of Denver.

106. Odent, *Birth Reborn*, p. 84.

107. Robert Howard, *Genesis (ASPO) Newsletter* (April/May 1983).

108. Ray, *Ideal Birth*, p. 75.

109. Ibid., p. vii.

Chapter 14

1. Candi Lean, "No Bloomin' Section," *Compleat Mother* (Spring 1986).

2. Poem by Caroline Sufrin, personal correspondence.

3. James Martin, et al., "Vaginal Delivery Following Previous Cesarean Birth," *American Journal of Obstetrics and Gynecology* 146 (1983): 255.

4. Jean Ricci and Mary J. O'Sullivan, *Obstetrics/Gynecology* Forum 8. no. 4 (July/August 1989): 3.

5. Marc Boucher, et al., "Maternal Morbidity as Related to Trial of Labor After Previous Cesarean Delivery: A Quantitative Analysis," *Journal of Reproductive Medicine* 29, no.1 (January 1984): 12.

6. Steven Clark, "Effect of Indication for Previous Cesarean Section on Subsequent Delivery Outcome in Patients Undergoing a Trial of Labor," *Journal of Reproductive Medicine* 29, no.1 (January 1984): 22.

7. Elliot Gellman, "Vaginal Delivery After Cesarean Section: Experience in Private Practice," *Journal of the American Medical Association* 249, n.21 (June 3, 1983).

8. Paul Meier and Richard Porreco, "Trial of Labor Following Cesarean Section: A Two-Year Experience," *American Journal of Obstetrics and Gynecology* 144, no. 6 (November 15, 1982) 672.

9. Harold Jerusun, "Vaginal Delivery Following Cesarean Section," *American Journal of Obstetrics and Gynecology* 75, no. 2 (1958).

10. Robert Mendelsohn from a radio conversation in Boston, 1986.

11. Jeffrey Phelan, et al., "Vaginal Birth After Cesarean," *American Journal of Obstetrice and Gynecology* 157 (1987): 1510–1515.

12. Tahilramany, et al., "Previous Cesarean Section and Trial of Labor," *Journal of Reproductive Medicine*, Vol. 29 no.1 (January 1984): 20.

13. Richard Graham, "Trial of Labor Following Previous Cesarean Section," *American Journal of Obstetrics and Gynecology* 149 (1984): 35–45.

14. Bruce L. Flamm, et al., "Vaginal Birth After Cesarean Section: Results of a Multicenter Study," *American Journal of Obstetrics and Gynecology* 158 (1988): 1979–84.

15. Richard Porreco and Paul Meier, "Repeat Cesarean—Mostly Unnecessary," *Contemporary Ob/Gyn* (September 1984): 55–60.

16. "ACOG Releases Guidelines for VBAC," *C/SEC Newsletter* 8, no. 3–4 (Fall/Winter 1982). Guidelines were revised in 1984 and 1988: Committee Statement, ACOG, 600 Maryland Avenue SW, Suite 300 E., Washington, D.C. 20024.

17. Graham, "Trial of Labor," p. 37.

18. Note: Every article on VBAC after multiple cesareans is favorable. Also, there is no limit to the number of subsequent vaginal deliveries "permissible".

19. Meier and Porreco, "Trial of Labor Following Cesarean Section" p. 671.

20. Phelan et al., "Vaginal Birth After Cesarean."

21. Tahilramany et al., "Previous Cesarean Section."

22. Irwin Kaiser, Albert Einstein College of Medicine, New York, personal correspondence, October 26, 1984.

23. Norman Gleicher, "Cesarean Section Rates in the United States: The Short Term Failure of the National Consensus Development Conference in 1980," *American Medical Association* (1980) 252: 3273–3276.

24. Personal Correspondence. See also Laurie Brant, "One Woman's Story," *Maternal Health News* 13, no.2:9.

25. Flamm et al., "Vaginal Birth After Cesarean Section," and Meier and Porreco, "Trial of Labor."

26. Meier and Porreco, "Trial of Labor," p. 677.

27. Ibid.

28. Carol Shepherd and Carol McClain, "Why Women Choose a Trial of Labor or Repeat Cesarean Section," *Journal of Family Practice.* 21 no.3 (1985): 210–216.

29. Meier and Porreco, "Trial of Labor" p. 677.

30. Ibid., p. 671.

31. Shepherd and McClain, "Why Women Choose a Trial of Labor."

32. Margaret Cantanese, "Vaginal Birth after Cesearean: Recommendations, Risks Realities and the Client's Right to Know,"

33. Paul Placek and Selma Taffel, "VBAC in the 1980's" 78, no.5 (May 1988): 512.

34. Everett Beguin, "VBAC: What are the Risks?" *Female Patient*, 13 (1988):16.

35. Gerald Bullock, "Apologies of a Reformed Obstetrician," unpublished manuscript, 1987.

36. Ivan Illich, *Medical Nemesis*, p. 90.

37. Lillian Hellman, *Pentimento* (New York: Signet, 1973).

38. Judith Goldsmith, *Childbirth Wisdom from the World's Oldest Societies* (New York: Congdon and Weed, 1984).

39. Carol Anne Dowsett, "A Personal Choice," *Military Lifestyle* (February 1986): 18.

Chapter 15

1. Sonia Johnson, *Going Out of Our Minds: The Metaphysics of Liberation* (Freedom, Calif.: Crossing Press, 1987), p. ii.

Chapter 16

1. Shirley Luthman, *Energy and Personal Power* (San Raphael, Calif.: Mehetabel and Co., 1982), p. 15. Originally by Olive Schreiner, *Track to the Water's Edge* in *Dreams*, Howard Thurman, ed. (Boston, Little, Brown, 1900).

2. Meredith Lady Young, "The Last Starfighter," from *Agartha, Journey to the Stars* (Stillpoint Publishers, 1984), p. 72.

3. Findhorn Foundation, *The Faces of Findhorn* (New York: Harper and Row, 1980) p. 175.

4. Sonia Johnson, *Going Out of Our Minds: The Metaphysics of Liberation* (Freedom, Calif.: Crossing Press. 1987), p. 348.

5. Ibid., p. 346.

6. "Rabbi's Message," *Temple Sinai Newsletter*, no.21 (April 1966). It is originally from David Grayson's *Adventure in Understanding*.

7. Ellen Cantarow, *Moving The Mountain: Women Working for Social Change* (New York: Feminist Press, 1980). ·

References

Arditti, Rita, Renatti Duelli Klein and Shelly Minden, eds. *Test-Tube Women: What Future for Motherhood?* Boston: Pandora Press, 1984.

Arms, Suzanne. *Immaculate Deception: A New Look at Childbirth*. South Hadley, Mass.: Bergin & Garvey, 1984.

Brewer, Gail. *What Every Pregnant Woman Should Know: The Truth About Diet and Drugs in Pregnancy*. New York: Penguin, 1985.

Brewer, Thomas, *Metabloic Toxemia of Late Pregnancy. A Disease of Malnutrition* New Canaan, Conn: Keats Publishing Co. 1982.

Caldecott, Leonie, and Stephanie Leland, eds. *Reclaim the Earth: Women Speak out for Life on Earth*. London: Women's Press Ltd., 1983.

Cassidy-Brinn, Ginny, Francie Horstein, and Carol Downer. *Women-Centered Pregnancy and Birth*. Federation of Women's Health Centers. Pittsburgh: Cleis Press, 1984.

Chesler, Phyllis. *Mothers on Trial*. New York: McGraw-Hill, 1986.

Cohen, Nancy Wainer, and Lois Estner. *Silent Knife: Cesarean Prevention and Vaginal Birth After Cesarean*. South Hadley, Mass.: Bergin & Garvey, 1983.

Corea, Gina. "Childbirth 2000" *Omni* 1 no. 7. (April 1979): 48.

Dematrakopoulos, Stephanie. *Listening to Our Bodies: The Rebirth of Feminine Wisdom*. Boston: Beacon Press, 1983.

Donahue, Phil. *The Human Animal*. New York: Woodward/White (Simon & Schuster), 1985.

Duda, Deborah. *Coming Home: A Guide to Home Care for the Terminally Ill*. New York: W. W. Norton, 1984.

English, Jane Butterfield. *Different Doorway: Adventures of a Cesarean Born*. Point Reyes Station, Calif: Earth Heart, 1985.

Gaskin, Ina May. *Spiritual Midwifery*. Summertown, Tenn.: The Farm, 1977.

Gerzon, Mark. *A Choice of Heroes: The Changing Face of American Manhood*. Boston: Houghton Mifflin, 1982.

Goldsmith, Judith. *Childbirth Wisdom from the World's Oldest Societies*. New York: Congdon and Weed, 1984.

Goodman, Linda. *Star Signs (A Practical Guide for the New Age): The Secret Codes of the Universe/Forgotten Rainbows and Forgotten Melodies of Ancient Wisdom*. New York: St. Martin's Press, 1987.

Herzfeld, Judith, *Sense and Sensibility in Childbirth: A Guide to Supportive Obstetrical Care*. New York: W. W. Norton, 1985.

Illich, Ivan. *Medical Nemesis*. New York: Pantheon, 1976.

Johnson, Robert. *He: Understanding Masculine Psychology*. King of Prussia, PA.: Religious Publishing Co., 1974.

Johnson, Robert. *She: Understanding Feminine Psychology*. King of Prussia, PA.: Religious Publishing Co., 1974.

Johnson, Sonia. *Going Out of Our Minds: The Metaphysics of Liberation*. Freedom, Calif.: Crossing Press, 1987.

Katz, Jay *The Silent World of Doctor and Patient*. New York: Free Press, 1984.

Keyes, Kenneth, Jr. *The Hundredth Monkey*. Coos Bay Ore.: Vision Books, 1981.

Koehler, Nan, *Artemis Speaks: VBAC Stories and Natural Childbirth information*. Published by Nan Ullrike Koehler. 13140 Frati Lane, Sebastopol, California 95472, 1985.

Korte, Diana, and Roberta Scaer. *A Good Birth, A Safe Birth*. New York: Bantam, 1984.

Leonard, Linda Schierse. *The Wounded Woman*. Boulder, Colo.: Shambala, 1983.

Lerner, Harriot Goldhor, *The Dance of Anger*. New York: Harper & Row, 1985.

Luthman, Shirley. *Energy and Personal Power*. San Raphael, Calif.: Mehetabel & Co., 1982.

Odent, Michel. *Birth Reborn*. New York: Pantheon Books 1984.

Olkin, Sylvia Klein. *Positive Pregnancy Fitness*. Garden City, N.Y.: Avery, 1987.

Panuthos, Claudia. *Transformation Through Birth*. South Hadley, Mass.: Bergin & Garvey 1986.

Panuthos, Claudia, and Catherine Romeo. *Ended Beginnings: Healing Childbearing Loss*. South Hadley, Mass: Bergin & Garvey 1984.

Ray, Sondra. *Ideal Birth*. Berkeley Calif.: Celestial Arts, 1984.

Richards, Lynn Baptiste. *The Vaginal Birth After Cesarean Experience*. South Hadley, Mass.: Bergin & Garvey, 1988.

Rothman, Barbara Katz. *Giving Birth: Alternatives in Childbirth*. New York: Penguin, 1984.

Rothman, Barbara Katz. *In Labor: Women and Power in the Birthplace*. New York: W. W. Norton, 1982.

Schaef, Anne Wilson. *Woman's Reality: Am Emerging Female System in a White Male Society*. Minneapolis, Minn.: Winston Press, 1981.

Starr, Paul. *The Social Transformation of American Medicine: The Rise of a Sovereign Profession and the Making of a Vast Industry*. New York: Basic Books, 1982.

Stewart, David *The Five Standards for Safe Childbearing*. NAPSAC International, Box 267, Marble Hill, Missouri 63764. 1981.

Index

About the Author

NANCY WAINER COHEN founded CSEC, Inc., the first and largest cesarean prevention organization in the country, in 1973. Since 1972, she has counseled thousands of women in the areas of cesarean prevention and VBAC (vaginal birth after cesarean—an acronym she coined). Cohen continues individual counseling and also speaks throughout the country to pregnant women, childbirth educators, midwives, health professionals, and consumers. Ms. Wainer Cohen is the co-author of *Silent Knife: Cesarean Prevention and Vaginal Birth After Cesarean* (Bergin & Garvey, 1983).